METABOLIC LIVING

CRITICAL GLOBAL HEALTH: Evidence, Efficacy, Ethnography
*A series edited by Vincanne Adams and João Biehl*

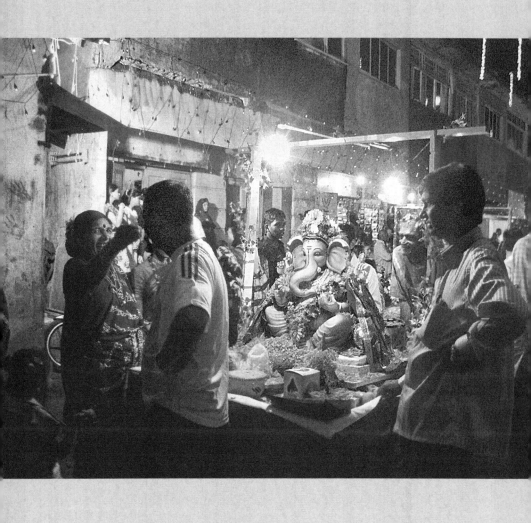

# METABOLIC LIVING

## Food, Fat, and the Absorption of Illness in India

Harris Solomon

Duke University Press   Durham and London   2016

Designed by Heather Hensley
Typeset in Chaparral Pro by Westchester Publishing Services

Library of Congress Cataloging-in-Publication Data
Names: Solomon, Harris, [date]
Title: Metabolic living : food, fat, and the absorption of illness in
India / Harris Solomon.
Other titles: Critical global health.
Description: Durham : Duke University Press, 2016.
Series: Critical global health: evidence, efficacy, ethnography |
Includes bibliographical references and index.
Identifiers: LCCN 2015039006 |
ISBN 9780822360872 (hardcover : alk. paper) |
ISBN 9780822361015 (pbk. : alk. paper) |
ISBN 9780822374442 (e-book)
Subjects: LCSH: Obesity—India. | Lipids in human nutrition—
India. | Food habits—India. | Malnutrition—India. |
Convenience foods—India. | Metabolism.
Classification: LCC RC628 .S656 2016 | DDC 616.39800954—dc23
LC record available at http://lccn.loc.gov/2015039006

Cover art: Man selling cotton candy. Daman Beach, India.
Photo by Gopal MS.

Frontis: Ganesh Chathurthi celebration

*For my mother, and in memory of my father*

# CONTENTS

ix    Acknowledgments

1    INTRODUCTION

27    *Interlude* Birthday Cakes

31    CHAPTER 1. The Thin-Fat Indian

65    *Interlude* Mango Madness

69    CHAPTER 2. The Taste No Chef Can Give

99    *Interlude* The Ration Card

105    CHAPTER 3. Readying the Home

141    *Interlude* Stamps

145    CHAPTER 4. Lines of Therapy

187    *Interlude* Waiting Room Walls

193    CHAPTER 5. Gut Attachments

225    CONCLUSION. Metabolic Mumbai

235    Notes
253    References
271    Index

## ACKNOWLEDGMENTS

I thank my teachers. In Mumbai, I am deeply grateful to all those whom I cannot name here but who taught me everything. The incredible individual I call Mary in these pages, who was my liaison to the neighborhood and my tireless research assistant, opened her community's doors to me and taught me to ask better questions. Raymond was selfless in his support and ideas. I also thank Chandrima Chatterjee, Cecilia Dias, Vikram Doctor, Naresh Fernandes, Leon Fonseca, Aakar Patel, Yogesh Pawar, and Ketan Vaidya for teaching me all the tiny details that cemented my love for Bandra and Mumbai. I had the incredible fortune to cross paths with Drs. Kalpana Swaminathan and Ishrat Syed, and I am grateful for their friendship, feedback, and passion for writing through mysteries of the body and the city. Many physicians shared their time and clinics with me, and I especially thank Dr. Arun Bal, Dr. Raman Goel, Dr. Shashank Joshi, Dr. C. S. Yajnik, and Dr. Vishali Naik. A special thank-you to Dr. Pallavi Patankar for her hospitality and reflections. Anita Khemka and Imran Kokiloo, in Delhi, and Maura Finkelstein, Ansul Madhvani, and Solomon Senrick, in Mumbai, offered havens of refuge, friendship, and unparalleled generosity. Antigoni Koumpounis was a soothsayer on the India journey since the beginning. I thank the faculty of the Department of Sociology at the University of Mumbai for hosting me during my stay, especially Prof. Kamala Ganesh for her support. Gopal MS conveys luminous everyday moments in Mumbai; I thank him deeply for sharing his art for this book's cover.

Catherine Lutz mentored me through this project's twists and turns. Cathy's clarity of thinking, shared in phone calls, e-mails, and meetings filled with laughter, offered steady guidance through fieldwork, writing, and rewriting. Across very large distances, this kept me going. Lina Fruzzetti taught me how to plot routes through India, protected me with blessings in the field, and challenged me to root my thinking in place. Daniel Smith taught me how to teach anthropology—and why that matters. Sherine Hamdy taught me to remain open to the unexpected. Lawrence Cohen shared immense kindness and thought and connected dots in ways that profoundly shaped my thinking. At Brown University, I also thank Paja Faudree, Anne Fausto-Sterling, Matthew Gutmann, Patrick Heller, Stephen Houston, Jessaca Leinaweaver, Patricia Symonds, and Kay Warren for their mentorship, time, teaching, and care.

My research in India was made possible by a Doctoral Dissertation Improvement Grant from the National Science Foundation, a Dissertation Fieldwork Grant from the Wenner-Gren Foundation for Anthropological Research, and a Doctoral Dissertation Research Award from Fulbright-Hays. At Brown, I thank the Graduate Program in Development at the Watson Institute for International Studies, along with the Population Studies and Training Center, for funding summer research trips to find my way. These sources of funding created opportunities to immerse and grow the relationships conveyed throughout the manuscript.

At Duke University, I have found a warm, wonderful home in the Department of Cultural Anthropology. Anne Allison, Lee Baker, Christine Folch, Engseng Ho, Ralph Litzinger, Anne-Maria Makhulu, J. Lorand Matory, Laurie McIntosh, Louise Meintjes, Diane Nelson, William O'Barr, Charles Piot, Irene Silverblatt, Orin Starn, Rebecca Stein, and Charlie Thompson keep the rooms of that home buzzing with intellectual adventure. Thanks to Pat Bodager, Kelly Furr, and Bernice Patterson for keeping an open door, always ready with an answer. My second home, the Duke Global Health Institute, has been supportive from the start, and I owe special thanks to Michael Merson, Randall Kramer, John Bartlett, Gary Bennett, David Boyd, Sherryl Broverman, Dennis Clements, Manoj Mohanan, Kathleen Sikkema, and Kate Whetten for carving out space to research, write, teach, and collaborate in new directions. Sumathi Ramaswamy and Ara Wilson have been fantastic interlocutors and guides. My gratitude also goes to Srinivas Aravamudan, Linda Burton, Rich Freeman, Deborah Jenson, Ranjana Khanna, Jehangir Malegam, Kathryn Mathers, Jessica Nammakal, Mark Olson, Angela O'Rand, Laurie Patton, Carlos Rojas, Kathy Rudy,

Philip Stern, Aarthi Vadde, and Priscilla Wald. I thank Jay Hammond, Libby Jones, and Dorothy Mangale for providing research assistance, and my graduate students for keeping ideas bouncing.

Jan Brunson, Sreeparna Ghosh, Susi Keefe, Andrea Maldonado, Andrea Mazzarino, Jessica Mulligan, Rebecca Peters, Katie Rhine, and Laura Vares taught me the ins and outs of graduate school. There was no wrinkle that Kathy Grimaldi, Matilde Andrade, and Margie Sugrue could not smooth. Carissa Diest, Lauren Gussis, Benjamin Junge, Timothy McCormick, Julie Piotrowski, and Shannon Shelton kept me laughing in ways only old friends can. I also thank my family in Indianapolis for keeping me grounded while writing. Lou and Sheila Rosenberg, along with Erin, Daniel, Mindy, Ruthie, Barry, Abe, and Jack provided many evenings of debate and delight. I owe special thanks to my friends and colleagues at Butler University: Elise Edwards, Betsy Erbaugh, Scott Swanson, Sholeh Shahrokhi, Ageeth Sluis, and Robin Turner.

For their close reading of and listening to various parts of the book and for their prodding toward different horizons of thinking, I thank Jonathan Shapiro Anjaria, Ulka Anjaria, Nima Bassiri, Sarah Besky, Crystal Biruk, Dominic Boyer, Mara Buchbinder, Jocelyn Chua, Veena Das, Joseph Dumit, Tim Elfenbein, Judith Farquhar, James Faubion, Kim Fortun, Michael Fortun, Duana Fullwiley, Angela Garcia, Susan Greenhalgh, Julie Guthman, Cori Hayden, Gabrielle Hecht, Cecilia van Hollen, Cymene Howe, Matthew Hull, Naveeda Khan, Stacey Langwick, Nadine Levin, Julie Livingston, Margaret Lock, Lenore Manderson, William Mazzarella, Townsend Middleton, Amy Moran-Thomas, Alex Nading, Kevin Lewis O'Neill, Aihwa Ong, Adriana Petryna, Shilpa Phadke, Sarah Pinto, Lucinda Ramberg, Eugene Raikhel, Laurence Ralph, Peter Redfield, Emilia Sanabria, Barry Saunders, Svati Shah, Bhrigupati Singh, Kalyanakrishnan Sivaramakrishnan, Tulasi Srinivas, Ajantha Subramanian, Kaushik Sunder Rajan, Sue Wadley, Ian Whitmarsh, Brad Weiss, and Mei Zhan. With incredible generosity, Megan Crowley-Matoka, Hannah Landecker, Elizabeth Roberts, and Emily Yates-Doerr opened up new avenues of thinking and writing. I owe a great debt to Jennifer Ashley, Kathleen Millar, Maura Finkelstein, and Tomas Matza for reading this manuscript from tip to tail, across time zones and continents, over the years. Their companionship has meant everything to keeping things moving. Audiences at Brandeis University, Columbia University, Cornell University, The University of Michigan, Yale University, and the Tata Institute of Social Sciences offered critical feedback that finessed the book's elements and ideas. Earlier versions and portions of chapter 2 appeared as "The Taste No Chef Can Give: Processing Street Food in Mumbai," *Cultural Anthropology* 30 (1): 65–90; and portions of chapter 5 appeared as "Short Cuts: Metabolic Surgery and Gut Attachments in India," *Social Text* 32 (3): 69–86. I thank the editors, reviewers, and readers for their feedback as this material developed into a book. João Biehl and Vincanne Adams have been wholeheartedly inspirational during this journey. My deepest thanks go to Ken Wissoker, my editor at Duke University Press, for his sparkling support and for making ideas materialize. I also thank Elizabeth Ault, Heather Hensley, Sara Leone, Thomas McCarthy, and Sharon Rodgers. The three anonymous reviewers of the book shaped it with spectacular insight and care.

My integrity of my father, Larry Solomon, continues to guide me. My mother, Dale Solomon, has selflessly invested in me her powers of curiosity about the backstories of people, places, and things, and has sustained me with her loving support. Turning wonder into words has not been easy, but Gabriel Rosenberg has made it possible by infusing his companionship, spellbinding intellect, and creativity into every page of this book. He is quite simply my *jaan*, my life.

Crosses

Crosses breach Bandra's paths. As signs of the large Catholic population
in this Mumbai neighborhood, the crosses stand up to ten feet tall. They
secure houses, garden grottoes, and alleyways. Some commemorate community leaders, on side streets and on main streets that used to be side
streets. Many others are known as plague crosses. They were erected to
ward off the plague during Bombay's 1896 epidemic, a mass mortality
that ultimately killed over 12 million people throughout India.[1] I counted
six plague crosses within a one-block radius of my apartment building in
Bandra. Changes in the city surrounding the crosses must accommodate
them: men would de- and reconstitute them brick by brick when municipal
crews widened the streets by a few meters. The crosses accommodate city
life: a quick prayer, a kiss on the way to work, or a smoky stick of incense.
On one of Bandra's main seaside roads, Carter Road, stands a cross simply
marked "1896" at its base. Painted with a thorny, flaming heart dripping
blood into a chalice, it displays a stark red against the orange of its marigold garland necklace, which someone refreshed daily. The crosses take on
gifts of fresh flowers even as the winds coming off the Arabian Sea fade
their paint.

One morning, I noticed on my daily walk that the plague crosses had
new across-the-street neighbors: metal signs, bright yellow and reflect-
ing the sun, stuck into the ground every ten feet. The signs advertised

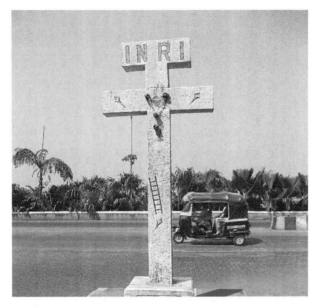

**FIG. I.1**
Bandra plague
cross

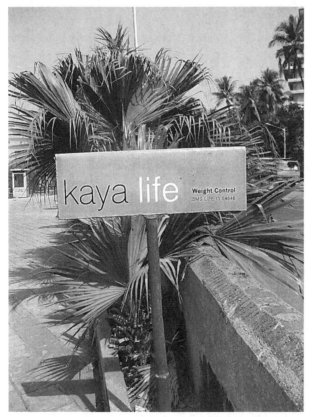

**FIG. I.2**
Kaya Life cross

a weight-loss company. They instructed their audience to send a text message with the word "LIFE" to a phone number for more information on how one might learn "weight control." Together, nineteen of these signs spanned the length of the waterfront promenade, insisting that too much food was a drain on life. A sentinel of bodily hazards had materialized again. These signs spoke of chronic disease.

Along with their older relatives across Carter Road, the newer crosses are straddling life and death in relation to disease. They interface bodies and the city. The plague crosses cement memories of residents felled by an infectious epidemic; the weight loss signs are part of a plan to forestall potential falls. Both are totems of events eventually called epidemics. Both mark out patterns of substances, environments, organisms, and illnesses. Death from infectious agents beckoned from the past on one side of the road, and life as fatness gestured from the other. Taken together they might seem like epidemiological bookends encapsulating a transition from communicable to noncommunicable diseases, from etiologies known to those contested, and from plagues of poverty to those of prosperity. But transitions are tricky.[2] Given the richness of life that unfolded around them, the crosses demand a more porous field for understanding patterns of disease than any solid line drawn across the street could provide.

At the time of the plague outbreak in Bombay—and still today—the crosses denoted mass death. The poet B. F. Patell described these circumstances in 1896:

One only race immune stands out,
Well known for high physique, no doubt,
A race of healthy, stalwart men,
Out of their shoes full five-feet-ten;
Aloof from natives and their ways,
Their cleanly habits worthy praise;
Their diet rich as rich can be,
Not "dal" and "bhat" with grains and "ghee,"
But beef and mutton, fowl and fish,
A pound helped out of every dish;
Wine, whiskey and cigars to close,
And nights of undisturbed repose;
Their dwellings open to the sea,
From all contamination free,

At Mal'bar Hill or Breach Candy;
Well-ordered homes of health and ease;
With "khidmatgars" [servants] and what you please;
The European race I mean,
Untouched who 'scaped Plague's horrors clean.

Food manifested connections between wealth and health: Foods "rich as rich can be" eaten by the pound for the "European race" who escaped, and *dal* (lentils) and *bhat* (rice) for the "natives" left behind (Patell 1896). In Patell's poem, as in this book, substances and environments set the terms of what can and cannot be absorbed to make life livable. Memory and marigolds, ghee and beef, fleas and fat: the city and its inhabitants are deeply permeable.

Absorption

Around the crosses, stories circulated about Indians in cities like Mumbai enjoying *too* much life, in the form of too much food, and becoming heavier and sicker as a result. In popular and scientific accounts, India was facing an epidemic of diseases of prosperity, especially obesity and type 2 diabetes. The country modeled global health paradigms that consider how the reduction of infectious, communicable diseases leaves bodies susceptible to modernity's morbidities such as hypertension, coronary disease, type 2 diabetes, and obesity. Often "Westernization" or "transition" abridges this dynamic, suggesting a generalizable West-to-East flow of prosperity and pathology.[3] These mediated illness explanations shared a coda of an urban "lifestyle" of alimentary indulgences and bodily sedentarism. Newspapers, television programs, and everyday conversations detailed the features of this dangerous pattern, usually as a face-off: between fatness as an older vernacular sign of wealth and newer aesthetic demands of thinness or between the harsh history and contemporary persistence of malnutrition and the spread of fast food in cities.

However hyperbolic or representative, these contrapuntal narratives posit that through food, some bodies have reached their limits of absorbing a changing world. Such narratives often contextualized the uptick in metabolic disorders amid India's economic reforms of the early 1990s. This reiterated the idea that postliberalization India is a laboratory of a massive urban middle class—a place where the market anchors possible futures in terms of consumer aspirations and anxieties.[4] Particular visions of metabolic order and urban Indian sociality converged, each making the other intelligible. The underbelly of the urban Indian middle-class fantasy simply seemed too big for a healthy, long life. Consequently, overconsumption became a salient explanatory glue for understanding relations between the body, everyday substances like food, and environments like the city.

In this book, I consider how people make connections between food and urban life to explain that absorption is taking hold as the grounds for experiencing and making sense of chronic illness. "Absorb" has a conventional meaning of soaking up or drawing in. It also has a figurative meaning: to preoccupy or rivet, in both its Latin root and its current English meaning. Throughout the book, I mark vernacular expressions of what is being absorbed and how. Often, these expressions employ variations to root morphemes that convey the action of taking for oneself (in Hindi, *le*; in Marathi, *ghe*). My own use builds on these meanings, with an emphasis on absorption as a dynamic process. Hence, by absorption, I mean the possibility for bodies, substances, and environments to mingle, draw attention to each other, and even shift definitional parameters in the process. In this usage, discursive and material changes both precede and follow absorption. As fat appears and as blood sugars blossom, people register relations to substances somewhere and sometime between desire and ingestion, bodily systems and environmental exposures, subjectivities and city life, and guts and drugs. Absorptions between persons and substances call into question how and to what extent the self and the world mix. Absorption allows us to see how ordinary objects like foods make metabolic illness stable enough to be operational and intelligible. From this perspective, bodies and cities are permeable interfaces of active traffic. This traffic—full of stops, starts, and dead ends as much as it is full of movement—offers insight into the connective permeability that undergirds India's rise in metabolic illnesses. A study of metabolic illness grounded in absorption, in contrast to one that assumes overconsumption as its starting point, can offer a thicker account of how people live through this phenomenon. I argue that attention to absorption can open up key questions in the context of chronic diseases connected to food: Who and what become the eater and the eaten? What is nutrition and what is poison? Who and what set the boundaries of inside and outside, delineating organism and environment?

Epidemiological and clinical studies suggest a varied landscape of prevalence and incidence of metabolic illness in India. For obesity, many researchers use proxy indicators such as the prevalence of type 2 diabetes or the incidence of cardiovascular disease (IIPS 2007). India's 2005–6 National Family Health Survey estimated obesity for the first time by calculating the body mass index for ever-married adults between 15 and 49. The survey listed the percentage of female respondents who were overweight or obese at 15 percent (29 percent of whom were urban residents) and male respondents who were overweight or obese at 12 percent (22 percent were urban residents). India is also noted to have the greatest number of diabetics globally, and ischemic heart disease leads as the nation's killer. For type 2 diabetes, epidemiological studies in urban areas place prevalence rates between 8 percent and 20 percent; for the state of Maharashtra, 6 million people are said to be living with type 2 diabetes.[5] It has been difficult to parse trends from these data and thus to quantify the problem.[6] Current figures about eating patterns in India are similarly porous. Regional variations are vast, social class, caste, and gender inflect food consumption patterns and nutritional status in complex ways, and obesity has multifactoral interactions of risk and realization with diabetes and cardiovascular disease.[7] Given the ambiguity of the numbers, the government of India has proposed testing blood sugar levels in a national surveillance effort.

In this space of calculated uncertainty, the relations I witnessed between persons, city spaces, desires, risks, and realizations of bodily states often hinged on matters of absorbing substances. My informants frequently began their stories about food/body/medicine connections from the starting place of the body's porosity. Whether it was a clinician holding fast to the "calories in, calories out" model of dieting, a neighbor talking about how different qualities of food fully please or fall short of one's hunger, or a biologist attesting to the idea that in utero exposures to environmental toxins materialize as diabetes later in life, these descriptions all posit concepts of shifting body/environment boundaries. Food and fat are the primary materials of concern in most of the stories in this book, but my use of absorption does not assume that once eaten, one thing converts unproblematically into another (i.e., fat into fat). As we will see, things eaten have travel companions in several complex nature-culture hybrids such as toxic chemicals, plastic shrink-wrap, diets, drugs, and surgeries. Agents of absorption could include persons incorporating food, food incorporating "healthy" qualities from food companies, or Mumbai's streets incorporating new forms of alimentary politics. Being absorptive meant incorporating a range of elements that shuttled between the worlds inside and outside the body. An analytic of absorption understands a seemingly bounded body to be twisted inside out, because bodies already are.

## Body/Environment Noodles

In Manuli, the area of Bandra where I conducted household research, the sea breeze puffs up the things left to dry on the beach under the watch of the plague crosses: laundry, boats from the morning's venture, and hundreds of the local fish called *bombil* (Bombay duck) roped together and hung on wooden frames. The wind snakes its way into neighborhood family compounds, where groups of shacks and more permanent concrete structures gather under tin roofing. My research assistant Mary's family compound was one of the oldest. Paying her a quick visit at home one morning before a day of interviews, I watched the wind rustle waist-high stacks of paper that lined her hallway. All of these papers were about food. Mary had accumulated recipes from cookbooks, women's homemaking magazines, and newspapers over decades. She also had accumulated an archive of weight-loss diets in the carefully curated, crumbly sheaves.

I had seen many collections of *things* in households in the neighborhood, like books, figurines, photos of family members and pets, and souvenirs brought back from places in the Middle East where many of the adult men worked on oil rigs. Neatly arranged stacks of papers weren't surprising in the accumulative sense. The surprise came in their means and ends as diets, an accumulation of ways to diminish. "You can borrow them," Mary told me. "But don't lose them. They're part of my dowry." She smiled at her own joke that the archive—and by extension, keeping slim—was her contribution to the household, the thing a wife brought to make married life livable. (In the years since that moment, if I want a recipe or ask about a diet plan, she still tells me to consult "her dowry.") I took a peek at some of the diets, whose stacks paved a walkable path through domestic space. Yellowing newspaper clippings exclaimed the virtues of meals selected for low cholesterol, low sodium, high fiber, veg-only, fruit-only, or rice-only. Magazine pages torn from 1970s editions of the women's magazine *Femina* extolled slimness and offered stepwise photo instructions to fancifully arrange sliced cucumbers to please the family and cut calories.

Mary pulled one sheet of paper out of a giant stack: a record of her visit to the neighborhood dietitian just down the street. It was the pregnancy weight from her first child that she had wanted to shed. She recalled stepping on the scale, free-listing her eating habits, and listening to the nutritionist dictate a diet plan that Mary scribbled down in a notebook. She showed me this record of regimen: she was to take in certain foods at certain times and to "burn it off" through regular exercise, all to restore the

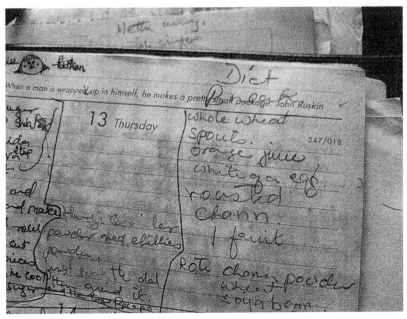

**FIG. I.3** Mary's diet

order of a thinner body. Calories in, calories out, foods to start and foods to stop. My instinct was to jump to a question about efficacy. I was going to ask, "Did it work?" but a squeal of delight interrupted us. Mary turned her attention around the corner, where her toddler nephew sat glued to a small television as he watched cartoons under the watchful eye of his mother, Mary's sister-in-law, Eliza. Eliza was getting ready to cook food for the small catering business she ran out of the house. She made money by catering tiffins (lunch box kits) for the growing number of young people (especially women) in the neighborhood who worked in call centers on the night shift, when eating happened at odd hours. Eliza fed newer forms of labor in the community, as people sat in front of computers under the watch not of crosses but of closed-circuit cameras.

A commercial for a new "healthy" whole wheat instant noodle had come on the television, provoking the nephew's joy: "I am healthy with a round twist, and I slip down your mouth!" squeaked a child's voice-over as noodles energetically swirled around in a bowl on the TV screen. The two women exchanged glances; Eliza remarked that it was impossible to tear her son away from these commercials, which magnetized his attention. Any time he saw these commercials, he would tell her that he wanted that food, now. The noodles danced in the bowl; we were supposed to imagine them dancing into our bodies. Of course we could—absorbing food is what bodies do. The papers in the hallway fluttered as Mary joined the boy on the floor and tuned in.


## Metabolism and Metabolic Living

The scene in Mary's house raises several questions: What is body and what is environment? Where does one end and the other begin? We might all have eaten the noodles, but how would our bodies register them differently? Who is feeding whom here, when a food company enters the picture? Bodies may share space and environments, but the complexity of the metabolism calls for a twist of these questions. Abiding ways to ask about inside/outside boundaries of body and world often rely upon the supposition that bodies in the same space are sharing the same world, made of up the same objects of concern. Yet the sciences and lived experiences of metabolism unseat that supposition. They demand a detailed look at the situated, absorptive interface of bodies and surroundings in which a condition like metabolic illness lodges inside a body. I call this visceral and thoroughly political interface *metabolic living*. Metabolic living is, as I define it, an actively ongoing process people endure to survive the porosity that all life entails. An anthropology of metabolic living attends to the practices of endurance in the face of absorption. To explore metabolic living is to explore the ways that people complicate and even dissipate boundaries across the skin and thus show how bodies and environments are mutually porous. Porosity requires work: work by persons who open up to or refuse materials like food, and work entailed in moving materials across uncertain boundaries. I investigate this work in a moment when the evidence it produces is both uncertain and prolific. In this context, the metabolism has accrued importance for understanding and expressing vitality and morbidity in urban South Asia and elsewhere.

To bioscientists, what the metabolism *is* currently is a matter of both historical and contemporary scientific debate that is being thoroughly re-scripted. Initially used to describe how food is digested and distributed as energy throughout the body, the metabolism is currently best understood as a set of physiological signals that regulate and produce energy, maintain cellular and organ function, and produce chains of changes that factor in to states of disease, well-being, and the heritability of biological patterns. The metabolism is distributed, meaning that it is a highly complex biological system that in humans operates at multiple scales of proteins, cells, hormones, tissue, organs, and neural connections. It distributes across forms of life, for the food we eat or do not eat is a product of the metabolic activity of plants and animals. One hears of metabolic rates, of metabolisms speeding up and slowing down, of "having" a metabolism. "Metabolic" can be an adjective to describe illness and disorder, although oddly and notably, "metabolic health" or "metabolic order" seems rarely invoked.

As clinicians and bioscientists alike consider conditions of relative health and sickness in terms of cascades of signals, the infinitive form "to metabolize" goes beyond the digestive system. It includes, for instance, how the body processes therapeutic drugs or how it experiences surges in neurotransmitters.[8] Sensorial stimuli, food, and environmental toxins belong to the domain of the metabolic as well, prompting us to think of life's risks in terms of exposure (see Landecker 2011). The domain of the metabolic bridges the organic and inorganic, the manufactured and the heritable, and the agential and the incidental.[9] The metabolism, collective and collaborative, blurs the lines between discrete entities (Dupré and O'Malley 2013). All of these things the metabolism is and does show it to be curiously agentive. The metabolism is at once a concept, an embodied thing, a mode of diagnosis and therapy, and a social rubric—all subject to intense debate. And when the metabolism appears to be sick or disordered, it becomes a salient analytic category of somatic trouble. The contingencies between "the science" and "the social" of metabolism are historically particular, and they too are absorptive as new ideas about the domain of the metabolic emerge.

The metabolism has produced its own pattern of social theory. For example, Marx and Engels described the "metabolism between man and nature" to elaborate on the exchange between organism and environment and correspondingly how labor could connect man to relationships of exchange (Landecker 2013a, 2013b).[10] Mid-twentieth-century cultural anthropologists questioned how a human metabolism reflected themes of energy, stimulus, and the circuit-like character of life force (cf. Fischer-Kowalski 1998; Bateson 2000: 409; Malinowski 1944: 91; White 1943; Harris 1978). In India, scholars of sociology and anthropology turned to collective metabolisms as a kind of political economy in order to explain the relationship between energetic forces and a world shifting toward modernity and prosperity.[11] For contemporary anthropologists of medicine and healing in India, somatic self-analysis and the body's possibilities for malfunction have appeared as metabolic phenomena insofar as they are about balance and regulation.[12] The above notions of the metabolism are highly varied in their analytic ends and means and range widely, from the literal to the metaphoric, in their application. What they have in common, how they open channels between the biological and the social, is that in all these ideas the metabolism prompts questions about the interface between bodies and the world. Metabolism has played out as an analytic in social science as a question of energy, but the conditions of exchange also are matters of permeability of organisms and their consequent capacity to change.

My understanding of metabolism and its inflection as theory has been fundamentally shaped by the work of the historian and sociologist of science Hannah Landecker. Her research offers a lucid account of the things metabolism is and promises to be, both historically and today, as science, medicine, and public health increasingly turn to it to understand not only metabolic disorders but also more general puzzles about how bodies and environments interrelate. Landecker argues that what the metabolism "is" is first and foremost a conceptual space. She shows that the metabolism is currently epochal as a form of bodily evidence because it encompasses the domains of the somatic and the substantive, inside and outside the skin: "Metabolism is a set—it does not consist in any one reaction, but is a cumulus of interlocking cycles. It is in cells and between cells, in organs and between organs. It is individual and communal. It is the interface between inside and outside, the space of conversion of one to another, of matter to energy, of substrate to waste, of synthesis and break down. A process-thing, it is always in time" (2013a: 193–94). Landecker explains that the metabolism hangs together as a concept of the past, present, and future as histories of science and philosophy move in and out of contact across geographic traditions and trends. I am interested in exploring how this concept can be a tool for ethnographic observation *and* a site of anthropological analysis.

Landecker's research shows how biology and philosophy reckon with the inside-outside-ness of metabolism. As the concept moves through the labs and hands and thoughts of different biologists, biochemists, historians, and philosophers, the "real" metabolism—that is, the one that is aggravating us all in moments of hunger, satiety, and possible states of endocrinological damage—does not easily allow what counts as "the environment" to stay outside the body. In one example, Landecker discusses the work of a key figure in the history of metabolic science, Claude Bernard. Drawing on Bernard's own reflections, she notes that for Bernard, "the animal's *ability to turn the environment into itself* through nutrition is constitutive of the argument that each organism, plant and animal, has the whole of life within it, and one is not 'made' to serve the other" (2013a: 204; emphasis in original). In this quote, Landecker offers a way to see how scientists have long called for a pause on the certainty that what is outside the skin actually stays there. The biological and philosophical work of Bernard and many other scientists and clinicians for over one hundred years now attests to the possible ways that the world outside the skin moves into and out of the body and effects changes. Landecker's rendering of this history provokes complex questions: How do we turn the environment into ourselves? Under what circumstances does the body twist inside out?

I address these questions through anthropology attuned to absorption. If absorption is the condition of possibility for metabolic order and disorder, I aim to elaborate specific social conditions under which absorption intensifies and diminishes. These are circumstances in which people must accommodate a world filled with nourishing and depleting substances. They make such accommodations as they feed themselves, their families, or their clients, in the case of street food vendors or domestic workers or nutritionists. They also do so as they prescribe drugs for ingestion, in the case of doctors, or as they swallow drugs with varying levels of trust or satisfaction, in the case of patients. Metabolic living is an ethnographic heuristic about the viable and lethal interfaces of substances and somatic experience we all face as we work on the routes and compositions of substances that go in and out of a body. My approach foregrounds how people reflect on the life-giving and life-draining power of this work and how the metabolism is a complex biological, semiomaterial apparatus whose epistemologies are in flux.[13] Landecker's research on the history of biochemistry reveals that over time, a dynamism among chemical substances in the body became "specific to metabolic life." I take a cue from this term for my anthropological research. My use of "metabolic living" relies on the word "metabolic" to point out the uncertain ideas and experiences emerging from the metabolism. I take seriously Landecker's argument that metabolism embeds specific, often circular, and conflicting histories of science and philosophy. To signal the ethnographic work I want the concept to do, I include "living" in the term. This draws attention to my informants' embodied additions to the metabolism's conceptual history and to their assertions that how much absorption is truly livable is an open question.[14]

Metabolic living bridges this book's key questions: Who and what is "in charge of" metabolic illness, in India and elsewhere? Is it a person's dampened willpower that makes her gain weight? Is it the deliciousness of fried street foods? Is it *ghar ka khana* ("home food"), lovingly (perhaps) and laboriously (definitely) prepared by someone like Eliza? Do food companies have a hand in the potentials of metabolic disorder as they market instant noodles to Eliza's son? Does the air in that room—Mumbai's sea breezes laced with heavy metals—have a part in the story? What delineates the boundary between the actions of insulin in a given body and that person's "adherence" to a doctor's prescription? Generally, these questions are asked as questions of blame and responsibility, and medical anthropology has productively examined blame as a window onto sociocultural fault lines.[15] Yet these are also questions about the relational power of absorption and, specifically, how material passages generate explanatory value as food, drugs, and diets anchor expressions of desire, fallibility, causality, blame, and resilience.[16]

Much like the brain, the metabolism has come to stand for personal pathologies—a tendency of metabolic realism and somatic personification.[17] That is, there is often a slippage between the stomach and personhood, such that it seems as if persons *are* their metabolisms, as opposed to *having* metabolisms.[18] This iterative difference converges with a moment in contemporary bioscience that is heavily invested in complexities and plasticity (see Landecker 2007; Niewöhner 2011; Malabou 2008; Papadopoulos 2011; Rees 2010). Further, it converges with increasing attention to chronic disease / cardiometabolic disease in global health. Further still, it converges with India as an idealized site of possible analysis and explanation of global chronic disease patterns. When "being" conflates with "having" at the population scale, the metabolic can determine public health risk. Stomachs can reflect the well-being of populations. Bellies can toll the bells of longevity. Guts undo nations. In this framework, we can see how the collapse of *being a metabolism* and *having a metabolism* dovetails with obsessions about middle-class overconsumption in urban South Asia.[19] Rather than rest on this collapse, I offer a different approach in order to trouble it. I show how people spotlight and disaggregate the patterns of substance, intent, and effect that biomedicine counts as metabolic in order to uphold the narrative that obesity and diabetes are a problem in India. Sometimes these patterns are open to rearrangement and a domain of open exchange and in other moments they appear to be a closed system. The book thus argues for attention to the absorptions of harm and care across political contours.

In its call for attention to permeability of bodies and environments, this book draws on an extensive literature in South Asian studies that addresses questions of relative openness based on domains of the home and public space and across persons, communities, and families (see Daniel 1984; Fruzzetti and Ostor 1982). Food and commensality have been central to these studies (Marriott 1968). From its inception, scholarship on food and eating in South Asia has been concerned with substance, exchange, and propriety. For example, this can be seen in anthropologist McKim Marriott's "cube" model of Hindu life paradigms that models possible arrangements between sentiments, temperatures, seasons, life cycle events, marriageability, and spatial arrangements of the home as they articulate with specific qualities of food (1989).[20] In contemporary India, across faiths and communities, the exchange of food is most certainly still enacted in the name of social hierarchy, but it is also done in the name of market expansion, class and caste dynamics, and the edification of a health problem. Scholarship on food in South Asia offers a means to think differently about biomedicine's assumed starting and ending points when it comes to metabolic illness. This literature also informs my analysis of what is constantly in play in my study of metabolic living in India: the persistence and continued history of malnutrition. Here I mean malnutrition in its general invocation as under- or inadequate nutrition. Often, though, physicians tell me that obesity is itself an issue of malnutrition, too—just one of *over*nutrition. This is a difficult claim to write about, because I want to capture that sentiment while being quite mindful of a question I encounter often: "Why study obesity in India, when there is so much malnutrition?" To be clear, this book does not attempt to dampen or deny the very real suffering that both under- and overnutrition cause. Indeed, obesity (in contrast to diabetes) has received little attention in medical anthropology based in India, not only because metabolic illness has been recognized as a recent epidemiological and cultural concern but also because of the lived realities of undernutrition and hunger.

This point also speaks to the broader representational and moral politics of an anthropology of biomedicine concerned with fatness and set in India.[21] At present, a dichotomy between the fat, overfed rich person and the starving peasant structures most discourses surrounding obesity in India. For example, it is quite common to encounter a contrapuntal narrative of haves and have-nots, marked by their embodied conditions of obesity and malnutrition. The problem with this setup is that the liberal subject of choice—here, the overfed body hungry for ever more options—anchors the play of good/bad or better/worse. Instead of reifying that dichotomy and keeping obesity and malnutrition conceptually separate,

I use stories of absorption to question the kinds of global health and social evidence produced in the shuttling back and forth between poles of deprivation and excess. I ask how appeals to consumption may, however unintentionally, exaggerate the distance between these poles, because metabolic illness is a concern not only for India's middle classes, although it has gained credibility through their bodies. There are significant concerns about obesity affecting poorer populations, in terms not of actual fatness but of the metabolic disorder that may not show up as extra kilos on the scale. Further, diabetes is understood to affect Indians across social strata. These concerns continue, rather than displace, the ways that malnutrition continues to work as a social and material fact.[22] Metabolic disease in India becomes a curious site, where malnutrition gains explanation not only from the usual realm of economists and policymakers but also from physicians, bioscientists, and food companies.

As a result of this move there are truth effects, such that food consumption gains increased attention only when perceived as a precursor of certain bodily conditions. The cultural figures of the middle-class housewife binging on *barfi* and the malnourished child must be understood in a reticular perspective; that is, one of many little nets rather than a binary. Absorption offers one framework for a reticular perspective. In this framework, the pleasures and vicissitudes of "food," "the body," and "the environment" emerge sideways to consumption and thus decenter it as a disease's only possible source of cause and consequence.

Methods for an Urban Environment

With an eye to the importance of location, one of my goals is to situate food and fat as a pattern constitutive of Mumbai as an urban environment. Doing so shows how specific body-city configurations connect science studies to area studies.[23] In the case of metabolic illness, Mumbai-as-megacity often is mobilized to prove a public health hunch: a city that is too stressful and polluted for healthy life, even as it offers the culinary temptations of cosmopolitanism.[24] Take, as an example, Carter Road's culinary rhythms unfolding by the plague crosses: fruit juice in the morning, sugarcane juice midday, and ice cream and *chaat* (snacks) in the evening. Day and night, they witness the tides of the Arabian Sea, Mumbai's porous milieu. My neighbors often pointed to the sea to remark on its receding coastline, ever-diminishing returns on fish, and ever-increasing concentrations of pollutants.

"The city" also materialized as crowded trains, disputes over living spaces, and hazardous roads that preventing walking and playing. My neighbors would tell me in one breath that only rich people got fat, that the neighborhood was not wealthy enough for obesity to be a problem, and that everyone in the neighborhood was dieting to lose weight. Men would slap each other's bellies. Women would greet each other with observations of how much one had "reduced" or lost weight (or to me, when I returned to Mumbai after time in the United States, they would remark how much I had put on). Mumbai's diversity added layers of richness to this problem but also dissolved difference in ways that made cultural moorings difficult to isolate. Religious, geographic, and linguistic communities would begin and end on one floor of an apartment building, in the building itself, or perhaps on a few city blocks: Goan Catholics here, Gujarati Muslims there, Marwari Hindus there. Of course, marriage matches went on, stereotypes persisted, and "regional" restaurants kept themselves in business with appeals to specific forms of culinary authenticity. But to conduct a project primarily about food in Mumbai required movements in and out of multiple communities and commitments. Thus, for readers interested in South Asia, in this book India and Mumbai appear in varying shades of uniformity and plurality, especially in biomedical settings that often demand homogenized bodies, symptoms, and treatments.

I conducted the research for this book in Mumbai from 2005 to 2012, in fieldwork periods ranging from two to eighteen months (the main research period was 2008/9). Fieldwork unfolded across three main subject domains. The first domain was everyday relations to food and health in a coastal, lower-middle-class neighborhood in Mumbai. This involved long-term, repeated observations and interviews with neighbors inside households and at neighborhood social occasions such as religious holidays and community events. The second domain concerned the diagnosis, treatment, and experiential narratives of metabolic illnesses—particularly obesity and diabetes—in two clinics in this neighborhood, one private and one embedded in a hospital. This second methodological arm involved interviews with and observations of nearly two hundred patients, eight nutritionists, and twenty physicians; data came from shadowing physicians in their clinical hours, up to five a day. If patients consented, I would then interview them at the clinic or at a place and time of their choosing; a typical interview lasted thirty minutes. My routes to metabolism did not include as many Ayurvedic consultative encounters as they did biomedical ones, but I do draw on the insights of scholars who have closely examined the links between food and Ayurveda, Unani, and other modalities in the South Asian landscape of healing (see, e.g., Ecks 2014; Halliburton 2009; Langford 2002; Nichter 1981).

Moving from the neighborhood into clinical domains raised questions about how endocrinology and its applied clinical practice hinge on the absorptive contingencies of fats, proteins, and carbohydrates. Clinicians may determine obesity by means of body weight or the body mass index (explained further in chapter 1), but they also declare a person obese using definitions of adiposity (a measure of visceral body fat) and dyslipidemia (abnormal levels of lipids in the blood). The clinicians and patients I observed also navigate the terminological contingencies that crisscross obesity and type 2, or "adult onset," diabetes, which is a condition of ineffective insulin usage in the body. One term is "prediabetic," meaning that a person's fasting glucose and/or glucose tolerance levels are between parameters of "normal" and "diabetic."[25] Another is "metabolic syndrome," a concept introduced in the late 1980s to describe a bodily state in which one is at increased risk for type 2 diabetes mellitus and cardiovascular disease (see Reaven 1988). Adiposity and dyslipidemia are key measures of metabolic syndrome in a clinical setting, as is the measurement of HbA1c, which is glycated hemoglobin (hemoglobin that has glucose attached to it). Inflecting many of these measures and states is insulin, a hormone secreted by pancreatic cells called beta cells. Metabolizing and storing glucose is what insulin signals cells to do. Diabetes arises when insulin is not present at adequate levels in relation to blood glucose levels and/or when cells do not respond to insulin's signaling actions. This latter state characterizes the dampened insulin response that is called "insulin resistance," which is considered to be a hallmark of metabolic syndrome (see, e.g., Joshi and Parikh 2007; Johnson 2013). My clinical observations showed biochemistry and endocrinology to be domains of knowledge that scaled into solid disease categories that medical experts, neighborhood residents, and food companies could all use to diagnose, narrate a history, or identify a market niche. These categories had remarkable staying power, even as I witnessed people explode them.

The third domain of fieldwork concerned the commercialization of food, which involved observations and interviews with food company marketers, street food vendors, and produce and meat vendors, some in the neighborhood but also spread out across the city. During my time in Mumbai, several national regulations concerning nutrition labeling and packaging changed, prompting meetings of specialists in food regulatory policies, food marketing, and food safety. These meetings allowed me to meet multiple individuals at once and then follow up individually in interviews. Yielding over thirty encounters, this methodological arm involved observing a day's work of a vendor; for food marketers in companies, it involved attending isolated meetings and select interviews with workers and company staff. Additionally, I attended multiple medical conferences concerned with metabolic illnesses in Mumbai, New Delhi, and Chennai that gathered hundreds of Indian physicians and allied medical professionals. At these conferences, I used convenience sampling to build a broader network of physicians, surgeons, and nutritionists across India to interview, so that opinions on nutrition and metabolic disease would be transferable to populations beyond my immediate neighborhood and beyond Mumbai. Thus, my fieldwork sites coalesced across three broad scales of the city: Manuli's home and street life, its nearby clinics, and more multi-sited spaces occupied by food companies, government nutritional regulators, and biomedical and public health conferences. I worked across these scales guided by the methodological maneuvers of Cohen (1998) and Rapp (1999), interested in the ways that "the clinical" or "the scientific" settles into forms of living.

I began my study in an area of Mumbai called Bandra; specifically, in an area of Bandra that is a small neighborhood I call Manuli.[26] I first came to Manuli, a fishing village, or *koliwada*, because of my real estate broker, George. He had shown me all around Bandra, where I wanted to be based for research because of its demographic diversity, its large number of family-owned and chain restaurants, and its significant number of weight-loss and metabolic disease clinics. We came to Manuli, and I was fascinated by its architecture and histories. We walked down its main street, just opposite the shore, and came to the church, whose founding parishioners date to 1575, a period when the Portuguese Jesuit presence in the area was strong. George lived close to the church and grew up in the neighborhood. He showed me an available flat in a building just up the street. It was a good fit, and the landlord, Francis, was pleasant and easygoing, two qualities I came to value deeply since I would be living directly next door to him, his wife, and their two children. My bedroom window directly faced a small clearing between homes and apartment buildings. I later learned that this space was the site of the jubilant wedding scene in the film *Amar Akbar Anthony*, one of several Hindi films with Bandra as its backdrop. Fifty years ago, it had been used as an open space to dry freshly caught fish. Now it was a makeshift garbage dump and passageway between the main road and the neighborhood's snaking back alleys.

The government sold the land around the clearing to a private developer who flouted building codes and built slum-like temporary structures anywhere with open space. Another neighbor later explained that many of the hutment inhabitants were Muslims who came from neighborhoods torn apart by the Bombay riots in 1992, whereas this side of Bandra—Bandra West—had remained largely unscathed. However, despite the cosmopolitanism of the neighborhood (including its criminal underworld threads, in the form of brothels and illegal land sales), it was regarded mostly as a *koliwada* of "East Indians." According to an ethnography of Mumbai's East Indians written in 1967 by sociologist Elsie Baptista, the East Indians were Hindu converts to Catholicism during the sixteenth century; they thus first became known as "Portuguese Christians" (although, importantly, Baptista captures both the multiplicity of the community's origin stories and how community members also reckon far earlier origins in the North Konkan region). Later, according to Baptista (1967: 25), the community adopted the name "East Indians" because "they wanted to impress upon the British Government of Bombay that they were the earliest Roman Catholic subjects of the British Crown in this part of India."[27] Many of my informants identified as East Indian, but I also interviewed a number of Catholics who traced their origins to Goa. Many of the Hindus in the neighborhood I interviewed were Gujarati or from the interior of Maharashtra, but an equal number claimed Mumbai as their "family place" of origin.

To meet people, I joined a neighborhood yoga club, which practiced at 6:30 sharp every morning in a small seaside park. Friends there introduced me to several leaders in the church, beginning with Mr. Gomes, who had assumed the role of the church (and neighborhood) archivist. Because East Indians had been in Manuli so long, he explained, there were rich food traditions that deserved documentation. Mr. Gomes suggested that I pursue my interests in food and health by linking up with the church's office workers. Another neighbor introduced me to the church social worker, Mary, whom he suggested could help me formulate a neighborhood survey of food consumption. In return, if I uncovered any "interesting" traditions or long-lost recipes in the course of the survey, I would share them, along with pictures of the foods, for a photo calendar the church was compiling as a fund-raiser.

A week later I walked down the street to the church to discuss this with Mary, who agreed to help with the survey. Assuaging my concern that we would be talking only to Catholics, she promised that we would speak with Hindus and Muslims who also lived in Manuli. "Mary knows everyone," an elderly woman in the church office assured me as she meticulously recorded the week's offerings. Mary was more than a neighborhood social worker, a position she held as a volunteer on top of her regular work as the church office manager. She was a tireless advocate for the neighborhood's residents of all faiths and the coordinator of Manuli's chapter of a *mahila mandal* (women's group). We agreed that I would accompany her on her "regular" work, which entailed listening to residents' concerns on many issues: trash pickup, sewage line hookups, food ration prices, school uniform costs, noisy neighbors, and municipal politicking. I shadowed her on her rounds through alleyways and sea-facing footpaths, through pukka homes and makeshift hutments, as she listened to endless complaints. She took on the injuries of others: no food or water access, botched admission processes for a family's child, claims to discrimination against Catholics. She connected residents to the proper channels for action, whether that entailed NGOs, the church, or the city government, or if immediate action was needed, she would directly phone the local corporator (municipal politician). In these visits and on their paths of redress, if the person we were visiting consented, I could ask my own questions.

Mary was a fixer and a fighter—she became my research assistant as well—such that she was generous enough to open some of her world to a foreign stranger even as she took on the heavy load of casework of the community's domestic and public disputes. As a result, my inquiries about food and health were inextricable from the everyday political complaints that brought us into homes and from the daily domestic work, like food shopping and cooking for her family, that Mary still had to do amid all her other occupations. To grasp the imprint of the clinical was impossible without understanding the neighborhood as a critical site of analysis, and its residents as differentially emplaced in obligations to kin and other residents (Das 2014). My position in these encounters was as a neighbor, someone who moved in and out. "He lives just over there," Mary would say as a means of introducing me to others; vague but close enough. This position, which I want neither to overexaggerate nor underplay, appears in my analysis throughout, such that I choose to use "neighbor" to describe my informants in the neighborhood.

Across my three domains of inquiry, I learned that food, whether as something eaten or something that triggered attention through its metabolites in a blood sample, was just one of many substances that infused metabolic stories. The knotty rope connecting food and fat revealed other ways of weaving elements—stress, family relations, labor conditions—together in patterns. Attention to the absorption of these patterns challenges the inevitability of individuated consumption as the penultimate stop on the dead-end train to healthism and medicalization. As we will see, the biomedical does not and indeed cannot always script the punch line when it comes to food and fat.[28] Biomedicine hardly has exclusive claims to matters of body weight in India. Certainly the usual suspects of weight-loss companies and health-advice columnists have stepped in to help amid obesity's epidemic invocations. Even Baba Ramdev, a famous spiritual leader to many in India, offers *motapa ke liye yog*, yoga for obesity, accomplished through breath work and posture combinations illustrated in pamphlets and DVDs. Health science is often part of these appeals, but there are many other appeals in play, such as those to fair skin and sexuality. Other healing modalities also are on the table. Mumbai's landscape of slimming clinics, Ayurvedic centers, and homeopathic stalls predates concerns about mass metabolic illness but now is differentially implicated in them. Inside and outside medicine, substances make patterns.[29] These patterns help illustrate the possibilities and limits of medicalization as one of medical anthropology's narrative tactics and make room for additional frameworks such as absorption.

## Writing the Metabolic

Anthropological engagements with obesity and diabetes have most often been concerned with health outcomes or the aesthetic dimensions of fat, with narrative illness experiences, or with the ways that disease categories concentrate and flourish (see Edmonds 2010; Popenoe 2003; Kulick and Meneley 2005). These studies suggest the importance of the materiality of substances like fat and sugar, but I would like to tread carefully in writing about these substances only in terms of their medicalization. Medicalization too easily assumes that biomedicine itself consumes life's pleasures (like food) and subjects them to the endgame of rationalization, measurement, cause-effect, and commodification. Again, we are back to an arrangement of power and agency in which persons are already patients, ready to avoid consuming objects that are already risks. By contrast, a focus on absorption points out actions of soaking in, working, and taking in stress and highlights the relational capacities of elements like pollutants, adulterants, sugars, and trans fats. Metabolic living means living through lipid assays, fasting sugar levels, inches on the waist, kilos on the scale, BMI numbers, diet foods, and wedding foods. Specific materials and specific bodies are needed to make a phenomenon such as "metabolic illness in India" happen (see Thompson 2005). It is the problematic movements and the constant redefinitions of body and environment that guide what we know to be a problem and how that problem surfaces viscerally and in public culture.

This distributive dimension of the metabolism presents several puzzles for ethnographic theory, method, and writing. First: How to conceive and discuss something that is simultaneously internally and externally connected to the body?[30] This problem features prominently in biomedicine, because the question of who can put the outside in is quite relevant to tactics of prescribing drugs and diets. One approach in medical anthropology, informed by science and technology studies, has been to think about how specific practices bring these divides into being. This kind of reasoning attests to the multiplicity and distribution of disease and names practices as central to understanding the many forms that disease can take.[31] I certainly agree that it takes many objects to constitute, order, and disorder the metabolism. Scraps of diets moving in and out of homes, exchanges of food at festivals, and scales recording changing body weights surely have multiple incarnations. Just as disease categories must be understood as multiply enacted, we might engage substances as plural and relational, as more than simply the "missing masses" of objects that satisfy demands to add the nonhuman back into human stories (Latour 2005; see also Mol and Mesman 1996; Mann et al. 2011). Bodies also operate in the plural in the domain of metabolic life. Those who feed, eat, breathe, and labor do so often in nonindividuated arrangements with immediate and extended families, friends, and communities. That is, categories such as "patients," "obesity," "diabetes," "food," "drugs," and "metabolic illness" materialize and overlap in lived experience, even as they fashion urban India as a site of mass illness in the imaginations and interventions of biomedicine and global health. This concern over distribution and plurality is as compelling to scientists as it is to those invested in cultural studies of science. With its focus on absorption, I contend that metabolic living is a framework that can accommodate such diversity.[32]

Yet a challenge of positionality arises, for the very topic of food conjoins ethnographer and ethnographic subject in that, as humans, both are metabolic persons. So much of my research unfolded around moments of eating or talking about eating. Expressions about bodies and health surfaced over meals or between my requests for recipes or in sidebar conversations about food that punctuated daily rhythms of my informants like taking insulin.[33] This is evident in the earlier vignette about the noodles. Whose visceral metabolism and whose analytical metabolism are at stake? I found that problems of metaphor and of possession overdetermined the field of thinking with and about metabolisms even while being able to do the research because I have one. Complex relations generate literal *and* metaphorical distributions of the metabolism. I pinpoint these distributions with Ed Cohen's discussion (2009) of metaphor in mind: "Recognizing and appreciating the transformational force of metaphor, both within science and within the world, means considering how metaphor matters, not merely as an instrumental manipulation *of* the world but also as a new way of living *in* the world" (38). Many people I encountered, from fishmongers to physicians, attested to the constellation of metabolic illnesses. They recognized that fatness did not always mean sickness, that stress was as much a cofactor for the development of disease as was familial genetic inheritance, and that the time frames of the "chronic" in chronic disease varied widely (see Manderson 2010). Some named problems specifically as metabolic, while others, working more metaphorically, pinned down bodily speed, corporate greed, or failed willpower as the conditions for obesity's possibility. People took care of their maladies, often guided by biomedicine, and so therapy in varying forms was an integral part of daily life.[34] The critiques offered by my interlocutors offer ways of engaging differently with metabolisms and thus with bodies of all sizes and makeups.[35] The metabolism at the center of these discussions, across observer and observed, is a distribution of conditions that expand and constrict a livable, bearable life.

Each of the chapters in this book elaborates such conditions. Chapter 1 asks: How does fat get into individual and collective bodies? This chapter is concerned with absorption between past and present times. It examines the feature of bodily plasticity by questioning the condition of "globesity," the supposed west-to-east flow of capital and consumerist desires that sparked India's collective weight gain. It maps historical and literary portraits of fatness in India and details how globesity presumes a national vulnerability through comparisons of bodies experiencing newfound prosperity. As claims of obesity's emergence in India impelled physicians to change national guidelines for the body mass index, overnight millions of Indians were suddenly considered overweight. This generated a problem of matching metabolisms to persons over generations. Public health policies and their biological rationales circulated popularly imagined oppositions of the cultural figures of the hungry, lower-caste rural person and the overfed middle-class urbanite. This subject became known in biomedical discourses and epigenetic science as "the thin-fat Indian": the body that absorbs prosperity into its very constitution, even as that constitution increasingly marks the attrition of life and health through chronic disease. The figure of the thin-fat Indian is a sketch of how metabolism is temporal.

Chapter 2 is concerned with absorption between persons and urban space. Moving from the scales of globe and nation toward the scale of the street, it addresses how metabolism is spatial and how biomedical sciences and the science of urban politics overlap. The *vada pav*, Mumbai's famous fried street food, connected biomedical concerns about the rising rate of obesity to violent local politics and multinational food company interests. In doing so, projects to claim and reform the *vada pav* define the grounds of the political life of an object beyond the act of its consumption. Using the concept of "gastropolitics," I first describe how a local political party branded its own version of the food and then show how corporate franchises inspired by McDonald's rendered the *vada pav* "safe" and "clean" through mechanized standardization. Rather than take the metabolism of fried food for granted, I de-emphasize its consumption and foreground the political circumstances that inform and animate it through observations and interviews at street-side *vada pav* stalls, at new corporations determined to standardize *vada pav*, and with nutritionists who condemn the *vada pav* as the source of Mumbai's obesity problem.

Chapter 3 introduces another key concept of this book: the blur between food and drugs. It is concerned with absorption between persons and markets. It considers the feature of processing and explores the social lives of processed foods to examine relations crafted between forms of domesticity, market forces, and discourses of bodily threat. Metabolism in this chapter is commercially gendered, through the sciences of food processing and food adulteration. On one hand, because many packaged foods were snacks, physicians and nutritionists derided them for being unhealthy and causing weight gain. On the other hand, their aseptic packaging offered a "clean" alternative to foods tainted by seemingly ubiquitous food adulteration scandals, which housewives in Manuli attributed to "the nexus" of the urban underworld, corporations, and corrupt politicians. During the 1990s, advances in food packaging created means to "protect" foods but also enabled companies to fortify foods with "extra" nutritional additives that could help prevent chronic disease. Packaged foods opened up new possibilities to keep families healthy while tightening relations between the home and the corporation. This raises questions about what it means to absorb food provided by an unfamiliar other.

Chapter 4 asks how metabolism is diagnosable and treatable through the sciences of diabetology, nutrition, and surgical amputation. It is concerned with absorption between persons and clinics. Ethnographically, it is anchored in the clinic and works through substances like calories, insulin, and blood sugars as sites of diagnosis and treatment. Morals of individual responsibility and addiction filter into ideas and practices surrounding obesity, and disease categories collapse weight gain into other pathologies along specific relational lines. For some clinicians, diets could shore up their patients' sense of personal responsibility, with weight loss as a visceral reward for moral fortitude. There were limits to diets, however, as I discuss in the case of prescribing drugs and in the practice of limb amputation for diabetics.

Chapter 5 concludes the book by examining the extent to which metabolisms are renewable and even replaceable through the science of surgery. It is concerned with absorptions between the body and willpower. It considers what kinds of treatment for obesity are possible when drugs and diet fail. The chapter explores the phenomenon of metabolic surgery, in which surgeons attempt to reconfigure the inner organs, such as the stomach and intestine, to "adjust" the invisible force of the metabolism. Overweight people turned to metabolic surgery to free themselves from the perceived frailty of willpower to triumph over consumption, based on the belief that their body could no longer be further disciplined by diet. The surgery promises to cure metabolic disease by targeting the metabolism as a biomedically manageable proxy for the will.

In writing and thinking about the metabolism and metabolic illness, I often return to "Epidemics of the Will," an essay in Eve Sedgwick's book *Tendencies* (1993), partly, perhaps, because of my own professional trajectory in public health, beginning with HIV/AIDS work years before I became interested in anthropology or obesity, and certainly because of Sedgwick's prescient sense of the demands an epidemic narrative selectively places on bodies and lives. In "Epidemics of the Will," Sedgwick discusses addiction to substances such as food and alcohol. She notes that to study and write about the issue, one cannot locate analysis in either body or substance. Rather, Sedgwick suggests the importance of what she calls "some overarching abstraction" (131) between bodies and substances that is the locus of a problem. In this book, the metabolism is indeed an abstraction, one often called forth as a metaphor. But it is also thoroughly material, a pattern of biochemistry, physiology, and habit.

I explore the narrative potential of the metabolism as a semiomaterial abstraction in the interludes between the chapters. The interludes recount scenes of people demonstrating absorption's political terms and thus the terms of metabolic living: how food can be an object of desire and revulsion, how diets produce problems and possibilities, how food ration politics is a complex machine, how meat imprints bodies and the city, and how medication has its saving graces and its limits.[36] Together, these scenes constitute an overarching abstraction that governs how bodies and substances pattern. The interludes are attempts to work through several challenges afoot in writing about the metabolism. One is the already mentioned tension between the material and the metaphorical. Another is the tenuous centrality of food to a given vignette. Given that this book proposes the need to think more expansively about connections between food, bodies, and environments, how might one write about food without over- or undermining its importance to people as they are, as food might change them, and as they change food? Like the numbered chapters, the interludes work through this question by narrating sites of absorption. Like a metabolism, the interludes are a set of signals.

These signals of the in-betweenness of substances, bodies, and environments demand careful handling. They need care in order to be meaningful for this book's specific case study in India and to be meaningful for the configurations of substances, bodies, and environments elsewhere. The fact that bioscience and biomedicine are not clear on what the metabolism *is* registers in everyday ways for people in terms of what and how to eat or of how they flip between one diet and another and in terms of the city spaces that shelter food-body disconnects. The thing that is supposed to absorb the world is really not well known, and the degree to which it is known is constantly changing. As these changes unfold, their dynamic sciences and lived experiences open up spaces to ask about the fundamental condition of metabolic living: that people reckon constantly with absorption.

Sugar coats the streets in September. One afternoon it was *Ganesh Chaturthi*, a Hindu celebration of the birth of Lord Ganesha that takes on epic celebrations in Mumbai. Later that same night, it was the celebration by Manuli's Catholics of the birthday of the Virgin Mary. Sugar crystallized as *modak*, sweet dumplings filled with coconut and jaggery, which are considered Ganesha's favorite. Sugar also materialized a birthday cake six feet long: "Happy Birthday Mother Mary!" it exclaimed. The coincident festivals forced some creative logistics for spaces of celebration on Manuli's main street. In the middle of the street, people hoisted a flag with a picture of the Virgin headlined with "Ave Maria." It marked the beginning of the novena. Around the flagpole, my Catholic neighbors gathered and recited the Rosary, this one especially to keep rain away during the days of the novena. The flagpole stood next to a shrine of the Virgin, which people lined up to kiss before making their way to the food tables.

Manuli had a tradition of circulating a large statue of the Virgin among households during this time. Mary, my research assistant, was in charge of this complex operation. Her family had hosted the Virgin earlier that day, with the shift from another home into hers heralded by the ringing of the bells and a Rosary recitation. When the bells rang at dusk, Mary had been explaining to me a way to cook chicken she saw on television (pressure-cook to two whistles, then panfry in a nonstick pan with only one teaspoon of oil, "so it's healthy"). She scribbled the recipe on a piece of paper and ran out to join her family to carry the statue of the Virgin back to her home. Once in her family compound, the statue of Our Lady was garlanded and placed on an altar. Incense filled the room, as did flower offerings, more Rosaries, and twenty minutes of a sung refrain:

Mother of God, star of the sea, pray for the wanderer, pray for me.

After the song, the food: soda and small cookies served by the men in a reversal of the gendered axes of food service observable during certain festivals.

The evening's celebration of Our Lady's birthday shared celebratory space with the processions of mobile *pandals* (carts) carrying forms of likeness of the deity Ganesha called *murtis* (incarnate representations). The carts wove through the neighborhood to eventually end at the sea, where the statues would be submerged in the water in the ritual of *visarjan*. Drums sounded constantly. Women accompanying the carts handed out *modak* to passersby—offerings and blessings on the move. During the weeks leading up to *Ganesh Chaturthi*, newspapers fill with warnings to paint the *murtis* with environmentally friendly paints. Neighborhoods and apartment buildings in Mumbai make and decorate their own *murtis*, often with plaster of paris. But this plaster doesn't fully dissolve, and the brilliant colors of the paints gilding it are usually made with heavy metals, turning the sea pink and orange and poisonous.

The processions continued apace. Marigold petals flew, as did chants:

*Ganpati bappa morya!* (Great Lord Ganesha!)
*Ek, do, teen, char, Ganpaticha jai jai kar!* (One, two, three, four, long live Lord Ganesha!)
Twinkle twinkle little star, Ganpati is superstar!

When the drums beat loudest, they signal the arrival of the *pandals*, turning the corner onto the main street (the penultimate stop before inching down the alleyways to the sea). The Virgin Mary's birthday celebration parted from the center of the street toward its margins to make way for the carts. Slices of cake and *modak* changed hands across faiths. It still mattered who fed whom, but the rules seemed more relaxed. The bland rice outer layer of *modak* hid powerfully sweet coconut on the inside. "You can be a shit person on the outside, but Ganesh will find your inner sweetness," a friend explained. Many of the Ganesha *murtis* on the carts were especially chubby, little surprise given how the fat elephant and his ties to prosperity move easily through public culture. Children invoke him in the nursery rhyme *kitna achcha mota haathi, us par baitha uska saathi* (the fat elephant is so lovely, we sit on him together), authors of get-rich-quick books emblazon their covers with his image, and even an Indian plus-size women's clothing company has reclaimed him in their ads. In medical conferences, I saw cartoons of a young Ganesh on PowerPoint slides about childhood obesity. Here, he symbolized the sedentary schoolchild who became fat being absorbed in computers and video games. Too much absorption with computers, too little with exercise. This was much to the consternation of his *chuha*, the mouse who serves as his vehicle, who in these cartoons struggled to shoulder Ganesh's chubbiness.

It began to rain. The table with the birthday cake folded up, and the street opened for a dance party. The *pandals* continued down into the alleys, toward the sea. *Ganpati Bappa Morya!* Chants and drums intensified. Sometimes the *pandals* would snag on the gates of homes or even the homes themselves. One man climbed onto a house's corrugated roof and peeled it off at the corner to allow the cart through the space. My neighbor Prakash pushed his family's *pandal*. It was a nice break, he said, from a night at the call center where he phoned people in the United States to remind them of their mortgage default and the initiation of foreclosure proceedings by the bank his voice represented. It was 2009, squarely amid the global financial crisis, and he was making these calls constantly.

Down to the sea, behind the gaze of the plague crosses. The tide was out. The worship ritual of *aarti* began: one of Prakash's relatives circled a plate with a small burning lamp in front of the Ganesha *murti*. Hands clapped in unison over and over. As fire and gazes concentrated, I attempted to be useful by holding umbrellas to keep people and the *murti* dry. When this part of the ritual finished, the submersion (*visarjan*) began. Men lifted the *murti* off the cart, climbed off the dock, and floated as it sank into the black water, plastered layers of fat dissolving.

The Thin-Fat Paradox

In 1999, two endocrinologists, Dr. C. S. Yajnik, from Pune, India, and Dr. John Yudkin, from London, published a side-by-side photo of themselves in the *Lancet*. Their report is entitled "The Y-Y Paradox." The paradox, named "Y-Y" after their last names, emerges from the bodies of the scientists themselves. They sit together, coexistent but comparative, quite peaceful, given how their bodies would ultimately anchor a controversy (figure 1.1).

The photo shows how the two scientists have the same BMI of 22.3, but Dr. Yudkin has 9.1 percent body fat, while Dr. Yajnik's level is 21.2 percent. The text below the photo explains the paradox:

> The authors share a near identical body-mass index (BMI), but as dual X-ray absorptiometry imagery shows, the similarity ends there. The first author [Yajnik] (figure, right) has substantially more body fat than the second author [Yudkin] (figure, left). Lifestyle may be relevant: the second author runs marathons whereas the first author's main exercise is running to beat the closing doors of the elevator in the hospital every morning. The contribution of genes to such adiposity is yet to be determined, although the possible relevance of intrauterine undernutrition is supported by the first author's low birth weight. The image is a useful reminder of the limitations of BMI as a measure of adiposity across populations. (Yajnik and Yudkin 2004: 163)

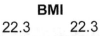

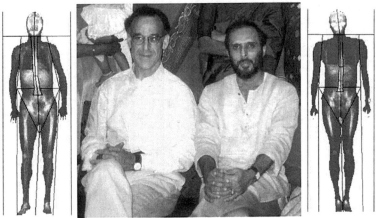

**BMI**
22.3       22.3

**Body fat**
9.1%       21.2%

**FIG. 1.1** The Y-Y Paradox of the Thin-Fat Indian, *The Lancet*, vol. 363, January 10, 2004.

In the Y-Y paradox, evidence emerges through a procedure, dual X-ray absorptiometry, that sends energy beams into the body to assess their relative absorptions by bones and fat. Fat inside the body, under the skin and around the organs, sends back a message: comparisons have their limits. Fat absorbs some kinds of evaluation (X-rays that will produce radiographs). But it resists other evaluative forms, producing "a near identical body-mass index" despite manifest differences in body fat between the men. Yajnik and Yudkin suggest that perhaps layers of living are the more accurate way to understand fat: in genes, in utero, in the elevator, in the marathon. In the Y-Y paradox, it is not fat itself that is anomalous. Rather, what matters are the absorptive interfaces between fat and the world. This chapter examines how those interfaces matter differently in making metabolisms uniquely Indian and the site of disease risk.

I learned about this *Lancet* article from my interviews with physicians, who suggested I look into the Y-Y paradox, which they referred to as "the paradox of the thin-fat Indian." This phenomenon gained its name in scientific literature (including that of epigenetics) that questions how histories of malnutrition in early life or in earlier generations influence the onset of metabolic disease in later life or later generations.[1] These puzzles materialize the puzzling body of the thin-fat Indian. This thin-fat Indian body can be thin *and* fat at the same time: thin morphologically but metabolically obese according to its impaired insulin sensitivity and elevated levels of lipids. In this figure of metabolic science, time and fat absorb each other.

Any person can exhibit the characteristics of the thin-fat body. The paradigm is intended to provoke several possible conclusions from the idea that thin bodies may be metabolically similar to fat bodies. One conclusion relates to the limitations of using size to determine metabolic pathology. A second is even more provocative: If thin and malnourished bodies can show the precursors of obesity, then brute associations of obesity to broad categories of social class and geographic area merit rethinking and refinement in relation to comparative temporalities.

The thin-fat Indian as a cultural figure and scientific theory engaged several theories and debates about metabolic science in terms of the physiology of weight gain in contexts of differential nutrition. The first, called the "thrifty gene" hypothesis, was developed by James Neel in a 1962 publication in the *American Journal of Human Genetics*. Neel suggested that the body had an inherent tendency to store energy as fat during times of sufficient food supply, which would ensure survival during times of famine. Because contemporary (mostly urban) life has brought about a constant supply of food, the body remains in a perpetual state of fat storage, driven by a "quick insulin trigger" generated after meals.[2] The second influential theory is called the "thrifty phenotype" hypothesis (also called the "fetal origins" hypothesis) developed by David Barker (2007), who proposed that a fetal environment shaped by maternal malnutrition would more strongly predict metabolic disease in later life. As anthropologist Michael Montoya (2011) has detailed, scholarship in population genetics, epigenetics, and evolutionary biology often appeals to such "thrifty" hypotheses even while other scholars deem the ideas unwarranted. The narrative arc of evidence here is that a lifestyle of modernity's excess activates an inner bodily force (formed either generations ago or in the fetal environment) and causes the body's energies to go awry. The words of a Mumbai physician I spoke with capture the layers of resource and failure built into these theories with a literal bang of a world working upon bodies: "Genetics loads the gun, but the environment pulls the trigger," he explained. This, even as he acknowledged that phenotypes do not map cleanly onto single genes (Sunder Rajan 2006: 191–92).

I found the photo of the Y-Y paradox compelling. As a configuration of two bodies from colony and empire, it does cultural work in asking the viewer to "see" a paradox of biology as a common thread between bodily histories. Famine and its political history consolidates in the peculiar similarities and differences between a British scientist and an Indian scientist.[3] If that thread is followed, the picture of the paradox poses something different than binaries of nature and culture, of kindling and sparks, of guns and triggers. The thin-fat Indian destabilized "thrifty" sciences even as it drew on them as resources. What mattered was not so much the distribution of triggers to nature *or* culture, to genes *or* environment—binary distributions that anthropologists of science and medicine have shown to be contingent, local, and enmeshed (Fullwiley 2011, 2007). The thin-fat body, made flesh metabolically, offered a different pattern of cause and effect than linear narratives of economic transition and resultant indulgent eating. A metabolic body informed the Y-Y paradox, and the Y-Y paradox discerned a metabolically unique Indian whose fat may be visible and/or lying in wait. The "and/or" already was accounted for by knowing the metabolism in terms of time. The thin-fat Indian crystallized past and present events outside and inside the body, as well as the rural-urban continuum grounding these events. "Thin-fat," not just "fat," demanded attention, because thin-fat demonstrates how the absorption of time becomes a trope for Indian bodies. These bodies, in turn, de- and restabilize everyday knowledges about somatic disorder.

Plasticity

The fat body in India is certainly not a novel medical concern, despite recent claims to "globesity" that pose a neat arrangement between India's economic transitions and bodily accumulation (see Arnold 2009). Globesity casts the world as a "biological public" in which a global health problem is both the defining feature of life and a teleological rationale for its own intervention (Livingston 2012: 31). The biological public of globesity is vulnerable because of its relations between inheritance and lived environment. However, the *plastic* fat body—the thin-fat Indian—anchors contemporary concerns in India around metabolic disease. This is a body that emerges from the sciences of epigenetics, wherein plasticity refers to an organism's ability to vary according to its surroundings. Specific to this chapter, the plasticity at stake is that which circulates in the Y-Y hypothesis and outside it, in terms of understanding how and to what extent environments are inherited and lived.[4]

Plasticity can be understood as the ability to give or take shape. Across the life sciences and science and technology studies scholarship that engages these sciences, plasticity is a feature of life that raises questions about what sort of sociotemporal worlds emerge at the interface of the material bodies and environments. As Hannah Landecker explains, the scientific narrative of epigenetics in relation to those variations is suffused with hope, for if it is the case that metabolisms are "open" to change during critical windows of possible exposure—by the mother surrounding a fetus, by toxins breathed in, by food eaten—then perhaps it is the case that plasticity is a pathway to solutions. "This may sound like biological fatalism in just another form," Landecker (2013b) writes, "but the great hope of epigenetics is the essential plasticity of the body: if the body is open to environment, then it is open to environmental intervention. Might we then be able to treat the metabolic diseases of adulthood—diabetes, obesity—by engineering the diets of pregnant women, infants, children and adolescents?" (179). Plasticity as a way of understanding life via the gut has several key correlates. It ties in with ideas about the brain, whose neuronal plasticity of cells and signal pathways also raises questions about the openness between the body and the world (Kuzawa and Quinn 2009; Malabou 2008; Wilson 2015). This linkage between the imprints of guts and brains also connects to debates in developmental biology, particularly in developmental systems theories of biology.[5] Like neural connections, metabolic connections do not and need not fit easily into arrangements of cause and effect or of biological determinism and social idealism. As Landecker points out in the same passage, the emergent sciences that scrutinize plastic connections can lend themselves to hope. My intent is to show how such a hope for change operates through specific tropes in the Indian context, where figures such as the thin-fat Indian manifest a pedagogy of plasticity. The thin-fat Indian is instructive, because its endorsement teaches that fat is an important substance of change over a lifetime, and that the parameters of health and illness are metabolic.[6]

In 2008, the body mass index, or BMI, for Indians changed. (BMI, a calculation of metric height over weight squared, is a measure of body mass, with the mass of fat most often of interest.) This change underscored how a substance like fat becomes a substance of time. While global standards diagnosed a person as "overweight" at a BMI of 25, the new Indian BMI diagnosed overweight status at a BMI of 23. More Indians came to be at risk for metabolic disease, and this occurred at thresholds different from those for other populations. Using this event as a backdrop, this chapter maps out the currents of plasticity running through it. First, I explore the creation of this Indian body mass index and describe the cultural and political work required to turn 25 into 23. The development of the Indian BMI points out the vernacular particularities of plasticity in the face of claims to a global trend of metabolic disease. The creation of 23 aimed to expand diagnosis of metabolic plasticity while giving it local grounding, such that metabolic disease would be more apparent to at-risk persons and their doctors.

Second, I describe what it takes to enumerate this intensified risk and how plasticity appears through the trope of the bad copy: the body that can only be comparable in its shortcomings. Third, I explore conversations in Manuli with my neighbors about everyday metabolic disruptions. I discuss expressions of *tenshun*, an embodied critique of the stresses that life poses to the impressionable body. The body of *tenshun* is open and malleable to the stressful times of the city—crowded trains, long commutes, violence, bureaucracy, and the everyday grind of family life in tight spaces. Sometimes persons are understood to be porous to stresses and to let them pass through without a hitch. More often than not, though, stress sticks and creates lasting damage. Lastly, I return to the Y-Y paradox and the figure of the thin-fat Indian. Discussions with Dr. Yajnik and his interlocutors elucidate what the thin-fat body can do for advancing understandings of metabolic disorder.

I came to understand that scales were productive ethnographic sites to work through the question of how plasticity's actions are recognizable to people in specific moments and through specific cultural figures. If the thin-fat Indian makes plasticity matter, scales offer observational and methodological inroads into those matters. Scales do this in at least two senses. As instruments for measuring weight, scales are technologies of truth, however partial. Historically, the domestication of the scale from public venues into homes was essential for mainstreaming the measurement of body weight. Without the technology of measurement, the moralities affixed to body weight simply couldn't adhere (Schwartz 1986). In another sense, as Anna Tsing explains, scale is a rule of analytic distance that can magnetize or distance us from a problem.[7] The national BMI created in 2008 certainly worked in these two senses of scale. It measured changes in bodies based on a standardization of body weight. It also put the previously used American/European index in the spotlight and anchored a series of extensive debates among biomedical experts about the relationship between risk and enumeration. A story of risk emerged at the dynamic interface of bodies, environments, and time. Concerns over obesity demarcated vernacular bodies through numbers, engaged claims about global epidemiological shifts, and accomplished both these moves by foregrounding a body whose temporal malleability enabled the accumulation of fat.[8]

## 25/23

An elderly man pulled up his white kurta with one hand, inserted a one-rupee coin with the other, and stepped onto the scale. The machine whirred awake. Its face spun green and red lights, and a slit in its front shot out a piece of paper. The man stepped off carefully, slid his feet into sandals, and gave the paper a cursory glance. He shared the results with his two companions. "It says 94 kilos, but I'm 64," he said with a chuckle. In a rush along with all the other commuters, the men (with surprising agility) hopped onto the moving train car arriving at that moment, leaving behind the guess-your-weight scale, one of the most ubiquitous features of Mumbai's local train stations. With visual dazzle, these scales print weight on one side of their readout slips and a fortune on the other. The scales measure bodily change at the intersection of curiosity, certainty, entertainment, and diagnosis.

Scales in the city come in multiple forms and are themselves plastic in their ability to give, take, and shift form. On street corners, men sit cross-legged behind bathroom scales, with a cardboard square laid out in front that announces the one-rupee charge for the passerby to step on and weigh in. Alongside human ones, other bodies are constantly being weighed. Vegetables, fruits, meats, and grains dance onto the scale at vendor carts and shops, where every nudge of the finger on the counterweight can add or subtract rupees from the total sale price. Scales have already determined how much of that food arrives at the market. In Manuli, fish is an essential element of life and work, and scales determine a fisher's remuneration for a morning's catch. Through a fast-moving business ritual on the beach, a distributor for the area weighs what each fisher brings in from the sea and credits the man's account by marking a scrap of paper. Only then will the fish make its way to baskets women carry up and down stairs of apartment buildings, calling out as both question and demand the morning's offerings that eaters will eventually absorb. As for human scales, new forms proliferated, too. One day, outside the Glamour movie theater, I noticed that the long-standing guess-your-weight scale by the ticket line was gone, only to be replaced by a machine that purported to measure BMI. In contrast to the playful ambiguity of train station scales, the BMI machine suggested scientific certitude behind a number combining both result and fortune. No spin dials of lights appeared on this scale's face; instead, a digital readout and a clear question printed in English: "Are you overweight?"

The potential for an answer to that question was at the center of India's story of mass metabolic disruption. In mid-November 2008, newspapers reported that millions of Indians suddenly became overweight. Waiting for the local train, I read a headline about this development: "You Just Got Fatter: What Is Overweight for Caucasians Is Now Obese for Indians." I bought several newspapers at a kiosk on the train platform and found other headlines: "Obesity guidelines rejigged for Indians"; "Fat's in the fire, Gov't brings more under 'obese' and 'overweight'"; "Think you are slim? New norms may make you obese"; and the instructive "How to remove BMI," which included suggestions for approximating actress Kareena Kapoor's famous and ever-elusive size 0 (begin the morning with a glass of warm water with a teaspoon of honey and a squeeze of lemon).

The news reports surfaced after a group of concerned doctors, epidemiologists, and nutritionists gathered in New Delhi to formulate a new body mass index especially for Indians. The group's rationale was that the global standard BMI did not adequately capture the unique conditions of metabolic illness in South Asians because of their unique forms of plasticity. These experts are certainly not generalizable as a medical mass. Some of the leading figures disagreed with Dr. Yajnik's hypothesis, while others embraced it. But regardless of their stance on the particularities of the thin-fat Indian, these experts eventually agreed that transitory body fat could materialize debates about the local biologies of metabolic illness in India (Lock and Kaufert 2001). The meeting trafficked in appeals to global trends in metabolic disease and asserted that India illustrated a particularly intense manifestation of mass metabolic disease because of the metabolic plasticity of Indian bodies. After several days of debate, the expert group produced a consensus statement that created an "Indian" BMI with lower thresholds for the major categories of risk.

A guiding idea here is, first, that the Indian body distributes fat uniquely, in particular areas of the body (such as the abdomen) where the presence, type, and workings of fat increased one's risk for metabolic illness. Put differently, fat is not fat in the eyes of biomedicine—what matters is the makeup of that fat: the *kind* of tissue composing that fat and its specific location. Fat on the arm is not the same as fat on the belly. Measurements of adiposity—the amount and composition of particular types of fat tissue called adipose tissue—arbitrate when and where fat is more or less concerning. There are several types of adipose tissue, and each has specific physiological properties. For example, adipose tissue can protect the organs it surrounds and also can be involved in a complex chain of events that regulate insulin. In the Indian case, the aggregated data leading to the BMI change was based on the idea that South Asians tend to accumulate abdominal fat, called "central obesity." This is not the same kind of fat as the subcutaneous fat on the arms. Abdominal fat is hormonally active such that belly fat has specific relationships to the overall levels of lipids and insulin in the body. These levels, in turn, are related to the risk of metabolic disease.

The calculation of BMI was developed in the early nineteenth century by Adolphe Quetelet, a Belgian mathematician tasked with estimating "normal" body size. For years it was simply one of many possible anthropometric calculations, but by 1970 it had been incorporated into the population and clinical sciences as a standard estimate of excess weight, beginning with a study of Norwegian children. Dr. Ancel Keys, who published a multicountry comparative study of obesity in 1972, gave the measurement the name "body mass index," although he was using the same calculation as Quetelet had 150 years before. During the decades following Keys's study, the BMI became a standard measurement of obesity. Institutions such as the US National Institutes of Health used it to define "thresholds" for normal, borderline, and abnormal conditions of body weight. This authoritative tying of BMI to definitions of individual obesity proceeded even though Keys had written that the BMI was not a useful *individual* diagnostic because it ignored any variable other than weight and height (Hacking 2006). Several doctors I interviewed agreed with the limitations of the "standardized" Western BMI. For most physicians I interviewed in Mumbai, BMI had been a well-known but relatively incidental calculation for health in India until the late 1990s. For example, a doctor who started Mumbai's first obesity clinic in the 1960s had long preferred to use body weight as an indicator because it was easier for patients to understand and track.

Others, like Dr. Modi, a diabetologist who practiced in Mumbai's suburbs, felt that the BMI didn't help diagnose the complex forms of comorbidity he encountered in his clinical practice. He described the age of diagnosis of metabolic disease as "down by decades" in his current practice, as opposed to when he was in medical school thirty years earlier. The archetypal patient with metabolic illness also changed. "It doesn't fit into the classical obese, sedentary type," he said. "You come across a nice-looking chap who's young and probably in his twenties or early thirties, an executive working somewhere, but very stressful work." He noted that this was an indication that "the phenotype is changing completely." As a result, obesity has to be differently defined, too.

Dr. Modi saw immense potential in changing people's mind-sets about what counts as overweight because it had direct implications for diagnosing metabolic illness. "I hope that day comes when a lean person *thinks* he has diabetes," he said. "But there are a lot of others who are sedentary or who are upper-body obese who should think about diabetes. For that, awareness is surely very, very high today. In urban India, awareness is very high, and patients *are* getting themselves checked on their own, without anybody recommending it. But I think there's a huge portion of people who still don't. It's a time factor in Bombay . . . everything gets pushed [aside]." Something was temporal about Indian bodies, and that something needed better measurement.

Dr. Anoop Misra, one of India's most prominent metabolic disease physicians and a figure integral to the ratification of the new measure, put the debate into the broader historical context of the rise of metabolic disease in India. He explained to me that in the early 1990s, diabetes received little attention in public media, and "obesity was nowhere in sight." Dr. Misra pointed to 1996/97 as a crucial period in terms of a turning point in the politics of estimation. It was then that the World Health Organization (WHO) reported that India had the world's highest number of diabetics, he said: "But despite WHO saying anything, still people, especially in the health sector, health policy managers, were not at all attuned, were not willing to agree that diabetes was increasing in India. So one expert, very bright guy, submitted one document to the government, and I made one, and we presented it to the government, but it was minuscule as far as diabetes control is concerned. And when you talked about diabetes, they would say, 'What diabetes? We have more of other diseases.'"

In 1999, several epidemiological studies in Singapore and the United Kingdom among diasporic South Asians proposed that compared with other groups, South Asians were developing diabetes, hypertension, and obesity at a BMI lower than the standard threshold for "abnormal" weight. They may have "measured up" as normal on the standard BMI scale, but their impaired metabolism suggested the inner workings of an obese or diabetic body. This apparent mismatch prompted clinical studies in India, and soon WHO set up a special subcommittee called Obesity in Asia to investigate the issue.

Initially, according to Dr. Misra, WHO didn't accept the report's findings of a differential "Asian" body response, "but debate started and was raging at the time." Dr. Misra himself carried out much of the debate, recalling (2003) that

in 2002, I was in the US, and then I went to São Paulo, and I debated against a professor from the US and this was a debate where the hall was jam-packed. And the debate was whether the BMI limit should be lower for Asian patients. I spoke for it, she spoke against it, and this debate was published in the International Journal of Obesity. And subsequently, a number of studies we have done have shown that Indians are developing diseases at a lower BMI than Caucasians, and that they have a lot more body fat, liver fat, muscle fat, that creates a lot of problems. If you name one adverse factor, the Indian population has more than the other races. In 2006, WHO set up another committee, which again looked at this particular point, and they couldn't come to a conclusion. [WHO] said, 'we can't have two criteria in the world.' And we said, 'well, we know the Indian population develops diseases at a lower BMI and there's a need to lower the BMI.'

Beginning in 2003, some hospitals began using a revised "Indian" BMI scale for their patients, even though WHO had not formally approved it. In 2008, over 150 metabolic specialists and dietitians across India gathered for a consensus conference in Delhi, debated the scale for two days, and then publicly issued a recommendation for the country to use a new scale. On the new "Indian" scale, a person is considered overweight if her BMI is 23 kg/m2, compared with 25 kg/m2 internationally, and she is considered obese if her BMI is 25 kg/m2, as opposed to the international standard of 30. The official qualification for bariatric surgery also changed, from the international standard of 35 kg/m2 down to 32. The consensus statement itself listed the rationale for the change, with reference to the benefits for type 2 diabetes mellitus (T2DM), cardiovascular disease (CVD), and levels of high-density lipoprotein (HDL, also known as "good" cholesterol):

WHY REVISIONS OF GUIDELINES FOR OBESITY AND THE
METABOLIC SYNDROME ARE NEEDED FOR ASIAN INDIANS

A. In view of rising trend in prevalence of obesity and related metabolic diseases, effective interventions are needed for Asian Indians immediately.

B. Since Asian Indians manifest clustering of cardiovascular risk factors and T2DM at lower levels of obesity, the diagnosis of obesity should be made at a lower level of weight for height than in non-Asian Indian populations.

C. In a consultation on obesity in Asians, the World Health Organization has decided not to take any firm actions on this issue, and has left governments of respective Asian countries to take a decision of guidelines for BMI. Hence onus lies on physicians and scientists in India to decide which are the best guidelines for Asian Indians. The current international criteria of obesity need revision for Asian Indian population.

D. If options of diet, exercise, drug and surgery are applied at lower levels of obesity, nearly 15% of the adult population of India (nearly 5–7 crore [50–70 million] people) will benefit and T2DM and CVD could be prevented in them. (Misra et al. 2011)

The consensus statement also defined metabolic syndrome in terms of fasting blood glucose levels, hypertension, triglycerides, and HDL levels. Additionally, it offered prescriptions for exercise and muscle development, with specific guidelines for frequency and duration of activities ranging from football to dancing.

The "extra" population now considered overweight was the centerpiece of media reactions to the new BMI scale. One article suggested that overnight, 70 million more people became "officially" obese (IANS 2009b). Another pointed specifically to the racial geography of measurement standards: "If the Western benchmarks told you that you were bordering on the obesity line, the Indian guidelines may, well, prove you to be obese. Obesity sure seems to be acquiring epidemic proportions. . . . Time to measure up, indeed" (Yadav 2008). Many of these articles quoted Dr. Misra, who emphasized how the new BMI guidelines would help identify at-risk individuals who would have otherwise gone unnoticed. In the refrain "time to measure up," the pattern of BMI numbers made obesity in India a public issue, particularly because the numbers affirm a sensitive body that tends toward illness. An Indian guideline could prove obesity and join India to a broader global problem.[9]

These developments add to deeper histories of how anthropometric estimation anchors what counts as political. Among several historical accounts, Nicholas Dirks discusses how beginning in the nineteenth century, the Ethnographic Survey of India emphasized anthropometric measurements because the British believed that there was far less "intermixture of races" in India than in other imperial holdings. As Dirks (2001) explains, "it was observed that anthropometry was a science that would yield particularly good results in India precisely because of a caste system that organized social relations through the principle of absolute endogamy," making India "the ideal laboratory for race theory" (214). The measurement of Indian bodies by colonial surveyors had both subtle and explicit effects on ideas about the "natural" divisions of populations, applied both within India and in other colonies of the British Empire. The emphasis on anthropometry in India did not lessen after Independence. Anthropometric measurements continue to be integral in demographic and health surveys, such as the National Family Health Survey, which now uses BMI for its estimates of under- and overweight respondents and whose results guide funding allotments for government and international public health programs. The BMI in India thus has a sustained history of connecting Indians to theories of race and indicators for international development programs, even though its application to obesity is a recent turn. Indeed, public health and clinical experts call upon the BMI to speak to its own history of generational patterning and bodily risk.

Historian of medicine Charles Rosenberg, in his essay "The Tyranny of Diagnosis" (2002), points specifically to BMI as an example of this "linkage" work accomplished by a diagnostic technology. The body mass index enables "bureaucracy, market, cultural identity, and other factors [to] interact around the creation of an agreed-upon disease threshold" (255). This linkage effectively pathologizes excess body fat and, at the same time, legitimizes treatment through pharmaceuticals and regulation through insurance by making the BMI a self-evident standard of disease. BMI turns body weight into disease, according to Rosenberg. More than simply mathematical meaning, the numbers of BMI communicate the spread of disease by quantifying comparative risk. I agree with Rosenberg about the power of linkage work in biomedical quantification, a topic medical anthropologists have explored across many different contexts. Given their interrogative character, we could read the numbers of the BMI as biopolitical mechanisms of classification, like those of the census.

Yet in light of the daily, deeply seated, and pervasive classificatory power of caste, religion, and place of origin in India, attributing similar power to BMI would simply give it too much credit. The BMI does not strike me as a clear-cut case of biopolitical heavy-handedness, whereby obesity is the unsurprising conclusion to a story of new economy consumerism and its medicalization. To sketch it as such would be to plot inaccurate vectors of a causal narrative in which fatness and pathology remain untroubled wholes and close relatives. This numerical narrative simply doesn't begin to capture the striking plasticity of the cultural figure of the Indian who could be both thin and fat, apparently healthy but internally sick, and uniquely sensitive to the potential for metabolic disruption. Indian bodies became differentially measured, and these differences pulled scientists and clinicians in new directions. The threshold of change—23 for the moment—could itself change if experts deemed it necessary. With the BMI, numbers could mark out metabolic plasticity and its shifts into risky territory.


The Bad Copy

I was curious about how claims to plasticity might emerge when bodies weren't the main topic of discussion. In most of my discussions about obesity, globesity, diabesity, and all the types of co-occurring problems with fat, it still seemed that the fat body was the scale at which "the problem" took form. I did not want to dismiss biomedicine as uniform, though: to call the BMI change a mere medicalization of the fat body fails to account for the complexity and diversity of medicine in talk and in practice when it came to metabolic illness. Looking for a different scale and possibly a different analytic standpoint, I sought out a medical diagnostics lab that trafficked in metabolic measurements.

When the local commuter trains leave Mumbai proper and cross into Navi Mumbai (New Bombay), it feels like a divide between urban and suburban. Gone are the buildings vying for space on the island city, replaced instead by stretches of highway and residential enclaves reminiscent of South Delhi's "colony" housing system. Green hills, visible without the city's usual dense belt of smog, background low buildings. The headquarters of ScanTech, one of India's largest medical diagnostics operations, is sandwiched between pharmaceutical factories in Navi Mumbai's industrial area. In ScanTech's waiting room, I watched a group of men work on a web page to list their activities for the upcoming World Diabetes Day. Ads plastered the cork board above the couch, announcing the company's diagnostic tests in big letters with titles such as "A Gland Plan" and "Think Thyroid!" This was my first of multiple encounters with ScanTech, whose work I observed at their headquarters, in their outreach activities, and in their public media campaigns championing medical diagnostics to learn of one's risk of metabolic disease. When a person has a blood or urine sample drawn for medical investigation, it eventually finds its way here.

On this visit, I spent the day with Dr. Nita, the head pathologist who oriented me to the lab by running me around the perimeter of two sunny rooms, cheerfully naming each machine by brand. The rooms were bordered by shelves of stacked red trays filled with plastic vials. Giant troubleshooting flowcharts were carefully tacked to the walls above each relevant machine. Dr. Nita, who trained at one of Mumbai's most prestigious medical colleges, became fascinated by pathology during her time there. When I told her the topic of my study, she said "globesity" was most certainly a problem for India. She remarked that she was on a bit of a mission to get her cousin to lose weight. "His stomach is so big, so bulgy," she said, but he wasn't doing much about it. The other weekend, she pestered him again, and he responded in jest with a rhyme: "*Nahin dekhya peth, toh kaisa lagega Seth?* (If my stomach wasn't visible, how else could I appear to be a *Seth*)?" By invoking the *Seth*, a subcaste of the Khatri caste associated with wealth and mercantile savvy, her cousin emphasized long-standing connections between a bulging stomach and reputation, profit, and power. (Perhaps, a friend suggested later when I related the rhyme, Dr. Nita's cousin was even inverting the diminished tie between a fat stomach and political power by uttering it as a joke.) As her own laughter quieted, Dr. Nita picked at her lunch tiffin. "India is a slowly growing economy" she said. "We used to be poor, but we're gaining power. But we're copying Westerners." She felt pressured to speak English in public and felt that if she wore "traditional" clothes or spoke Hindi, she wouldn't be considered "up to standard" by her peers. "We're losing everything. OK, so they're a superior race, but you just can't copy them. We're getting fat. And they don't force it. It's not them."

I initially took Dr. Nita's frustration as another in a long list of rues about westernization in the tone of postcolonial critique, as a commentary on the native body's place in relation to a colonial other. I had heard this remorseful refrain often. An endocrinologist I interviewed in Delhi lamented that India had been the *sone ki chiḍiya*, the golden bird, a civilization of prosperity and good health chipped away by the idealization of "outsider" ways of life.[10] One of my neighbors in Manuli, John, who built ovens for a local bakery, told me, "We're copying the West, but doing a bad job of it, and it's killing us," referencing his daughter's refusal to eat *poha* (beaten rice) for breakfast and insistence on Kellogg's Corn Flakes. Things were moving too quickly in Mumbai, John explained. "Western ways" of eating and living take adequate time for adaptation, but he saw everyone taking the *fatafat* (quick, shortcut) route in their desire for burgers and pizzas. There was desire behind these changes, and that desire didn't sit squarely in colonial attempts to "develop" populations through health, nor did it work exclusively as the yearning for modernity. When Dr. Nita said that the West was the "race" to be copied, she underscored that the act of copying wasn't forced by outsiders: "It's Indians who feel that they have to be that way," she said. She described a cultivation of ideals that resulted in mimicry's ruinous consequences for the body politic. *"We're getting fat"* was a process that developed through an intimate and sustained coexistence with others. *"It's not them"* pointed to local dimensions of weight gain. Dr. Nita spoke of a transnational comparison in which local bodies accumulated life's changing pleasures, which eventually fueled metabolic disaster. The figure of accumulation here was the bad copy, which is "bad" because it marked absorptive accumulation with unwanted side effects. The effects proved copying to be open ended rather than predictable. Unexpected changeability anchored this postcolonial explanation, but it also upheld epigenetic explanations similarly premised on generational forms of copies gone awry. The bad copy condensed sites of science and of history. If the thin-fat Indian became a *process* that replaced the *product* of a fat body, the bad copy can be similarly understood as processural rather than static.

ScanTech was one site that bridged excess weight to pathology, but with the weekly, if not daily, circulation of health news about lifestyle diseases, I began to wonder how health reporters assembled their stories around fat's pathological potential. How and to what extent did news stories write plasticity into circulation? I began cold-calling journalists whose health reporting I followed. One of the reporters I spoke with, Kapil, wrote for India's most widely circulated English-language paper. His stories frequently came across my newswire, in both their original English form and also translated into Hindi.[11] Kapil had been a diabetic for seventeen years and frequently faced misunderstanding in terms of what type 2 diabetes entailed. This inspired him to direct his health care reporting to focus on diabetes and, over time, on obesity as well. He wrote for "the average Indian," who he felt was educated (regardless of whether he lived in a city) and who was aware "that today's times are all about consumption and materialism." Whether rich or poor, middle class or working class, all Indians were united by "the curse of the thrifty gene." "We're made to adapt to famine," he explained, but when things go awry, the "famous Indian potbelly" emerges. And now diabetes was a household name, with obesity close behind. People were becoming more aware of the problem but had yet to adapt their own habits to sync with their already adapting bodies.

Kapil spoke at length about copying, *bad* copying specifically: "We blindly ape the West," as he put it. Like Dr. Nita, he placed responsibility on Indians themselves. Blame put on the West, on outsourcing, or on multinational companies was misplaced for him. "First *we* need introspection," he said. To rely on stories of call centers affecting a country's health care profile was merely media buzz. It deflected from what he called a typical Indian response of fatalism and "flouting the rules for your own body." "What is essentially required," he concluded, "is good self-management," an appeal that structured his news stories. Good self-management began with good information, he felt. Thus it was common for his stories to be laced with statistics: not only would he write that India was the "Diabetes Capital" of the world, but he would also cite global mortality statistics and contrast them with those emerging from India. Kapil did scale work in his journalism. In these stories, being unaware was as threatening as the disease itself. For example, in one story, by noting that 50 percent of people with diabetes don't even realize they have the condition, Kapil wanted to emphasize that the scope of the problem was not always so clear. He also made an effort to write about children. "Indian children are being cursed with obesity, and we don't know what to do about it," he said. Chubby kids are seen as well fed, "but people don't realize that every inch they add to their children is worse for their health." This concern materialized in his writing in warnings that ended many of his articles: "Sedentary lifestyle, dietary indiscretion, physical inactivity . . . are you passing on the perils of modern life to your children as well? Think about it."

I asked if he thought his articles resonated with his readers enough to inspire change. He was doubtful; the handling of diabetes and obesity was too piecemeal right now. "No one in India understands how chronic disease patients need motivation," he said. "You cannot just keep a person under abstinence. Just telling them to avoid bread and potatoes isn't going to work." He felt India needed "comprehensive" education and hoped that at some point, his own writing would settle into the larger public health matrix. But until then, he found it difficult to be optimistic. "This is just the start of the epidemic," he said. "By the time we wake up, it will be too late." Kapil's appeal could in one sense be read as deeply inflected by neoliberalism through its emphasis on information, awareness, and self-management. However, I also heard an emphasis on the emancipatory power of science, which has long been central to Indian national narratives of progress and transformation (see Prakash 1999). What was specific to Kapil's news stories and others like them was the way in which epidemiological science sat comfortably alongside images of chubby children and potbellies. Chronic disease was a powerful canvas on which to sketch evidence of plasticity through numbers, parables, and calls for self-awareness.

Both Dr. Nita and Kapil centralized the figure of the bad copy. Because Indian bodies are understood as intensively dynamic when it comes to metabolic affairs, any behaviors transposed locally will not stay rigid. The bad copy's body buckles, and comparisons crash. These accounts differ somewhat from the effort to turn 25 to 23 in the case of the new BMI scale. In the BMI transformation, experts recognize that copying is not an avenue worth pursuing. Instead, the plasticity of the vernacular needs to be the grounds of accurate measurement. Doctors make comparisons with the hope of cultivating a sense of risk—recall Dr. Modi, who wants thin persons "to think that they have diabetes." It is less nominal comparison at work across figures of the bad copy and the figure of 23 than comparisons of the specific in-betweenness of plasticity.

This in-betweenness illustrates what literary theorist R. Radhakrishnan calls "the third space" of comparison. For Radhakrishnan, the act of comparison involves a de- and relocation: from the point of origin of each artifact in question to a comparative space. "Any act of comparison," he writes, "is predicated on an unavoidable deracination and a yoking together that one hopes will not be violent. The two works to be compared are deterritorialized from their 'original' milieu and then reterritorialized so that they may become cospatial, epistemologically speaking."[12] There is a spatial dimension to distributions of comparison. It is not a jump directly between the poles of comparison: between the United States to India, in many accounts of globesity, or between a unified West or East. Rather, comparison entails a jump from both origin points into a third "cospatial" domain. What I want to flag here is how plasticity is the ground for the cospatial domain, to use Radhakrishnan's terms. Plasticity becomes a kind of risk informed by appeals to the historical (in reckonings with a malnourished, supposedly past agrarian body) and to the contemporary (in nods to environments of highly moralized behaviors and living styles). When plasticity is foregrounded, the medicalization of weight needn't hew closely to the biopolitical absolute of number. Sometimes the demands on the plastic body exceed anything measurable by numbers alone.

## Tension

Plasticity became apparent through appeals to biomedical risk, but it also had everyday reverberations. In particular, the trigger for the body's change was a key concern in my daily conversations about the relationship between bodies and the city. Its most common invocation was in terms of stress, or more locally, *tenshun*. *Tenshun* articulated the body's porosity and instability in relation to its variable environments. The potential for the body to change was ever present, and it was not particularly strange to relate this changeability to particular events and environments.[13]

My neighbors rarely took claims of globesity at face value. They did not articulate (and by extension, they warned me against interpreting) *tenshun* as a culturalist response. Overattention to media glitz or folk categories, they assured me, was as sure a route to missing the point as any. Giving a flashy concept with a flashy name too much credibility missed the pathologies in plain sight: people in India *were* showing signs of obesity, often in tandem with other kinds of maladies: diabetes, thyroid problems, hypertension, cardiac disease. How to take *tenshun* seriously, then? What was fat and what was stress, and when were they pathological pairs? A person could be *mota* (fat), *charbi* (fatty, oily), *tandu* (potbellied, used especially for lazy cops), or *jharia* (a Gujarati word for "chubby"). There was the commonplace English-inspired euphemism *healthy*, and people often pointed out the irony of a word used to mean a big size in present times when to be fat was to be sick. The word *motapa*—fatness at the level of the population, translatable as "obesity"—was hardly uttered outside clinical settings, and print media in Hindi and Marathi often simply used a direct transliteration of *obesity*. For diabetes and cardiovascular problems, *sugar*, *BP*, *pressure*, and *blockage* were the most common terms conversationally.[14] Universally, though, something was amiss in sugar levels and body weights and most often expressed that the body absorbed stresses of living.

Conversations with my neighbors would often turn to matters of tension whenever I asked about fat. This first occurred when I spoke with Rose, who lived down one of the many snaking alleyways leading from Manuli's main road to the sea. She kept her front door ajar, fashioning it into a coat hanger for my soaked rain jacket, and led me and Mary from the kitchen/eating nook into the living/bedroom stacked with neat piles of clothing and papers. Photos papered over the peeling blue paint on the wall. Born in Goa, Rose married a man who was raised in Manuli and moved there soon after their wedding; she didn't mind because Manuli reminded her of a busier incarnation of her home village. Now thirty-five, she spent her mornings at the nearby home of an older woman who is the head cook for a bakery. She and "Aunty" made all of the bakery's snacks, including meat cutlets, pan rolls, potato chops, and veg cutlets. Fish cutlets used to be one of the bakery's specialties but are no longer offered because of the drop in Manuli's fish supply, which Rose attributed to environmental pollution.

Rose ate lunch at Aunty's house during her workday, meals that she described as "rich" (so rich, Rose said, that Aunty was scolded by the doctor that her oil usage was giving her children what Rose called "diabetes pressure"). When she returned from work at 4 PM, Rose prepared dinner for her husband, who is a rickshaw driver, and her two children. She tends to cook Goan food but also makes East Indian curries that she's learned from the neighbors. While they ate "lighter" food (fish and chicken) during the week, they ate "rich" food like beef on Sundays when the family gathered together. Rose suggested that people shouldn't be too fat: "Slim is best," as she put it. "Too much fat isn't good for your health, and it can give you diabetes pressure. It comes through the family. In my family, we've all got it. My mommy and daddy died from it, diabetes pressure. My big brother died of the same thing—diabetes pressure. He had gone to Goa and died on the beach. That hot sun, no? He never knew that he fell down. And [in Goa] there are all these foreigners, and one fellow saw him and ran to catch him. But by that time he slipped and he went [out to sea]. After four days they found his body. My big brother. That diabetes pressure. So now we tell the children to take care."

Although she hadn't gone to a doctor to confirm it, she suspected that she too had tinges of this disease that she couldn't see but could sense otherwise.

In the stories of her brother's death, of Aunty's children, and of her own bodily dynamics, Rose articulated a condition I heard invoked repeatedly in Manuli to describe co-occurring general malaise: *tenshun*. *Tenshun* could be a symptom, cause, or effect of diabetes pressure, or "diabetes-BP."[15] Rarely did diabetes or high blood pressure occur alone, but their self-treatment was often the same: avoiding sweets and salt and taking pills: "*Ek hi tablet, bas*"—Just one tablet, that's it, explained Mr. Manikar, a retired fisher who traces his family history in Manuli back a hundred years. These pills could range from vitamins to drugs for hypertension or diabetes. Usually, it took more than one tablet to do the trick. Mrs. Rodrigues, whose one-room home was filled with chirping songbirds in tiny cages glowing from a neon crucifix in the corner, once unceremoniously dumped hundreds of pills onto the couch when I asked about stress and its association with weight. The link is all *sochte se, tenshun se*, she said, pointing to the pills: from thinking, worrying, and tension.

This was a sentiment shared by Father Matthew, one of the priests at Manuli's church; I interviewed him in his upstairs office in the church rectory. Father Matthew grew up in Mumbai, in Vasai, and began our conversation by assuring me that he used both food and tablets to control his diabetes. He pulled open a desk drawer and showed me a small baggie filled with *methi* (fenugreek) seeds, a common home remedy for diabetics. His routine was to swallow a few before going into Mass and try to endure the harsh, bitter taste they left in his mouth all day. His doctor diagnosed him as diabetic when he started feeling constantly "giddy," "sleepy," and felt "warmth in his legs" that wouldn't go away. Father Matthew thought it might be diabetes; he had heard about the symptoms. He had been a school principal before taking up the position at the church, and the all-day cascade of parent, teacher, and student needs caused him immense levels of stress. He wasn't surprised when he was diagnosed. The doctor gave him a long list of food restrictions: no beef, no pork, little alcohol, low salt, no high-sugar fruits like chikoo or mango. All sweets were off-limits. "But everything is normal now," he said, "because I took the doctor seriously." As a priest at a church, he now feels far less stress. "They say it's *tenshun* that does it," he said in describing how disease actually manifests. People may have it in the family (through heredity, he said, although his parents died young when he was three years old, so he has no idea if his diabetes is familial). He also railed against the sedentary lifestyle he feels urban Indians are now inclined to lead: "table work" he called it, anchored by computers and television. This is what makes children fat: rich children are spoiled with food, and even for families who aren't rich, the parents both work, bribe kids with food because they're so tired, and plunk them in front of the computer or the TV. He said that as a child, they would eat simple meals of fish curry and rice and then be unleashed to play outside. But children don't play anymore, he said, and it's making them sick. People don't have control over food. At the root of all of this is *tenshun*.

Disease-causing tension could emerge from any number of circumstances or misfortunes. Another volunteer in the church office, Winnie, felt frequent *chakar* (giddiness, dizziness) from her tension. She was diagnosed with high blood pressure and had been told to be on the lookout for symptoms of diabetes. This all began when her husband's small shop was robbed. His was the main source of income for them; he was missing a limb and therefore qualified for a government-subsidized street-side shop that sold cold drinks out of a small refrigerator. Her tension was high following the robbery, as she was unsure about how they would sustain themselves and their children. After consulting with a doctor, she learned to take her "pressure" pills: "If I miss one, I feel giddy, hyper, and angry," she said. "My children see it immediately; my speaking and my behavior and my body patterns change immediately, and the children know that I haven't taken my tablets. I don't know what I'm doing, but the children know."

Like many women in the neighborhood, Winnie took on work as a cook for families that could afford to pay for household help. This was a stressful job, too, because the couple she worked for was very strict about their food. They themselves were trying to lose weight. They closely monitored Winnie's dishes; she was to avoid using more than minimal amounts of ghee, oil, and salt. Despite the oversight, she felt that her employers appreciated the work she did; an added bonus was that cooking for them with little salt, oil, sugar, and spices was rubbing off on the cooking she did for her own family. Nonetheless, she still had to carefully watch her weight. She first started having "body weight problems" in the course of rehabilitation for her "drinking problem." "I was drinking," she explained, "and then I had to go through rehab. They gave me lots of detox tablets . . . so after stopping the drinks and taking [the] detox medicine I put on the weight." When I asked what the "detox tablets" were, she explained that one was for sleeping and others for cleaning out her blood. The medicines made her hungry. The diet at the rehab center was vegetarian, and she began eating large amounts of rice in order to satisfy her hunger pangs. Even though her time in rehab was years prior, she still is as careful with her diet as she is with her blood pressure tablets.

Just as it was a precursor or effect of metabolic distress, *tenshun* was also a mode of diagnosis. One morning while I waited for Mary in the church's main office, one of the volunteers, Eileen, expressed interest in our household interviews. Eileen was a retired elementary school teacher who still tutored in an evening program for poor students at the nearby convent school. A lifelong resident of Manuli, Eileen remarked that it seemed that everyone in the neighborhood was showing signs of cardiovascular distress and weight gain. On one hand, she found Manuli a relatively peaceful place—the same expression of cosmopolitanism I heard often, with descriptions of Hindu, Muslim, and Catholic neighbors living in relative harmony. "Even during the riots [of 1992], it was peaceful here," she emphasized. But something was happening that put the neighborhood on edge, in a semipermanent state of stress. There was no time to take care of oneself, because the pressures of city life diminished opportunities to give the slightest thought to self-care. The result, she observed, was a startling prevalence of diabetes, "BP," and weight gain. "Even the younger ones, I've noticed, they've got diabetes," she said. "There's one young man in our building who developed [type 2] diabetes. Now how can that be? How could he develop that? Maybe because of his eating habits? Or stress?" Eileen pointed out the demands of time on metabolisms. Her observation was one I would hear repeatedly: young people were developing metabolic disorders in ways unseen a decade before. Diabetes had not so long ago been a problem for the elderly; now it was increasingly common to hear stories in daily conversation, in the news, and in clinical reports about how twenty-somethings were the new sentinels.

Eileen herself was a diabetic, and her doctor had her watching her weight. "It happened after I lost my husband," she said. Her husband had died from a heart attack, she explained, brought on by high blood pressure that he had left unmedicated: "You're supposed to take the tablets continuously. He had stopped taking the tablets for ten days or so, but I didn't know. So I found that he had skipped on then. And with the heat, he just dropped. So of course that was a shock. And when I went for a checkup soon after, I found out that I had diabetes. But now it's under control. I take tablets—the insulin. Only one a day. I don't have any rice, potatoes, or sweets. I'm not fond of dairy, but it's out anyways. But I don't do much walking or exercise. There's just no time."

Eileen explained that time—more accurately, the lack of it—was perhaps the reason everyone was so stressed. The temporality of tension is a semipermanent state of stress. Stress came to define the rhythms of living, eating, developing symptoms of illness, and working on the body in response to those symptoms.

These narratives of *tenshun* expanded beyond the bounds of an ethnomedical category and its possibilities for interpretation and relay as such. I shared stories from Manuli, like those of Rose and Eileen, with Dr. Misra. Did his patients use the language of stress or *tenshun* to describe their maladies? Did tension's association with metabolic disruption manifest in clinical spaces? He responded: "Many times. The problem with stress is that it's not been studied properly. Last year we started a study, where we looked at diabetics who had major stresses over a three-month period, and we had psychologists do this study, case control. The study has yet to be completed, but many people relate diabetes to a particular incident, someone dying in their family. One particular event makes a strong determinant of diabetes. . . . I've had a good exposure to all socioeconomic strata in this country. For low income people there's stress over finding money to eat, to buy medicines. But stress is increasing, especially in urban settings. For young people, sometimes we can't find any cause of diabetes, and they're thin, but they say they have stress from their jobs."

Like Dr. Misra did, another diabetologist I interviewed also blamed stress for hormonal changes that manifested as diabetes in the blood and as extra weight on the body; stress makes "everything go haywire," as he put it. A psychiatrist interviewed by the *Times of India*, in an article headlined "Stress Leaves City on the Brink," agreed: "We experience aggression, suspicion, and hatred on a daily basis . . . [which] could have a cumulative effect some time later" (TNN 2010b). A wide range of biomedical research on stress hormones and sugar levels, as well as the public media coverage of such studies, pointed to weight gain as one such delayed effect. "Don't know why you are putting on so much weight?" asked one article. "Blame the stress at work and at home" (Sinha 2007). This division between stress at work and stress at home was inflected along lines of gender and social class. Stress at work was a threat to men, especially young men, who worked in offices. "Work" in this sense meant a certain kind of middle-class work—sedentary work accompanied by stressful commutes on city trains. Health insurance advertisements played on this definition, and I often saw ads plastered on buses with large photos of men in collared shirts, headlined "Who will care for his health?" This was elaborated on March 8, celebrated in India as International Women's Day, when newspapers produced more troubling news about stress and obesity experienced by women. The Associated Chamber of Commerce and Industry, a private industry public relations group, claimed that 68 percent of women between twenty-one and fifty-two in its survey of working women "were found to be suffering from lifestyle ailments" such as obesity. The pressures of work—"work" meaning office work in the survey's case— "have led 53% of the respondents to skip meals and go for junk food" (IANS 2009a). The putative mechanism was that workers were simply too busy to feed, thus care for, themselves. For women, the implied lines of care extended to husbands and children. News articles announced that "the Indian woman is not okay" and questioned the real advances women in India could make in time-demanding formal work sectors if their advancement came at the cost of their longevity (Gianani 2009).

Moments of measuring *tenshun* pose a body that accumulates the stresses of life, more so than an extra portion of food, and open up a critical concern about the costs of the middle-class life and the naturalization of self-care. If taken as a mere folk category, *tenshun* can only relate the native to the natural. The effort to critique epidemic exclamations in India to "prove" something about global health can easily render the figure of the peasant a testament for and against globally consolidated biomedicine.[16] Further, this effort can obscure the ways that, historically, diabetes in India was understood as a condition of weakness coincident with a tropical environment (Arnold 2009; Abu-Bakare et al. 1986). But taken in the register of plasticity, of the ability for biological material to reshape itself, *tenshun* scales somatic resilience and vulnerability to everyday events. When metabolism met with troubled times, any number of effects were possible.


## A Tale of Two *Lancets*

The picture of the Y-Y paradox stayed with me as I listened to people describe tension as the ground of plasticity and plasticity as the ground of fatness. To understand more, I visited the Indian Y—Dr. Yajnik—at his research center in Pune, Maharashtra. When I arrived, Dr. Yajnik gave me a tour of his research outfit, which occupied an entire hospital floor. In addition to a clinical area, where the hospital's diabetologists regularly saw patients, his team had offices where they conducted large-scale epidemiological and intervention research studies. The central thrust of the team's work is to attempt an intervention among young women prior to pregnancy. The team has worked with roughly six hundred people in villages surrounding Pune—villages that have seen considerable economic growth in the last decade, in part because of the global market for sugarcane. Prior to speaking with Dr. Yajnik, I met with some of the clinicians and epidemiologists on the team. They described noticeable shifts in housing in the villages over the last decade, from huts to structures made of cement, along with an increase in mobile phones. In this city hospital, the village loomed large.

Dr. Yajnik's engagement with metabolic disease began in medical school, when he pored over American textbooks and came to think of Indian patients as "very different" in comparison to the indexed, "normal" diabetic patient in the textbooks. But even at that time, in the 1970s, he was seeing diabetes among lower-middle-income people. The hospital where he was doing a rotation had a ground floor OB/GYN center, where low-birth-weight babies were born; the diabetes center was on the fourth floor. At a colleague's prompting, he began to wonder how the two floors might be connected by more than an elevator. In medicine, he said, if you don't understand something, you appeal to genetics to explain it. WHO, for its own part, had absolute authority over medical standards. Unsatisfied with easy explanations and skeptical of universal medical measures, he listened to a colleague, who advised him that he should explain to WHO how Indian bodies were different. His research team received funding from the Wellcome Trust to start a small study that did intensive measurements—not just body weight but also skin-fold caliper testing, and they found that "Indian patients had more fat." This was the start of the thin-fat rationale. They distinguished *obesity* from *adiposity*. Obesity is a weight/height measurement; adiposity is a body fat percentage measurement.[17] By 1991, they were coming to the conclusion that "central rather than generalized adiposity was the problem." Indians accumulated fat in the midline, and it was fat in this specific location that was cause for concern. Here the very substance of fat came to matter prior to its medicalization as obesity. Adiposity was the elemental site of plasticity.

In response to his early findings, Dr. Yajnik said, "everyone told me that [the effect] was genetic. And I said, 'Yes, but *how*?'" This is where his colleague David Barker entered the picture, with the adage that "genes learn how to behave when they grow in the womb; the message is conveyed by the mother." Together, they began to think about "how things happen before you're born." Barker's idea was that low birth weight in babies was a precursor to diabetes in later life. The Pune Maternal Nutrition Study worked on this proposition by measuring weight, length, and more detailed anthropometrics. The study concluded that Indian babies were eight hundred grams lighter than English babies (the comparison was done at Exeter), but subscapular skin-fold measurements of body fat were the same across the two populations. This meant that the thin-fat characteristic was present at birth. That left Yajnik's team with a conundrum: if the genetic patterning of type 2 diabetes was assumed to be relatively similar across the world, then their findings opened up possibilities for alternative explanations.

"Our idea was that the thin-fat Indian was epigenetic," Dr. Yajnik explained, referencing the phenomenon of changes in gene expression that are heritable across generations. This change is attributable to environmental conditions, such that fat can be a survival value in some contexts but in others it could be harmful. The research team turned its focus onto what Yajnik called "hidden hunger"—micronutrient deficiency. This was in contrast to manifest hunger, which was about proteins. But micronutrient deficiency was seen as a major contributor to (poor) fetal growth. A mother who is micronutrient malnourished can give birth to "small, fat, and thin" babies. These babies could conceivably grow into a population of obese and diabetic adults. The "small, fat, thin" type of body morphology helped clarify the details of rural starvation. Yajnik's team was trying to argue that hunger was not simply about the quantity of the food but also was a matter of food quality. The consumption of quality foods, in terms of nutrition, did not always match expectations. For example, they observed more protein and folic acid deficiency among upper-middle-class people in Pune than in their comparison groups in the villages around Pune. He said this was a possible side effect of vegetarianism among upper-caste Hindus, and led to a conclusion that across several socioeconomic strata, mothers were giving birth to "thin-fat" babies. This was a finding he had difficulty mobilizing in the face of strong public discourses about the rise of obesity in the middle class. It may be that the urban middle classes demonstrated signs of metabolic disease, but his research showed that rural people faced similar challenges, too.

The original cohort of women that Dr. Yajnik worked with now has children who are approximately seventeen years old. The team is working with them, too, conducting research on nutrition and performing metabolic assays. Their aim is to monitor this generation before the young women become pregnant. They will also monitor the babies born to the young women, thus producing data on three generations. I began to grapple with the nature of intervention at hand here: It is an engagement with metabolic plasticity that is not pegged to putting someone on a diet, a presentist intervention, but rather is aimed at future generations. As one of the researchers explained it: "By the time I'm born, I'm born with a certain risk [for disease]. Anything you ask me to do—like dieting—will have some effect. But what about our children?" In contrast to the claims of globesity that centralized the spread of obesity across territory, the claims generated in this research space concerned the spread of obesity across time. Metabolic living's geographic coordinates had temporal locations. So too did the various commemorative plaques on his wall from medical meetings over decades. He moved down the line of them to explain the shift in scientific terminology that governed the names of the associations themselves: from "fetal origins of disease" across several other iterations to the now more current "developmental origins of health and disease" (which casts "health" as one of the many possibilities of life.)

I asked Dr. Yajnik specifically about the proliferation of the term "globesity." "It's a short-term view of things," he replied, "without any reference to susceptibility. Now, one way to say it is that we will remove all the McDonald's. So will all the diabetes and obesity go away? No. It will be replaced by something else. And therefore it's important to change your susceptibility. The diabetes prevention trials of today have completely ignored susceptibility." Ultimately, what Dr. Yajnik and his colleagues argue for is the plasticity of the human body and its sensitivity to specific kinds of nutritional change. He showed me slides on his computer of a clay potter who sets up his wheel only a few kilometers away from the hospital we were sitting in. It was the same clay, Dr. Yajnik explained, that was shaped into any number of different types of vessels. So too with the human body: plastic, malleable. "Plasticity actually tells you that when an organism begins as one cell, it has an opportunity to go in different directions; that is determined by the environment and so that is the environment-gene interaction which leads to the phenotype," he said. The same clay makes up the metabolism of all humans, but their environments can literally shape it into different forms. What mattered in the end was "programming," which is the restriction or opening up of plasticity. In a given environment, does the body lean toward a balance in nutrients and a state of relative health? Or do imbalances in micronutrients drag the body into states of illness? "The answers are more complex than blaming the food industry or prescribing exercise," he said. If one looked to the thin-fat Indian as a particular kind of material phenomenon, instead of reifying either malnutrition or overnutrition, one could see different (and for Yajnik, more nuanced) symptoms of the *potential* to be sick. As I got up to leave, I noted that what was remarkable about his research was that he seemed to bridge the under- and overnutrition streams of discourse about India. He smiled. "It's not a divide," he said. "It's a coexistence." With an eye to this kind of chronicity, malnutrition was in parallel to adequate or overnutrition, not in an anterior position.

Other physicians, epidemiologists, and scientists I spoke with had varying points of agreement and disagreement with Dr. Yajnik's research. Dr. Mehta, a biochemist studying metabolism-regulating properties of Ayurvedic remedies, felt that the thrifty-genotype hypothesis was simply historically inaccurate. To him, it erased the history of Indian wealth before colonization by substantiating a false narrative history of starvation that was only recently remedied. "India was rich, obese, and alcoholic when the British arrived," he said. For Dr. Mehta, "thrifty" hypotheses had postcolonial reverberations.[18]

Dr. Mehta's claim to fat's historical trajectory and its relation to colonial medicine is apparent 140 years before the introduction of the Y-Y paradox, in the same medical journal that Dr. Yajnik appears in. Here, a different relationship emerged involving India, body fat, and evidence. In 1859, British Assistant Surgeon Dr. W. G. Don wrote a case study about "a very remarkable example of perverted nutrition" in Bombay for the

*Lancet.* I came across this *Lancet* article in searching through medical journal archives for historical instances of biomedical case studies of fatness in India. In this 1859 article, "Remarkable Case of Obesity in a Hindoo Boy Aged Twelve Years," Don included an engraving that was "a very good representation" of a photograph of a boy "known in the streets of Bombay under the sobriquet of the 'Fat Boy'" (Don 1859: 363) (figure 1.2).[19]

In the article, Don, recounting the story of the twelve-year-old boy named Shakarm, described him as follows: "His father and mother both died several years ago, and he is now a beggar, living on the bounty of the many charitable citizens of Bombay. In his second year he became very fat, and the obesity has increased with his growth, year by year, till his whole body is now encased in an immense mass of solid adipose tissue, which hangs in pendulous folds over his chest and hips, and the flexures of his limbs. He enjoys excellent health, and has a moderately good appetite, living chiefly on dhal (peas) and rice. He has no complaint whatsoever, except a difficulty of breathing when he subjects himself to any very rigorous exercise" (Don 1859). In Don's presentation of the case, Shakarm grows fat from accumulating the charity of others. His fatness emerges gradually, "year by year." Don offered some sense of scale to the case: He measured Shakarm's weight at 206 pounds, his arms at 48.5 inches, and also provided measurements relating to the "girth" of the boy's chest, abdomen, thigh, calf, arm, and foot. To be clear, I read the sketch of Shakarm alongside the Y-Y paradox figure without presuming any historical continuity. Shakarm's is the body that is measured, but to recall Don's assessment, he is also a boy estimated to enjoy "excellent health." It was manifest fat that merited curiosity rather than a direct attribution of sickness to fatness. The curiosity around the Fat Boy becomes visible in a sketch emphasizing adiposity, the extent of fatty tissue. The moral currents surrounding the "discovery" of the Fat Boy, however, seem different. He is, in Don's estimation at least, healthy.

Other epidemiologists had their own senses about bodily histories. One epidemiologist I spoke with, Dr. Kartik, noted that earlier in his career, he doubted Barker's work and as a result was unsure that Yajnik was accurate in his claims about the Y-Y paradox. But over time, Dr. Kartik has come to accept it. His own spin on it is what he calls the "life is shit" hypothesis: "I conceptualize it such that when life is shit, people age quicker, like the wrinkles in your face or the hair going grey. In the mind, you carry these conditions. Like with heart disease, your arteries are aging. So anytime in your life, whether early life, midlife, or later life, when you

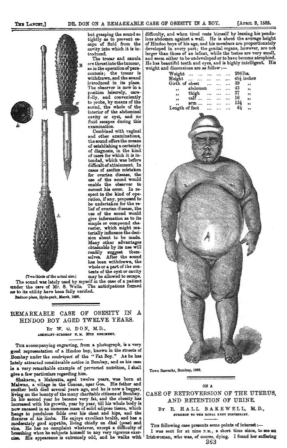

**FIG. 1.2** "Remarkable Case of Obesity in a Hindoo Boy," *The Lancet*, vol. 73, February 1859.

go through a period of time when life is shit, your body systems are under attack and either you age quicker or your energy resources are diverted toward survival, so they draw away [from other systems]. It's like any other machine. If poor early-life circumstances are there, I think they'd have an impact on [the body]." Dr. Kartik took a phenomenon like *tenshun* and scaled it to particular stages of the life course, such that one carries stresses with visceral effects, from damage to the circulatory system to depleted energy levels.[20] These were matters of how the metabolism—and by his extension, life—could accommodate events.[21]

Dr. Kartik also explained to me that the theory of the thin-fat Indian seemed accurate from another angle: that of simple visualization. He echoed a central idea behind the BMI consensus statement that fatness in

Indians is different and that one can see it. Indians express "a different kind of fatness," he noted. These days, he said, "I can walk into any room in India and everybody will be fat. But it's a different kind of fatness; next time, watch carefully. You don't have to go to high-end restaurants, just go to a small street-side restaurant. It's not the American kind of fat." He gestured to the table next to us, in the cafe where we were meeting. "So even this table on our left, when you get up, just watch them. All of them are fat. But it's a different level of fatness; it's not apparent. Can you see that guy in the blue shirt? He's fat." Dr. Kartik assured me that I probably wouldn't notice this otherwise: that the man in the blue shirt had central adiposity that would go otherwise unnoticed by the observer looking for general adiposity in order to visually diagnose fatness. With an eye trained to fix attention on the body's midline, one could actually see the thin-fat Indian in process and could visualize plasticity in action.

This act of visualization and identification ("just watch them") first struck me as a sudden break from the register of plasticity structuring the conversation thus far. It was an odd moment that reminded me of Dr. Don's visualization of fat on Shakarm's body. Yet Dr. Kartik still specified the uniqueness of the fat in question; it was, as he put it, "a different kind of fatness." The thin-fat Indian is a capacious figure indeed, open not only to the demands of biological theories of metabolic plasticity but also to historical reckonings of body morphology and their attributions to social class. Put differently, the thin-fat body is a semiomaterial form open to biological memory work in a context of tensions between city and village (Nandy 2007). "Metropolitan culture," Ashis Nandy writes, "[is] primed to relate to the village through memory, primarily the memory of an abrogated or superseded village" (159). Cultures of medicine and expressions of general well-being are no exception. At the same time that this city-village comparison unfolds, the "Indian" BMI also compares Indian bodies to their Western counterparts. The thin-fat Indian is absorbing the legacy of rural life and a legacy of mistiming, even as it heralds the potential of urban Indian bodies as both alarming and encouraging.

Out of Proportion, Out of Time

Although concerns about obesity often hinge on the changes *between* states of thinness and fatness, this chapter has stayed with "thin-fat" to reflect on how harms can coexist *across* bodily morphologies and temperaments.

In the new BMI scale and in the narratives of tension, people craft a story of how something is amiss with absorption. The Indian metabolism is a site of scientific inquiry, of illness experience, and yet as it is measured and evaluated it reveals its own limits as it proves to be unexpectedly patterned. Plasticity justifies the claim that obesity is difficult to recognize in Indians, and so a new scale must be created. Such plasticity is sometimes amenable to measurements like body weight or blood sugar levels and can easily be captured by numbers. Yet amid these measurements, sensations of disease remained, most notably the sense of stress. These sensations, not easily captured by numerical measurements, are nonetheless crucial to mark out in order to better understand the conditions of chronic disease's expression in everyday terms. I am not claiming expressions of lifestyle or *tenshun* should be stacked against the BMI in a question of accurate modes of diagnosis for metabolic disease.[22] Rather, expressions of stress paint a different picture of illness: one in which the challenges of life in the city are ever present and permeating bodies. We see different economies of recognition of plasticity: in numbers, in phenomenological expressions, in the indignities of approximation, and in generational temporalities of harm. The Indian body mass index works through a specific set of relations between persons and the world, wherein Indians are set against the West and its standard measurements. As a result, the new BMI measurements conjure up a rural, malnourished state, even for urban middle-class Indians.

Expressions of stress are similarly symptoms of absorptions between environment and body but tend to highlight the city as a stressor. In these modes of diagnosis, the city and the village coexist in relation to the plasticity of the body. As Dr. Yajnik attested, it's coexistence, not a divide. I would qualify his statement even further: obesity is a coexistence of *harms*, actual and potential. For all of its potential problems and for all the varying degrees of agreement that biomedical experts had with Dr. Yajnik, there was a broad consensus that the BMI could be a scale of patterned distribution that we should take seriously, far more seriously than claims to globesity. Sciences of the thin-fat body could coexist because they could selectively absorb each other, just as fat and time did.

My broader aim in this chapter has been to narrate the disruption of metabolic living from the standpoint of the temporal body and its plasticity. The dynamic ability of fat to take shape, to cause controversies, and to make bodies particular to a place while still being comparative globally has material precursors and aftereffects. I took up scales as sites to work through the powers of time. The comparisons grounding scales of metabolic disease involved material patterns of fat: how fat emerges—literally—in specific body parts, and how fat bodies constitute patterns in the aggregate. Scales translate plasticity's potential into patterns and affix attention to specific moments of living. This is why I have described scales as events. A scale may weigh a person, comparatively, against previous versions of herself or against future possible sizes. Scales also produce temporal and spatial truth claims, such that historical conditions of malnutrition inflect risks of metabolic disease, and the spatial friction presumed between India and overconsumptive Western worlds creates a sense of national metabolic vulnerability.[23] Scales articulate the Indian case and the transferability of this case to a broader global picture of obesity's intensification.

Scales of plasticity arranged certain individuals as at risk for fatness, set fatness in terms of sickness, and fixed contemporary India as (to some) a surprising home of chronic disease. To match metabolisms to persons and places took complex work. Once on the scale, to be 23 was to express a vulnerability to certain orders and disorders of time in the very same body. New possibilities to make sense of disease causality proliferated, as did tales of triggers: the elements activating metabolic dynamism. Specific sensations, knowledge, and technologies of time are necessary to activate and arrange the cultural figures that come to the fore in a problem. As much as symptoms attest to the complexities of disease categories, I argue, so too do they illustrate common concerns that Indian bodies are uniquely sensitive to elements of the world and that living with these elements shapes the risks of ill health. It is plasticity, expressed in scientific theories and daily conversations alike, that connects symptoms to persons, persons to diagnostic categories, and individuals to epidemics. At different scales, we see how metabolic disorders are in some senses highly ordered. Plasticity works to make metabolisms deserving of concern in terms of how a person becomes a specific kind of body where time can take its toll. Expertise like *tenshun* and expertise like the Y-Y hypothesis attend to bodies, environments, and ways of knowing their porosity somatically and visually.

Writing in the context of the United States, Lauren Berlant has described obesity as "slow death." "Obesity," she writes, "is an effect of the intensity with which so many people need more and more mental health vacations from their exhaustion" (27). Berlant specifically points to the environment in which this takes place and notes that "the stress we experience in environments that are already absorbing the best part of our energy and creativity is so enormous that we are forced to ask whether we can even *imagine* this world as a world organized for health"(32).[24] The symptoms of chronic metabolic distress in India, whether evidenced by the BMI or by mundane invocations of stress, point to some similar conclusions. Berlant usefully shows how environments are absorbing people's energies in several forms of labor, affective and otherwise. Yet prior to eating or noneating, the limits of metabolic distress can also emerge amid the politics that move food through the city.

*Mango Madness*

"Tell me I can still eat mango," the woman greeted the dietitian. In clinical encounters, mangoes were a bargaining chip. A mango was the element of suspicion most doctors had in mind when patients came in with inexplicably high blood glucose levels. One physician I shadowed, Dr. Nair, often half seriously accused patients of mango madness in her diabetes clinic. In the summer, her mango inquiries saturated her rapport with patients and in turn my observations of this relation.

Mangoes interrupted fieldwork in small moments. During an interview with a nutritionist named Poorvi about her thoughts on the emergence of metabolic illness, the door flew open and her assistant rushed into the office to pull Poorvi aside for a few minutes. When Poorvi returned to the room, she apologized for the intrusion. "I wrote an article for [the Mumbai daily newspaper] DNA on *aamras* (mango juice) and its importance," she said. "I gave them a recipe, but they've added half a cup of sugar to the recipe I provided. They just did it on their own, thinking that it's a nutritious thing to add half a cup of sugar. And there's probably nothing I can do about it; it's likely already gone to press." Poorvi reached for the phone and, after a few transfers, reached the newspaper's health editor. "Hello," she said, "this is Poorvi speaking. [*Pause*] What's *my* problem? Someone's added a recipe that says '175 grams of sugar' in it. How can we do that? I didn't give any sugar in my recipe. Tell them *aamras* needs no sugar, just mango pulp. Please, don't add sugar. You want me to what? Send you the recipe? Just keep it the same *but don't add sugar!*"

Visibly upset, she hung up, turned to me, and sighed: "They don't want to do anything about it." Her article outlined a healthy alternative to *aamras* made with pureed mango pulp, no sugar, and a touch of skim milk. But the (incorrect) recipe attached to the article would make just the opposite: a sweet, creamy mango milkshake at odds with the tempered enjoyment she had tried to put forth.

Mangoes and Mumbai go hand in hand, especially during the mango season (roughly April until September). The most buzz-worthy type of mango is the fragrant Alfonso variety (*Hapoos*), and it was always a guessing game as to whether one's fruit wallah had the real deal at understandably inflated prices or was just substituting another kind. Mangoes appear everywhere: signs at restaurants read "Mango Madness!" and mangoes blend into local delights ranging from *aamras* (the drink that plagued the dietitian) to forms of gifts (a kilo of mangoes as a thank-you for a business transaction or special favor). Newspaper columns penned by journalists pay tributes to now forgotten or near-extinct varieties of the fruit (and how this one from Kerala or that one from Tamil Nadu *really* tops the Alfonso). Even after the seasonal uptick, mangoes' indelible imprints remain in orange stains on clothes but even more fully in language that genders and sexualizes the body's fleshy contours, in everyday conversation, and in slang shouted on the street and volleyed in songs.

In Dr. Chitre's clinic, there were moments where I felt transported from the room's plain table and chairs to a confessional booth whose screen had a pulpy mango pressed against it. A sixty-three-year-old priest came into the clinic one morning. "I broke my diet," he said as he sat down across from her desk. "Mangoes?" the doctor asked. "Yes, mangoes," he replied, looking down. Dr. Chitre explained to me—and I suspect, as an object lesson, to the priest as well—that June/July is a terrible time for diabetics. They all "break" carefully cultivated diet regimes for mangoes. It means that a patient will have to adjust the insulin carefully. Some of her patients just amp up the insulin without consultation. She sees the consequences: they overcompensate with the insulin during mango season but forget to recalibrate once it ends. As he sat in front of us, the priest's metabolism crystallized in his exceedingly high postprandial blood glucose levels: dangerous. Dr. Chitre explained to him that so far, ketones were not showing up in his lab reports—and that's good. If they were, she'd have to admit him to the hospital and start him on a saline drip. "Mangoes are *finished*," she said to him firmly. She increased his insulin dose in the afternoons. "Also, you have to cut down on your meat," she said. "No red meat. Chicken is OK, fish is OK. But once the kidney is affected, it's always affected, and we can't revert back." Mangoes were metabolic provocateurs, and handled without care they could impart permanent damage. Better offered as gifts to others who worked on your own sugars: "I'll bring you a mango next time," the priest promised the doctor.

Photographers wound through booths draped in white linen while men in orange shirts lifted crispy spheres out of sizzling oil. On a dry November evening, an elaborate festival celebrating Mumbai's quintessential street food, the *vada pav*, belied its humble constitution: a chickpea-battered, deep-fried, spicy mashed potato patty (the *vada*) tucked into a slightly sweet soft bread roll (the *pav*). The evening festival, called the *vada pav sammelan* (vada pav convention), was sponsored by the Shiv Sena, a regional political movement that promotes the rights of Hindu Marathi-speaking people born in the state of Maharashtra, whose capital is Mumbai. Since its founding in 1966, the Shiv Sena has focused on the rights of the *Marathi manoos* (the native-born Maharashtrian) through a variety of performative acts against "outsiders," ranging from South Indians living in the city to migrants from the northern states of Bihar and Uttar Pradesh. The festival took place in Shivaji Park, the site of the Shiv Sena's first mass meeting and a symbolic center of the party's power in the city.

As an influential bloc in Mumbai's municipal government, the Shiv Sena consistently lobbies for "reservations," or reserved job vacancies, for the Marathi manoos. Unhappy with the progress of instituting these reservations, the Sena took the vada pav into its own hands as a potential street-side job creation project. The party announced its own version of the food as the "Shiv vada pav" and embedded this old-new commodity into what Gyan Prakash (2010) describes as "the nostalgic 'tropical Camelot'"

(23): an Indian megacity built on the tenuous grounds of heritage, cosmopolitanism, violence, and consumerism. The Shiv Sena, however, was not alone in this newly intensified focus on the vada pav. Corporate start-ups had begun to sell branded vada pav in McDonald's-like restaurants, claiming that street food was dangerously unhygienic and that mass-produced, uniform versions of it would be cleaner and safer. The iterations of the vada pav attest to the ways that food is part of what Hansen and Verkaaik (2009) call "urban charisma"—the affective myths and corresponding political relations emanating from the city's iconic sites and stock characters. As one vendor told me, "vada pav is the lifeline of Mumbai. You can't live here without vada pav." This seemed a striking statement, especially when considered in light of assumptions that street food was harmful to the body in terms of metabolic disruption. What does it mean for the relationship between food and politics, then, if the vada pav is a "lifeline" necessary to "live here"? In addressing that question, I work through its underlying proposition that a city can have a metabolism and thus lives metabolically.

## Killer Vada Pav

For public health authorities, it was perhaps no surprise that that the vada pav was hardly a vehicle for life, a "lifeline" to live in the city. Rather, it was a "killer" primarily because of its high calorie count, and the killing could be stopped only by stopping its consumption. The figure of the obese person—especially the obese child—anchored many stories about the risks of vada pav to Mumbaikars. For example, a front-page article of the city newspaper DNA told the story of eight-year-old Abhay Gunjal, who at fifty kilos (110 lbs) was taunted by his classmates, who called him Motu (fatty). Abhay wouldn't eat "anything that is home-cooked or healthy," his mother told the reporter, and favored vada pav instead. The article cited a survey conducted by A. C. Nielsen in Mumbai, Delhi, Chennai, Kolkata, and Bangalore that found Mumbai to have the worst scores in terms of children's unhealthy snacking: "75% of children surveyed in the five metros consume unhealthy snacks, especially before dinner. . . . Mumbai leads this trend with 95% of the children in the city bingeing on pre-dinner snacks" (Suryanarayan 2009). To stem the tide of childhood obesity emanating from the overconsumption of vada pav and other fried street foods, the article quoted nutritionists who encouraged parents to emphasize "nourishing," "substantial," and "wholesome" food habits. But parents, the article concluded, feel helpless and "blame urban lifestyle and the Western influence." Adults had little power against children's hungry desires. An image alongside the article visualized the threat of vada pav in terms of calorie counts. It showed a child with a large belly holding a burger in his outstretched hand, each component representing a "killer" food, with the vada pav on top.

Building on the "killer" theme, other articles similarly called the vada pav "junk" or, more viscerally, "heart attack food" (Nandakumar 2007; Patel 2009). As with the image of the burger, here too they trafficked in calorie counts and grams of fat to discredit the vada pav. In similar language, official public health surveys located vada pav in the crosshairs of a scope searching for obesity's cause. Of special concern was a strong epidemiological association between the vada pav and childhood obesity. KEM Hospital, one of the city's largest, determined in a February 2010 survey that 15 percent of 3,200 students surveyed in eleven of the city's government schools were overweight. An article citing the survey noted that the survey also found that 82 percent of the surveyed students who purchased their lunch instead of bringing it from home opted for "junk" street foods, like vada pav. A physician who worked on the survey put it plainly: "If this dietary pattern is not changed, then we are staring at an obesity wave" (TNN 2010a). When put in a broader context of the vada pav's machinations, though, it seemed that city residents were riding several waves of object relations that could be as much a source of life as they were the source of life's attrition.

In this chapter, I argue that projects to claim and reform the vada pav define the grounds of the political life of an object beyond the act of its consumption. A close examination of the food's different manifestations and relations helps explain the kinds of unruliness coursing through food and persons that are workable and livable. I approach this by reconsidering the notion of "gastropolitics," defined by Arjun Appadurai (1981) as the "conflict or competition over specific cultural or economic resources as it emerges in social transactions around food."[1] In suggesting that the moment of an object's consumption does not exhaust its politics, I aim to direct attention to specific events where gastropolitics stabilizes or devolves at the relational interface of food and urban sociality. Gastropolitics is partly about contests over the identity of eaters, but the eater is not the only cultural element whose recognition is at stake. Connections between ordinary objects and repetitive forms of labor—from family-kept street carts to automated potato cutters—blur the boundaries between authenticity, pleasure, and risk even as they mediate instrumental consumption. These complexities suggest that gastropolitics is multiple, ephemeral, impactful, and forged across persons and things. To assume that gastropolitics is uniform and stable would be to obscure key object relations forged outside those between eater and eaten. Further, an analytical overreliance on the act of eating dampens the extent to which food's received qualities, such as specific flavors or degrees of cleanliness or contamination, materialize out of dynamic techniques of city life. Tensions between taste, hygiene, and street politics can reveal the multiple forms of harm and protection at play in questions of survival in the city. Mapping these tensions reveals several kinds of body politics that might remain underexplored in accounts of street food premised solely on "public health," where biomedically defined virtues of health are the ultimate measure of life.

Instead of beginning with "public health," which risks joining an assumed state of well-being to an assumed public that free-floats spatially, I instead anchor my analysis in circumstances when a city holds together or falls apart. I do this by entering into conversation with several thinkers in urban studies who have proposed that a city should be understood metabolically. Challenging notions of hydraulics, inherited from urban modernism, that cast cities as homeostatic systems of self-regulation, urbanists such as Matthew Gandy (2004) suggest that "relational perspectives differ fundamentally from the linear flow–based models of urban space associated with concepts such as 'industrial metabolism,' 'ecological footprints' and other functionalist conceptions of urban space" (374; see also Swyngedouw 2006). I agree with these efforts to rethink the historical deployment of the metabolism as a lens onto urban dynamics. However, to declare the city a specific kind of metabolism is itself a historical statement about the science of body-environment connections. Scholars of urban metabolism risk overlooking the contingencies of the biomedical science that the concept itself recruits in their assessment of urban politics.

The case of the vada pav is an opportunity to reckon with the question of how the city and the body suffuse each other amid changing notions of what bodily and environmental metabolism is and does. I am interested in ways to understand the efforts to remake the vada pav at scales ranging from recipes to specific places on the street to family relations. The urban studies scholarship on urban metabolism described above tends to uphold "the metabolism" as something already given as a model for urban sociality.

This line of thinking poses a given object of urban infrastructure (such as water or electricity) as lying in wait for its consumption. Yet food and eaters and the many people that come between them do not line up so easily. Efforts to remake the vada pav show that the figure of the choosy eater is sometimes stable but only in certain circumstances. Consequently, I am interested in the conditions that allow and disallow confidence in understanding precisely what is metabolic about the city.

My way into this discussion is through a focus on relations that seem to be instances of the city's ur-objects—specifically, its beloved snack—pleasing and harming the body. Street food was the coda for many public health concerns about obesity. I was struck by how strong an object analysis this was: that a single thing could cause so much bodily damage. This object analysis on the part of public health authorities uniformly deemed consumption the problem. But what if the arc between fast food and metabolic illness was framed differently, from the standpoint of permeability and porosity? What does the blame game of obesity look like when the vision of consumption public health might assume is not taken as already evident? What kinds of elements and environments can be said to compose a city and its politics? Rather than take the materiality of food for granted or exaggerate materiality to the exclusion of sociality, I engage an object by de-emphasizing its consumption and foregrounding the circumstances that inform and animate it. Gastropolitics, I argue, is a key feature of metabolic living, and personal, familial, and neighborhood histories condition the terms of the "social" and "political" that make up gastropolitics. These historical and ongoing operations center on the question of what kinds of people and things are licensed to coexist on Mumbai's streets.[2] *Food* becomes *street food* not only out of a politics of located consumption but also out of a politics of relations that no one "chef"—whether party scion, street vendor, aspirational businessman, nutritionist, or even the food itself—can solely bring to fruition.

## The Object of Gastropolitics

I employ the term "gastropolitics" rather than "food politics" for several reasons. The term has an important intellectual lineage and continuing resonance about commensality in South Asia that I do not wish to dismiss (see Alter 2000a, 2000b, 1999). For example, from Appadurai's exploration of gastropolitics, Parama Roy (2010) extends the political valence of the concept further, whereby it is a lens onto the contingencies of postcoloniality:

"Who eats and with whom, who starves, and what is rejected as food are fundamental to colonial and postcolonial making—and unmaking," she explains (24). Gastropolitics also usefully illustrates the permeability of domestic and political spheres, as Jon Holtzman has demonstrated in his study of African pastoralist groups (2009). From its inception through its continued applications, the term has been concerned with relationality, commensality, and propriety.

I thus draw on this concept for reasons particular to my field site. But I also engage gastropolitics as a conceptual intervention to broaden the rather narrow scholarly focus on individuated consumption in food studies across regions, wherein eating tends to be the conceptual gatekeeper between food and identity politics (Mintz and Du Bois 2002; Sutton 2010). An analysis confined rigidly between consumption and identity making cannot account for the vendor's keen observation of the mutual entanglements of food and urban life that make vada pav a "lifeline" of Mumbai. This is because an overreliance on consumption takes food as a uniform object, thus sidestepping food's material contingencies and their resultant power effects. The vada pav is a single recognizable object to eaters yet crystallizes multiple political visions such as party solidarity, entrepreneurism, and urban hygienic order. In contrast to consumption, gastropolitics is a sharper lens onto the materiality of these visions and their uneven contours of power over livelihoods.

In relating the object of food to urban spaces, anthropologists have observed how making, selling, and eating street food can be understood as a way of what Judith Farquhar (2009: 561) calls "peopling the city," an embodied form of claiming urban space. From this perspective, street food is a compelling ethnographic object because it accompanies persons through memories and ideals of the city, favorite tastes, notions of authenticity and belonging, and client-vendor relations. Situated in urban spaces, then, food is part of the generation of urban political infrastructures (see, e.g., Anjaria 2009, 2006; Anand 2011; Anand and Rademacher 2011; Hansen 1999, 2002; Mukhopadhyay 2004; Rajagopal 2001; Varma 2004). Indeed, the material centrality of food to everyday life has long been a concern in South Asian studies, as discussed in this book's introduction (Appadurai 1981, 1988; Conlon 1995; Khare 1992; Iversen and Raghavendra 2006; Nandy 2004; Osella 2008). Often, as already described, the thrust of the analytic concern has been how food can substantiate identity relations such as caste systems and class standing. The articulation of a "Mumbai" identity and imagination certainly emerges through eating vada pav.[3] Even so, the food's popularity also turns on other objects (spices, street carts), practices (sharing street space, the labor of continuing family histories of food vending, mass-producing a snack) and their linked genealogies. I draw on ethnographies of food and eating, especially in India, and reframe them by focusing on the material contingencies of food itself, particularly through vignettes about efforts to standardize it. I do not suggest that the vada pav does the bulk of the Shiv Sena's political work but, rather, that the food offers a compelling case study worth exploring for its resonance in other streetscapes where material objects bind vernacular disputes. Ethnographies of urban politics and ethnographies of food and eating have many possible points of convergence in this light.

However, I would like to tread carefully with street food. It is a seductive but nonetheless singular material anchor that risks object overdetermination. Therefore, as this chapter works out a material gastropolitics, it also addresses broader problems in addressing the ethnographic specificity of viable person-object arrangements that must exist alongside public health intentions to eliminate fast food. These arrangements include employment, violence, and everyday survival. I suggest that gastropolitics is a conceptual frame that can accommodate a more nuanced ethnographic engagement with materiality and, specifically, the material forces that interlink bodies and their surrounding space. Recent ethnographies have richly articulated how space and place inflect the politics of food (see Paxson 2013; Weiss 2011). Guided by these works, I am interested in pursuing a more general challenge for anthropologists engaged with object controversies. I follow Yael Navaro-Yashin's assertion: "The relation people forge with objects must be studied in contexts of historical contingency and political specificity."[4] Simply put, the relation between street food and urban politics is an entanglement whose materiality cannot be taken for granted. By moving beyond the confines of street food as a bounded entity, it is possible to map the reach of gastropolitics into livelihoods, community injuries, dreams of urban renewal, and transnational enterprise.

Historically, food has been integral to Mumbai's complex political projects, and the vada pav as a site of study must be situated in the Shiv Sena's comprehensive reaches of power across local and regional articulations of Hindu nationalism, gender, and urban consumerism since India's economic liberalization (Appadurai 2000; Mazzarella 2003; Rajagopal 2001; Sen 2007). Arjun Appadurai (2000) explains that the Shiv Sena is one of the many parties linked to the Hindu nationalist coalition called the

Sangh Parivar. Formed in 1966, the party's platform combines language ideology (Marathi), regional primordialism (a celebration of the regional state of Maharashtra), and a commitment to a Hinduized India (*Hindutva*, the ideology of a land of Hinduness). The Shiv Sena Party's founder, Bal Thackeray, is often regarded as the embodiment of this platform. Thomas Blom Hansen (2002) has argued that the Shiv Sena's enduring power derives from its "permanent performance" of politics and that we must pay attention to how "governance has become organized around competing languages—biopolitical rationalities as well as various forms of sovereignty (legal, person, etc.)—both within and beyond the state" (233). The decline of Mumbai's textile mills, whose owners, union leaders, and workers have had tangled relations with the Shiv Sena, has also been integral to the party's power dynamics (Finkelstein 2015). Malls and movie theaters have replaced many of the mills, providing ample sites to examine the dynamics of investment capital and consumer desire for India's "new" middle classes and their thorny relationship to the Shiv Sena.[5] Collectively, these studies narrate the Shiv Sena's physical and ideological claiming of streets through neighborhood-level events and agitations. They show the efforts of the Shiv Sena to isolate specific qualities of the street in order to stabilize it enough to launch schemes like the Shiv vada pav. I add to this work an analysis of metabolism, which necessarily bridges materiality to events and experience. From this perspective, the symmetries between "the food in Mumbai" and "the Mumbai in food" are not given. Rather, their differences materialize through efforts to transform the boundary potentials of food, street, and body.

The vada pav itself has a long-standing tie to the Shiv Sena in terms of food's dynamic links to the city's urban geography.[6] For example, the Shiv vada pav festival exemplifies the iconographies that are essential to the Shiv Sena's constant public performances (Bedi 2007: 1535). Also notable are the forms of exclusion and inclusion that take shape around objects. A friend explained to me that in the 1960s, some Shiv Sena protest signs read "*Idli dosa bagao*" (stop *idli* and *dosa*), referencing the two iconic snack foods of Tamil Nadu, as Senaiks attacked South Indian Udipi restaurants when party founder Bal Thackeray accused South Indians of taking jobs that "rightly" belonged to the *Marathi manoos*. Object controversies also shift the political economy of urban public space. For instance, in the 1990s the Shiv Sena created an employment scheme based around *zhunka bhakar*, a Maharashtrian porridge and bread dish. That effort has largely been understood as a failure in terms of popularizing the food: many *zhunka bhakar* outlets in the city now serve Chinese food instead. (As an employment scheme, however, it was moderately successful.) These examples illustrate that the vada pav has many short-lived gastropolitical antecedents. What I want to flag in these instances and what I describe for the vada pav is that it takes *both* human and object investments to materialize gastropolitics, however long the political formation may last and to whatever degree the formation emerges as a health threat.

### *Jai* vada pav!: Potatoes and Protection

At the Shiv vada pav *sammelan*, potatoes took center stage as the marker of an urban political formation based around a competition for conformity. The political vision guiding this competition was one in which a standardized food and a standardized cart would anchor the presence of the *Marathi manoos* on the city's streets. The Shiv Sena Party leader, Bal Thackeray's son Uddhav Thackeray, invited twenty-seven of the city's vada pav vendors to the *sammelan* at Shivaji Park to fry up thousands of free vada pav and advertised the event widely. The winning recipe would become the official recipe of the Shiv vada pav, which the Sena planned to launch several months later. The Shiv vada pav would be sold in thousands of dedicated food stalls across the city, based on the premise that Sena supporters could receive jobs as vendors. The Sena positioned the Shiv vada pav as the bellwether of taste and hygiene, because the food stalls planned for the Shiv vada pav were made of stainless steel to ensure sanitation and "clean" frying. They hyped this party-line brand using the narrative that the vada pav was the food that nourished party members during violent protests in the 1960s and the food that energized Sena constituents during harsh economic times. They also invited marketers from McDonald's and Coca-Cola to add a slick consumer appeal to the enterprise through logo and food cart design, each of which materialized a vernacular and transnational standard.

Inside the festival grounds, the organizers set up billowing fabric walls. Metal detectors funneled the crowd into semiorganized lines; once through, women in orange saris handed over score sheets printed in Marathi. Booths lined the perimeter of the grounds, each representing a different vada pav vendor. I started from the corner booth and moved down the line, eating three vada pav in succession. The first didn't seem freshly fried. The second came immediately from the oil, crunchy on the outside. The third had the best flavor, slightly citrusy and sweet; months

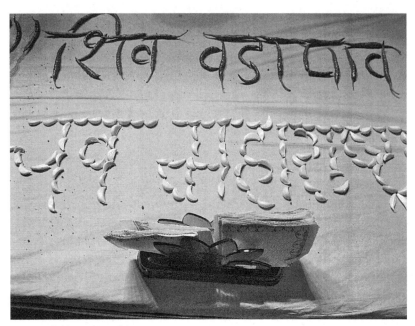

**FIG. 2.1** Chilies and garlic

later I learned that this would be the winning recipe. Each booth was uniquely decorated; one especially creative vendor spelled out "Shiv vada pav" in Devanagari script using green chilies and "Chav Maharashtracha!" (taste Maharashtra!) using garlic cloves (see figure 2.1). Each time I sampled a vada pav, the vendor or an assistant gently reminded me to give them a good score. As I made my way around the booths, growing full very quickly, two twenty-somethings with cameras approached. They were from Saamna, the Shiv Sena daily newspaper. Wearing jeans and T-shirts embossed with trendy American clothing design brands, they clicked a photo of me enjoying "the Bombay burger," as they called it.[7]

A boom of fireworks reverberated through the space. Hindustani musicians began a concert on the stage at the front of the festival grounds. Amid chants of "Jai vada pav!" (praise vada pav!), a series of party members gave speeches, each trumpeted by a man dressed as a Maratha warrior blowing into a long ceremonial horn. The "guests of honor" took the stage: senior executives from McDonald's and Coca-Cola, and Uddhav Thackeray himself. The emcee of the program asked the McDonald's and Coke execs to stand and unveiled the official Shiv vada pav cart to another round of horn toots. On the left side of the stage, drapes fell away from a round dais, and beneath it spun the prototype cart gleaming with stainless steel. The backdrop of the stage glowed from the spotlights: enormous photographs of Uddhav smiling and of his father, party founder Bal Thackeray, pictured with his fists clenched. McDonald's and Coke logos were interspersed among these larger-than-life photos of the party leaders. Uddhav presented each of the execs with a miniature version of the street cart, prompting more horn toots and applause. The cart was a critical sign as the standardized interface between the winning recipe, the entrepreneurial vendor, and the authentic cosmopolitan consumer. Two speeches wrapped up the event. In the first, Mumbai's mayor, Dr. Shubha Raul, extolled the vada pav as the city's cultural treasure, whose added benefit was its nutrition, because it contains vitamins and carbohydrates. Uddhav Thackeray concluded the evening with his keynote speech. He explained that India's regions are best characterized by their food and that the Shiv vada pav will do that work for Mumbai and for the people of Maharashtra.[8] Fireworks exploded as his speech ended. Above the stage a giant sign made of sparklers reading "vada pav!" in Marathi burst into flames and officially concluded the event. The spectacle illustrated the Shiv Sena's tactics of corporatism, taking the party beyond mere communal politics and rudimentary violence. The cart and other objects mattered here, because it was through material appeals to removing microbes and enforcing hygiene that the Shiv Sena connected transnational corporations to its employment generation strategy.[9]

Over the ensuing year, the Shiv vada pav continued to make headlines. The Shiv Sena fought battles with other constituencies in the municipal government, which decreed that vada pav street carts would violate hawking regulations. City news columns poked fun at the endeavor and noted that the glossy production of a new street food was nothing but another instance of a Sena publicity tactic. To add insult to injury, the opposition Congress Party announced plans for its own politicized street food: the "Congress poha", a traditional spicy snack made from beaten rice flakes (Desai 2009a, 2009b, 2009c). Others followed suit: Ramdas Athavale, the leader of the Republican Party of India (Athavale), said that if the Sena would have Shiv vada pav, his party would have "Bhim" vada pav to honor the Dalit intellectual and political leader Dr. Bhimrao Ambedkar (UNI 2009). The Sena's politicization of the vada pav inspired a host of other possibilities, each trying to standardize a food to advance the party line.

Although the festival made the vada pav seem like a natural member of the Shiv Sena family, both published and oral histories of the food point to a more complex ancestry. I was struck by the variety of origin stories told about the food, and though no one story ever stood out as a singular truth, they nonetheless converged on the food's roots in Mumbai's unique history of immigrant communities. Vikram Doctor, one of India's most influential food writers, traces the origins of the pav (the bun) to either the Portuguese, who first settled the islands of Bombay, or perhaps to later Goan and Irani immigrants, who opened Bombay's first bakeries. Doctor explains that the vada (the potato ball) most likely comes from Maharashtra and notes that potatoes themselves are of British origin dating to the nineteenth century. Over time, potatoes spread to the city, and "sliced thin or mashed they were dipped in chickpea batter and deep fried as a snack" (Doctor 2008, Doctor n.d.). Putting the vada and the pav together was "the real inspiration," according to Doctor, and entailed adding "enough chutney to moisten the pav and add spice to the blandness of bread and potatoes." Doctor echoed a story I had heard often: that this inspiration of joining potato and bread came from a street vendor named Ashok Vaidya, who lived in central Mumbai. Once Vaidya began selling the vada pav in the 1960s, it quickly became popular. Shiv Sena officials noticed the food's symbolic potential, encouraged party members to set up vada pav stalls around local party outposts (shakhas), and thus connected the food to the party's visibility on city streets after its beginnings in struggles for Maharashtrian empowerment in the 1960s.

A city beat journalist, Dhruv, anchored the origin point of the vada pav in earlier events. During Partition, he explained, large numbers of Hindus arrived in the city from Sindh Province in Pakistan. Jawaharlal Nehru decided to keep the Sindhis in a town a few hours from Bombay with a barracks complex originally built by the British for Allied soldiers during World War II. The town, Ulhasnagar, is now also known as Sindhunagar because so many Sindhis remained in the ensuing years, despite promises that their shift there would be temporary. Dhruv said that Ulhasnagar had a rail yard for the cleaning of trains and that Sindhi residents would board newly washed trains bound for Mumbai or Pune for daily work. The Sindhi commuters carried their own food, especially spiced potatoes and bread, which he noted were staples back in Sindh. The inspiration for the vada pav was born out of this commuter practice, Dhruv explained: "One day a man came along and thought, 'why should eking out a living be so difficult?' He wanted to sell food to his own people on the train. So he put mashed potato into a ball, and sandwiched it between bread. The only problem was that the potato would chunk off and fall out of the bread. People complained, especially because many of them wore white kurtas, which kept getting stained by stray potatoes. So the man realized that if he battered the potato ball, and then fried it, it would keep the potato chunks intact and the Sindhi kurtas white. You can still get a vada pav without the batter in Ulhasnagar, even today." Once this battered potato ball sandwich took up residence in Mumbai, the city's diverse residents changed it over and over again with different chutneys, spices, and chilies, especially with the Maharashtrian staples of garlic, peanut, and chili. "But its origin was in Partition," Dhruv emphasized. "Khane mein mitti ki khushbu hai" (that food has the scent of the soil in it), he said. "A taste of the people it comes from."[10]

Although different in its beginning, Dhruv's story joined Vikram Doctor's and others I heard in terms of the vada pav falling into the hands of the Shiv Sena. Dhruv emphasized that the vada pav grew out of Mumbai's textile mills, which were primary sources of employment for city residents up until the 1980s, when strikes and economic reforms forced mill closures. When the mills closed and people needed income, they sold vada pav outside the mills. According to Dhruv, because the remaining mill workers would pass their former colleagues on the streets selling vada pav, to buy it from them meant "Here is my brother, laid off, and I will support him." As city police and municipal officials sought to chase "informal" economic endeavors like street hawking off the streets, the Shiv Sena stepped in and offered hawkers protection. Each shakha would take in "protection money" and had a minimum requirement dictated by party officials. It began as a few rupees each day but over time would indebt street vendors to the Shiv Sena in amounts of hundreds or even thousands of rupees a week. Protection could bring a street cart or a business under the watchful eye of the local shakha, which would informally monitor any potential vandalism and forestall official fines during rounds by the local police.

Protection also connected street-level politics to broader questions about the relationship between "proper" food and the future of an imagined body politic. When I later interviewed Vinod, a Shiv Sena–affiliated municipal representative, for his perspective on the Shiv vada pav, he began by saying, "The vada pav has been there since the beginning of the Sena. It's parallel with the Sena's history. It's about employment." He explained that because of a dearth of jobs in the late 1960s and because "at the time, Marathi lads were not so enterprising," party founder Bal Thackeray brought them together at a mass rally. "Balasaheb (an honorific of Bal Thackeray's first name) told them, 'If you can't do anything, just sell vada pav and earn some money for your families.' So they did. It's outside every shakha, and it's employed Marathi people." In this history of the vada pav, Bal Thackeray's innovation helped "the Marathi burger" gain fame because of its association with the Sena. Its simplicity made it successful, and its success supported thousands of families in times of hardship. Vinod pointed out the mill workers strike of 1982, when vada pav fed striking workers: "The vada pav has changed generations of families," he claimed. Because a vendor can sell thousands of vada pav a day, he can make a profit upwards of 5,000 rupees. "Some are crorepatis [millionaires] now," Vinod said. Yet the business of vada pav remained diverse, something that had gone relatively unnoticed until corporate start-ups entered the picture. During this time, Vinod had been in Delhi as a member of Parliament (MP) and often had fellow politicians beg him to bring vada pav back from trips home to Mumbai. One day, Vinod encountered a journalist eating aloo boonda, a fried potato patty snack believed to originate from South India:

> I teased that journalist, telling him that I felt sorry for him because he wasn't eating authentic vada pav. He replied, "Fine—so give me some real vada pav." I realized how much people liked it. Even Amar Singh (the former Secretary General of the Samajwadi Party) wanted it. So I organized a Delhi vada pav party. I flew vendors from Mumbai to Delhi, and they made fresh pav just for the occasion. All the stars, all the government babus, came to my house just for this. I came back [to Mumbai] and Balasaheb asked me why so many people in Delhi liked vada pav, but the demand wasn't as visible here. So Balasaheb met with vada pav wallahs and we did a survey, and found out there are 5,500 vendors in the city. Balasaheb and Uddhav (Thackeray) said, 'Let's brand it. It'll be the same taste, and the same size.' And Balasaheb named it 'Shiv Vada Pav.'

I pressed him on the association with McDonald's and Coke—what did he think there was to gain by putting the vada pav in the same frame as global fast food? After all, the Shiv Sena had famously protested McDonald's in 2001 over allegations that the company was using beef extract in its French fries. "The vada pav is not fast food!" Vinod rebuked with a dismissive hand wave. "It's got mirchi (green chili), haldi (turmeric), and kothimbir (coriander)—it's healthy food!" "Healthy," for Vinod, expressed the vada pav's generative qualities. Not only would the food standardize the employment of the Marathi manoos, but it also would reform entrepreneurial possibilities, cleaning the streets by filling them with stainless steel vada pav carts imprinted with transnational corporate logos. The Shiv vada pav illustrates how transnational capital is hardly anathema to vernacular politics; rather, corporate interests coalesce around a basic material like potatoes. The material basis of vada pav—potatoes and spices—enable this food's capacity for corporatization. However, the simplicity of these materials and their resonance with persons as basic staples also enable Vinod's remark that the vada pav was food, not fast food, and thus make the odd pairing of the Shiv Sena and McDonald's possible to dismiss.[11] Across origin stories and employment schemes, through reforms and resignifications, potatoes composed the gastropolitical infrastructure of the street along with people.[12] This infrastructure had an authentic taste, and stainless steel corporatism would be the vehicle of its amplification.

### "The Tiger Still Roars"

Despite Vinod's praise of the vada pav, I wondered how stall owners themselves expressed a relationship between the vada pav and vitality amid this impulse to create an ideal, uniform version of the food. If the Shiv Sena aimed to protect the *Marathi manoos* through the Shiv vada pav, how—if at all—did the sellers themselves engage these aims? Beyond the pomp of the *sammelan*, was the Shiv vada pav rebranding effort simply the publicity stunt its critics assumed it was? The Shiv vada pav promised a spot of entrepreneurial ascendance on the Mumbai streetscape and participation in a project of corporatized standardization. Even as the Shiv Sena's party line emphasized the flavor of the vada pav as the crux of the ideal city, vada pav sellers themselves exposed the fragility of this claim in order to control public space via food. For the sellers, too, the vada pav cart was a political sign, and the street corner was a critical political space that was deeply connected to informal enterprise. For one seller I met, the practice of standardization was one in which he sold his own family's classic recipe, which he believed drew in regular customers who favored both its taste and its long-standing presence on the street.

A friend had mentioned to me that an elementary school classmate, Mahesh, had taken over his father's long-standing vada pav cart. We linked up over the phone; Mahesh told me that he'd be happy to tell the family's story. His father had some health problems that might make communication difficult, he said, but I would see for myself that these challenges didn't stop his father from assuming his post behind the vada pav cart, as he had done for forty years. On the first of my visits, Mahesh picked me up on his motorbike at the Shiv Sena headquarters and angled through alleyways to his home, a low building in the heart of the neighborhood of

Dadar. His mother, who was preparing lunch, welcomed us as we came in via the kitchen. His father sat on the couch in the living room but stood up to shake my hand before leaving the room, passing three enormous trays of potato *vadas* that circled the television.

Mahesh watched my gaze stop at the vadas, perfectly rounded and yellow. He said that there were approximately 1,200 vadas in the trays, rolled out a few hours before my visit. He described his typical schedule. A day in advance of making the vadas, either he or his mother places the order for the oil, the *besan* (chickpea flour), the salt, and the potatoes. Early the following morning, they cook and check the potatoes to make sure that there are no rotten bits. "It takes a light hand to mix everything," he said. Machines mixed the mashed potatoes too vigorously and created too much starchiness, which would thicken the soft inside of the patty. Before rolling out the cart from behind the house, they ensure that his father has the right amount of cash in the box for making small change and that the cart is well stocked with packaging and with chutneys. From start to finish, it was a family operation—and a standardized one on its own scale.

As his father walked outside to check on the cart, Mahesh rummaged through a cabinet and brought out laminated newspaper articles about his father and the vada pav cart to help narrate their linked history. His father, Alok, started the cart in 1968, "when Balasaheb (Bal Thackeray) told the *Marathi manoos* to take up the vada pav," Mahesh said. Mahesh admired Bal Thackeray for the protection he had given to the family. In 1968, when Alok started selling vada pav for ten paise, Bal himself told him, "If you have any problems, tell me." Alok had manned the cart from 8 AM until evening virtually every day in the forty years since. "We also used to sell samosas," Mahesh said, "but the veg prices went up and we didn't want to compromise on quality." They used green peas, carrots, and other vegetables, but high prices meant they would have to double the price of the samosa. Two days prior, they raised the price of the vada pav to seven rupees, and he admitted that a few customers complained. But most of their customers understood how expensive vegetables had become and that Alok was a veteran vada pav wallah who wouldn't raise prices without considerable deliberation.

Mahesh started helping his father sell vada pav when he was eight years old. He suffered for this: neighborhood kids teased him, and his classmates and teachers insulted him, telling him that the son of a street food vendor could never be "up to standard" on the ladder of educational and career achievements. He set out to prove them wrong and eventually completed his bachelor's degree and started his own small business. He discussed his plans to open his own vada pav stall, which would sell Shiv vada pav, because he was the vice president of the Shiv vada pav initiative. Yet although the more senior members of the Sena saw public vitality and consumerism connected via the employment and sustenance of the *Marathi manoos*, Mahesh was not fully convinced. His move toward selling Shiv vada pav was a relatively recent one, even though his family had been longtime supporters of the Shiv Sena. A few men from the Shiv Sena's higher ranks contacted him and asked if he wanted to help lead the effort to popularize Shiv vada pav. He agreed and helped organize the *sammelan* by sorting through thousands of applications from vendors, hoping to make it to the final cut of twenty-seven who would compete.

However, Mahesh and other party members had different visions for Shiv vada pav. He thought it made more sense to sell the masala, or spice mix, instead of the food itself: "That way, housewives could make it at home, and because the masala stays fresh for a long time, it will turn a fast profit." He led me back into the kitchen and opened a stone urn underneath the stove. It was filled with a green-yellow masala paste, the centerpiece of the family's vada pav recipe. Yet the organizers of the Shiv vada pav venture didn't agree on selling the spice paste. They wanted to train people to make the food and sell it on the street, Mahesh explained. This made sense in terms of employment generation but came with its own risks: "The minute that person leaves the job, then someone else has to be trained. If they had chosen to market the masala packet, it could have netted more profit." For Mahesh, basic ingredients, more than the "soft" outcome of skills transfer to party supporters, paved the way to value. Taste diffused through uniform, portable spice packets was the most productive path toward standardization, he felt. Thus while Mahesh was in many senses the ideal *Marathi manoos* to take up the Shiv vada pav, his close engagement with and aspirations for the food's material particularities destabilized the Shiv Sena's corporatized vision.

In the early afternoon, we went outside to help Alok push the cart down the street toward the main road, an intersection just blocks from both Mahesh's home and the busy Dadar train station. First, we stopped at a collection of small hutments across from the nearest Shiv Sena *shakha*. Mahesh explained that they rent one of these small spaces to fry the vadas, and Alok had an assistant who had worked with him for decades to do the frying. Inside the closet-sized room, a fuel tank and a large black iron *kaḍai* (wok) left little room for anyone else. We continued to push the cart to the

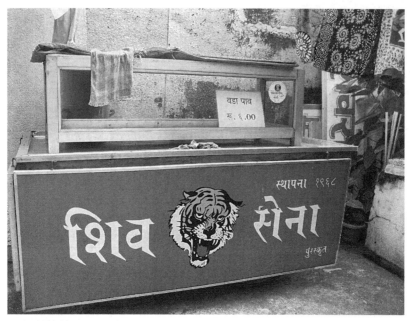

**FIG. 2.2** Alok's cart

main road until we reached the corner. Mahesh hung signs on either side of the metal cart: bright orange, with the Shiv Sena name and its official logo of a snarling tiger. It was Alok's original cart from 1968, with a few tune-ups (see figure 2.2). "The tiger still roars," Mahesh said cheekily, anchoring the vada pav as the transmitter of occupations delineated through kin.

Alok readied the cart with shaky hands. He unlocked the money box, made of weathered wood and covered in gold and red swastikas. He straightened his hat, orange and embossed with the Shivaji bow and arrow. The cart's preparation surface was carefully organized: a pile of newspaper squares for to-go orders, a small katora (bowl) for string to wrap the newspaper packets, larger bowls for the wet green chutney and the dry red chili chutney, and a tray for the pav, which Alok pulled from a burlap bag and stacked neatly. He silently motioned for me to touch them, grabbing my hand by the knuckles to nudge it into a pav: still warm. The cart officially opened at 3 pm, marked by the arrival of Alok's assistant who walked the half-block length with the first batch of vadas. There was already a short line of people waiting. Alok prepared the vada pav, gave it to the first man in line, and blessed the money he received in a ritual that consecrated the day's first business.

I stayed with Alok as Mahesh ran back and forth between the cart and the house to ensure a smooth flow of supplies. His customers were as diverse as the city itself. Schoolgirls begged Alok to rush their order in the seconds before their bus arrived (they needn't have worried, because upon its arrival the driver himself bounded out of the bus, cut the line, and announced "jaldi jaldi ek dena!"—"Give me one quickly!"). Several people were on their way either to or from the nearby Hindu Siddhivinayak Temple. Men and women, across classes, faiths, and age groups, clustered around the cart. "You feed everyone," Mahesh said, and this seemed to be the case, as some pavement dwellers approached the cart with coins in hand. Mahesh pointed out the corner's geography of street food: "There's a guy selling sev puri there, across the street. Down the block, there are sandwich guys . . . they're bhaiyyas (North Indians), and to some extent it's affected my business, but I let it go." He didn't feel his profits were too affected by the North Indians who were selling competing street foods across the way and did not see the choices of consumers as being terribly high stakes. If people wanted a sandwich or sev puri and the money went to the bhaiyyas, so be it—"it's their money," Mahesh said. The question of consumption was moot, because even in the face of competition there would always be someone lining up for vada pav.

A few hours later, Mahesh led me across the street to visit the pav bakery. Around the corner from one of the city's better-known sugarcane juice stalls, a wooden half door led to the small main office of the bakery. Passing it, we followed the alleyway through hutments until we reached a larger structure that held the ovens, two glowing rectangles cut into the back wall. It was a warm day outside, but inside the room it was searing. At least fifteen young men were inside: prepping the baking trays, inserting them into the ovens, removing the baked pav from the ovens, and packing them into bags. We helped a few of the men with the packing and then carried the bags filled with fresh pav back down the alley, across traffic, and down the block to Alok's cart.

He asked about my favorite Hindi movies and then expressed a preference for Marathi-language films. "They're not overacted," he explained. "There's subtlety to them," compared to "corny" Bollywood films. I asked his opinion of *Mi Shivajiraje Bhosale Boltoy* (This Is Shivaji Raje Bhosale Speaking), a popular 2009 Marathi film about a downtrodden middle-class Maharashtrian who receives life lessons from the spirit of Chhatrapati Shivaji Maharaj (the seventeenth-century Maratha ruler and present-day Shiv Sena icon). "It's brilliant," Mahesh said. "When the Muslims and the others were going to invade India, Shivaji won against them with only four hundred Maratha warriors. Think of it: Such a small number against such a large enemy. It aroused courage in other people, too, or at least it should." I responded that it also took courage to maintain civility in such a diverse city. After all, we had just left a street corner that captured a moment of cosmopolitan commensality. That cosmopolitanism was hardly secure. Mahesh began talking about the 1992 Bombay riots that pitted Hindus and Muslims against each other: "I saw horrible things. A man lit on fire in front of the train station, at 10 am in broad daylight. Street kids that took knives and were stabbing people. Horrible, horrible things. It was a dark spot on the city. But Dad was out there with the cart, after the curfew ended. No one had food, and so people lined up for vada pav."

To Mahesh, his father had fed the city during one of its darkest hours. Mumbai's cosmopolitanism might seem self-evident on any given day at Alok's stall, surrounded by vendors from different areas of India selling other regional specialty foods, but the memories of brutal violence couldn't be erased from the street corner or distilled out of the cart. As the Shiv vada pav stood to meld global corporatism with vernacular flair under the sign of the future city, for Mahesh specific historical events were still material. Street food generated life and money, even as its historical harms lingered, and his family worked through those harms one sale at a time.


"We Give the Street Taste, Without the Danger"

When Mahesh described his own soon-to-open Shiv vada pav stall, I had asked if he thought his product would incur competition from the number of small corporations that had branded their own versions of the food, such as the popular company Jumbo King vada pav. He scoffed: "They have an expiry date! I want fresh food, not food with preservatives." He described "those" vada pav as anonymously sourced, prefrozen, and laden with preservatives. I had heard similar sentiments from Nitin, another Shiv vada pav seller I interviewed; like Mahesh, he came from a family of vada pav sellers stretching back decades. "That's not the way," Nitin said of corporatized versions. "Freezing them, having expiration dates . . . it needs to be fresh, and homemade. The taste changes when you keep it on the shelf." The tenor of gastropolitics for the sellers I interviewed settled on freshness—which meant immediate frying on the street and the seller handing the food directly to the customer.

Despite these sentiments, corporate brands of vada pav had become an increasingly regular sight in Mumbai's train stations, in malls, and on the streets in the past five years. By appealing to fears about poor hygiene historically and presently attributed to the city's streets, these companies imagined streets sanitized via a standardized taste. Fans of vada pav could enjoy a city filled with cosmopolitan flavors but could avoid the health consequences stemming from a love for microbial food. If street-side vada pav emerged through a gastropolitics of freshness, corporatized versions of the food operated through a gastropolitics of clean uniformity, yet they still had to account for the raw materials of the street in the pursuit of maximizing customers. In this process, we see a self-regulating subject of choice emerge. It emerges such that the "consumers" idealized by companies are persons who accommodate the politics of the vada pav's constitution as part of complex urban political sensibilities. In doing so, the street of the consuming subject is a sanitized one, free of microbes. It is also one ideally free of vernacular political parties who use food to angle for power. Urban metabolism in this context is highly dependent on direct absorption between maker and eater, with a little help from industrial food processing.

One day in my neighborhood I noticed that my locksmith had an outside wall of his store painted with an advertisement for a vada pav brand called Maza; the tagline was "Vada pav No. 1." I hadn't seen this company's version of the food before and began asking friends and neighbors about their thoughts on it. Through a neighbor's connections, a few weeks later I walked into Maza's head office through a bright red door at the back of a sprawling suburban industrial complex. Parth, the marketing director, ushered me into a conference room. With an expression of friendly concern, he asked if I had read Eric Schlosser's *Fast Food Nation* (2005) and if my own interests paralleled Schlosser's investigative intents. At Maza, he said, they weren't engaged in exploitation, as Schlosser had critiqued in his study of the mass production of meat. Rather, in mass-producing street food, Maza was in the business of selling "the essence of Mumbai," which the vada pav exemplified. "The first thing visitors to Bombay want to do is see the Gateway (of India) and to eat vada pav," he explained. Street food was elemental to the standard itinerary of urban immersion.

The head of operations, Mr. Anand, joined us in the room and placed an "original" Maza vada pav in front of me to try. It was sweeter than I expected; Mr. Anand explained that the sweetness came from the wet chutney, which had more dates and *gur* (jaggery, or palm sugar) than many other recipes. He listed some basic ingredients—chilies, garlic—but most were unique to the "company special recipe" that took six months of testing to develop and standardize. Mr. Anand narrated the Maza story as I chewed, introducing it by proclaiming that "the vada pav has graduated from the street corner, and has grown up." "Graduating" the vada pav from the street corner put it squarely in a narrative of progress where vernacular objects and their desires must be improved and perfected by corporate expertise. The marketing team wanted to embrace how Indians were "experimenting" with flavors and hoped that several spins on the "traditional" flavor, like "Szechwan," would lift the vada pav out of the familiarity of the Mumbai streetscape and into more globalized aesthetics while still retaining its powers of deeply local nostalgia. A material intervention was needed to mature the palate and the city.

The impulse to perfect and sanitize the street dated back to Maza's founding and continued to structure the company's operational rationale. Mr. Anand's involvement in the company came from his desire "to do something for the middle class" and "to make people into entrepreneurs." He had been a part of several business ventures, but Maza's approach to vada pav was appealing to him because of its emphasis on employment and training. The Maza vada pav seller played an important role in maintaining social cohesion. "It's just like McDonald's," he said. "You give food to the masses. You generate employment. And if you don't employ people, they'll get led to crime, to terror—they'll go and plant a bomb somewhere." In 2004, he and his business partner wondered about doing something with street food after feeling "disgusted" by the lack of cleanliness they saw on a daily basis. To answer their central business plan question—"Can we make it like McDonald's?"—they turned to standardization. Standardization, Mr. Anand claimed, was Maza's unique contribution to a broader project of cleaning the streets. "There are no food laws in India," he complained. "*Filthy* is the vision for foreigners who come here. Even [the Mughal emperor] Babur marveled at the lack of hygiene when he arrived here centuries ago!" Through appeals to contagion both past and present, Maza's franchises galvanized an ethic of standardization to forestall public disorder and added another connective layer linking food, bodies, and risk. Like the Shiv Sena, corporatization was the ideal, and food's bare materials would be the ideal's vehicle.

In contrast to the Shiv Sena, however, Maza had to reconcile a different arrangement of objects and environments. To standardize a street food, Mr. Anand said, one can't simply operate on a vision of pure sterility, because the dangerous microbes that cause food-borne illness also are the crux of tasty street food. In the home, he said, microbes multiply in food but not enough to make you sick. By contrast, the street posed a more serious problem, "because bacteria multiply more there." Indians are well aware of this and can taste it: "With street food, even if it's vegetarian, those bacteria give the food a taste of non-veg, a taste that no chef can give." The challenge, then, is to corral the disorder of the infectious streets without sacrificing taste. He felt that Maza was unique among vada pav enterprises in accomplishing this feat: "That non-veg taste in the food, that's the taste of risk. We market that. We give the street taste, without the danger." In this rendering, the threat of nonvegetarian food was as profitable as it was problematic.[13] Microbes were the problem and solution to making risk profitable.[14]

"Even some political parties have become interested in vada pav," Mr. Anand said, to emphasize the craze around the food. As he changed the subject to discuss the machinery they used to process potatoes, I had attended the Shiv vada pav event in Shivaji Park. He sighed. "It's been a challenge, a controversy," he said. "We are avoiding certain parts of the city and are moving to the interior [of Maharashtra]. Basically, we're staying away [from the Shiv Sena]." Maza's troubles suggested that there were limits to the corporate interests in the vada pav that the Shiv Sena was willing to engage. Maza did not meet the minimum standards of name recognition and media magnetism in the ways McDonald's did. In order to stay out of the Shiv Sena's way but still grow business, Maza focused on "new markets" as yet untouched by Shiv vada pav, such as small towns in the interior of Maharashtra. Maza signaled their nationalist stance by choosing colors indicative of both the Indian flag and their company's guiding philosophy: red for *garam* (hot/freshly fried); green for *mirchi* (spicy); and white for clean.

Like the Shiv vada pav, Maza hyped its product through the virtues of standardization and transnational tie-ups. Maza linked up with a multinational food processing company, headquartered in Illinois, that operates an Indian subsidiary that processes and freezes chicken and vegetable products for Indian McDonald's outlets. Now this same food-processing outfit processes Maza's vadas. "We're like McDonald's in the 1970s—small and family-owned," Mr. Anand said, even though that small scale created conflict with the Shiv Sena. He was proud that Maza was the only small company in India to use such a globally standardized production process. He felt assured of the company's success because "in India, everything becomes an imitation of the West. Malls, restaurants—everything gets copied." Maza sat at the crossroads of vernacular indulgence and standardized, "copied" versions of transnational consumer outlets that were an increasingly integral part of consumer desire.

Mr. Anand left to take a phone call, and Parth took me into an office cubicle to show me a DVD recording of Maza's production process. In a dark warehouse, men and women in green rubber suits and galoshes hosed down open crates of potatoes. They tumbled the crates of potatoes into a mechanical peeler, which carried the peeled potatoes to another machine that steamed, boiled, and cubed the potatoes. The cubes rattled along a conveyor belt, under the watchful eye of men standing on either side of the belt who pick out "the bad bits" for quality control. The "quality" cubes fell into industrial-sized mixers, and a woman poured in a cauldron of spice paste. After the mixture cohered, she transferred it to a die-cutting machine that punched the mash into uniform disks, six at a time. The disks moved onto another conveyor belt, received a wash of *besan* (chickpea flour) batter squirted out of hoses, and the excess dripped through a grate. The coated vadas then entered a vat of hot oil for a four-second "par-fry" process. After another quality check, they moved into a box to be cold-blasted (an element of the individual quick-freeze food preservation process). More workers counted out the quick-frozen vadas into plastic bags, counted the bags into cartons, and moved the cartons into a cold room. The cartons would be shipped to Maza stores, where employees would reheat the vadas and dress the pav with chutneys. The five-minute video featured the vada pav as an object that was the product of other objects, in an arc stretching from potatoes to profit.

Maza made standardized corporate perfection a virtue discernible only through taste, but like the Shiv Sena, the company could not subtract the lived materialities of the streetscape from their political calculus. The street was dangerous but also tasty, and only standardized mechanization could capture that taste and its opportune qualities while sanitizing its corresponding risks. Yet as Shiv vada pav sellers Mahesh and Nitin both explained, this kind of standard seemed anathema to real vada pav. Dhruv felt similarly of corporatized vada pav: "It's not *real* vada pav," he said of products like Maza's. "The chaos of the street, the individualized taste of each vendor, *that's* vada pav. *That's* street food. You can't make it uniform everywhere." Even though all of these vendors worked through modes of standardization in their own right, the Shiv vada pav still was held to be closer to the street than Maza's version. Maza was seen as a force of object uniformity, and uniformity was risky in matters of taste. Uniformity everywhere, though, was exactly what Maza pursued. Their version of vada pav sanitized the local in order to make it marketable. The imagination of a standardized city, from this perspective, entailed a city of consumers who redirected their choice of vada pav from the street to the storefront. Maza needed only to reverse-engineer the matter of the street to successfully infuse the food with virtue.

## Prescribing Alternatives

Alongside these concatenations of the vada pav, concerns about metabolic disease suggested other interventions. News articles cited nutritionists and mothers concerned that children were drawn to vada pav. Nutritionists suggested that in order to avert this desire in children, a mother must ensure that "On all the five school days, each meal should be different." She should "grate vegetables, soya granules, or even paneer in the chapati dough to ensure at least one [of the child's] meals is nutritious" and acknowledge that because "children love snacking," she should "habituate [her] child to eat fruits." Drawing children away from vada pav could cultivate a habit that would benefit them later in life: "If a child makes healthy eating choices in childhood, chances are that he/she will make similarly wise choices in adolescence and adulthood," the article asserted (see Pandya 2010).

Perhaps it was easier to change children's habits than those of adults, as I did not witness any aversion to vada pav among adult patients in the many nutritional consultations I observed in a Bandra metabolic disorders clinic. This thoroughly disturbed Rashmi, one of the nutritionists I shadowed, who had a particular distaste for the food that I discovered one evening when a man diagnosed as diabetic and overweight came into the consultation room. A labor migrant from Chennai, he had come to Mumbai to work on transport ships. As he unloaded papers and pills onto the table, he expressed his primary complaint to Rashmi: "My pills aren't good ones," he said in Hindi. Rashmi asked him to recount a detailed list of what he ate on a typical day. He began with breakfast: two vada pav. Rashmi recoiled. "Never, never eat vada pav," she said with vocal emphasis on the "never" (*kabhi nahin*). She wrote this down in Hindi on a prescription pad, adding that he should eat more salad instead. Weight loss was his primary goal, she explained, and vada pav was not a wise route toward that goal. With her head down and double-underlining her proscriptions against vada pav, Rashmi didn't see his smirk.

In the clinic, I often witnessed dietitians proscribe the vada pav and prescribe an alternative snack. Most patients clearly understood that as a fried food, vada pav wasn't the healthiest choice. Yet it was such a regular part of diets that omitting it meant omitting an element of one's daily rhythm, as a patient in her midthirties explained on another visit. The woman, who had polycystic ovarian disorder (PCOD) and had gained a significant amount of weight, assured Rashmi that she ate *ghar ka khana* (home food) for dinner but got hunger pangs around 5 PM and "felt called" to eat vada pav. Rashmi suggested eating oats for breakfast to help stabilize her blood sugar and quell potential afternoon hunger pangs. "Oats? Yuck! Never!" the woman protested. Rashmi tried a different tack: "During teatime at home, you can eat dry snacks, nothing with oil—try puffed rice." The woman put a hand over her mouth, stifling a laugh. "What about my vada pav?" she asked. Rashmi replied that vada pav was out of the question. "I'm going to die with this diet," the woman said. "I can't believe I have to do this. You have no idea." Rashmi seemed duly annoyed: "I'm not asking you to starve," she said to the woman. "You just need to learn how to compensate." To balance, or "compensate," as Rashmi called it, entailed careful thought about the vada pav's ingredients and their relative demerits compared with potentially "healthier" choices. These choices needed to derive primarily from foods eaten in the home in order to truly avoid harm.

The impossibility of eating only home-cooked foods in lieu of vada pav prompted several middle-ground options. One day, I noticed a giant sign out front of my neighborhood bakery: "Try Baked Vada Pav! Healthy!" I entered the bakery and purchased one; at fifteen rupees, it was twice to three times the price of vada pav from the street. It was spicy but bone dry—unsurprising considering it had been baked hours before. The *pav* was whole wheat, the bakery attendant told me. A "healthier" one, he said.[15] A different solution was to eradicate the vada pav entirely, a tactic some schools pursued by calling in nutritionists to revamp lunch menus. In these schools, the vada pav and other fried items disappeared completely, replaced instead by dal and fresh fruit. The convent school in Manuli attempted this approach and even conducted nutrition training sessions for students and teachers. Months later, when I asked my neighbors if their children had stopped eating vada pav after the intervention, they reported that the kids simply walked outside the school at lunchtime and happily availed themselves of the vada pav sold across the street. Doctors I interviewed were disturbed by such disobedience. At one medical conference I attended, a physician showed a giant photo of the vada pav in his Power-Point presentation and fumed for ten minutes about "burger culture" stripping city residents of their life potential. In the hands of public health authorities, the vada pav was as contagious as Maza made it out to be but spread the ills of a fat stomach instead of an upset one.

More than an indulgence or a snack, the vada pav also was a quantifiable item for public health authorities: more about numbers than about taste. To think and speak of the vada pav in terms of "health" meant thinking and speaking in terms of calories and fat grams. Through statistics and standards, public health officials isolated an association between a single food and a burgeoning epidemic by taking a different approach to vada pav's contagious character. Choice would be the intersecting point between doctors concerned about obesity, Shiv Sena Party leaders, and start-up companies like Maza. Each had different ends in sight for the food and the kind of profit it could bring, but the means converged on similar terms: a political agency that was, as political theorist Chad Lavin (2009) writes of contemporary food politics, "all but unthinkable except in the terms of consumerism" (57). Like those of the Shiv Sena and Maza, public health renderings of vada pav also engaged the question of violence but bracketed the link between violence and the city in favor of the violence done to the body through obesity. Commercial expertise couldn't erase that violence; the only way to expel it was to introduce biomedical authority to expel contagion from the city.

## Political Ripples

Over time, infighting beleaguered the longevity of the Shiv vada pav. In 2011, a son of a state minister began his own "Chhatrapati vada pav" outlets to compete with the Shiv Sena's Shiv vada pav. Reporting on this development, one journalist commented: "I believe there might be many others out there like me who prefer their food without any political colour" (Anandan 2011). A limit seemed to be in play; people wanted just the food without its "colour." During a visit to Mumbai in the summer of 2012, I was curious to see how the vendors I knew had fared amid these political concatenations. I walked past Nitin's vada pav stall, just a block from Shivaji Park, and he was nowhere to be found; his Shiv vada pav stall had turned into "Mumbai vada pav" according to the new sign. (A friend explained to me that he never made much money from the Shiv vada pav enterprise and sold it off). I walked further into the heart of Dadar and toward the corner where Alok kept his cart. Mahesh was there, doling out vada pav during the afternoon rush hour. He never started his own Shiv vada pav cart after all. He had married and was starting a catering business. Alok, his father, was quite ill, and Mahesh needed extra money to pay the hospital bills. "Business is stable, but everyone's struggling," he said. "Thankfully, Dad built up the business for so long, so everyone knows him and comes here." I also spoke with Parth, from Maza, and learned that Maza had expanded to 150 outlets across the country. When I asked about the rise and fall of the Shiv vada pav, he politely noted that Maza "was not in the business of competing—we're in the business of meeting demand." Maza, he said, wanted to bring the taste of Mumbai to the rest of India and was now expanding its stores to Chennai, Hyderabad, and Bangalore. Maza's success hinged on baking the taste of Mumbai's streets into a vada pav that could transcend the city itself—all the taste, sheathed in plastic to protect it from vernacular squabbles as it wound its way from factories to stalls on streets of different cities.

In his expansive monograph, *The History and Social Influence of the Potato*, first published in 1949, Radcliffe Salaman follows the political ripples of the potato across temporal and geographic expanses ranging from pre-Columbian Mexico to World War II–era England. Salaman (1985) describes the unimaginably colorful pathway of such a humble vegetable: "It was not to be expected that officials or laymen realized that in urging the use of the potato they were calling into action an instrument charged with dynamic possibilities" (xxxiii). I have detailed such calls into action through an exploration of the differential gastropolitics of the vada pav. The critical signs of the vada pav cart, the street food vendor, and the food itself each underwent transformation—whether enrobed in plastic or doled out by hand, whether spiced aggressively for a favorite customer or seasoned uniformly for the standard consumer. So too did relations between persons, taste, and risk realign, each time expanding the scope of gastropolitics, from Alok's cart to newer iterations such as Maza's storefronts and the Shiv vada pav recipe. Different economies of gastropolitics crystallized different object entanglements: more peaceful or more profitable, more freshly fried or more reheated from deep freeze. The instability of the vada pav emerged out of power channels created within municipal mechanisms of governance (in the case of street-side food vendors who must be approved by the city government), and outside of those mechanisms (in the case of the Shiv Sena's or private companies' branding of the vada pav). Sometimes the food materialized urban authenticity, while in other moments it magnetized corporatism. Across the enactments of the food, absorptive overlaps between persons and the environments of Mumbai's streets held events and objects together.

I have attempted here to foreground the material contingencies of fried food by backgrounding the eater and to show how the case of street food can open up metabolic living to historical-political dynamics borne out in human relations. In the controversies over the vada pav, we see that urban charisma is corporeal, concrete, and contextual as much as it is mythical. Urban charisma bleeds through food, the body, and the city; in fact, in many circumstances it bleeds the very distinction between them. The meanings of food to the city—indeed, how food can materialize as the city's lifeline—are vibrant even when the act of consumption is not made primary, either by informants or by the ethnographer. These meanings illustrate the kinds of value that food can have within, outside, and at the margins of medicalization. They underscore the power of porosity between cities and bodies as food changes hands, and they raise the question of what it means to be fed by another.

Despite the amount of dieting I encountered in Manuli, far more people relied heavily on the support of social services to sustain the bare minimum of daily nutrition. When Mary had some schedule conflicts for our interviews, she suggested that I accompany Leo, another member of the church's social service outreach program, as he did his rounds. Leo was in charge of direct disbursement of money and food to some of the neighborhood's poorest families. A retired bank teller, Leo said that the money the church offered wasn't much but it helped people buy food to stay on their feet. Most of the recipients worked intermittently and had no security net. He quickly looked over paper-clipped bundles of hundred-rupee notes, and we set off down the lanes of the neighborhood. His normal routine was to distribute the money and then to walk the beneficiaries to the ration shop to buy food to ensure the donation went to its intended purpose.

The first house we arrived at was an old shack, sparkling clean on the inside with one small room for living and one curtained-off area for cooking. A very old woman lay on a mattress in the middle of the floor. The old woman's daughter, herself "around 60," she said, showed Leo the newest list of prescriptions the doctors told her to get for her mother, who was diabetic. I recognized the older woman from the neighborhood—I often saw her wandering around during the day, looking lost. "She's very confused," her daughter admitted. "She'll walk away when I'm not watching."

Leo offered the daughter a small packet of cash, and she thanked him. She insisted that we pray. She recited her Hail Marys and Our Fathers in Marathi; Leo said his in English. I stayed quiet. She opened her eyes at the end of the prayer, looked at me, and added, "Mother Mary, bless this one too," repeating my name into the roster of those to bless and protect. Finished, she and Leo laughed at the oddity of a foreigner tagging along on charity rounds. As we walked on toward the next home in what would be six visits that day, Leo said to me that it wasn't just the money that kept the families fed. "It's the joking, too," he said. "It's the feeling that they're not alone in the world." To Leo, the government's programs to provide minimal rations were a start, but hungry families still needed supplementary support, in terms of finance but also in terms of companionship. The worst thing was not just to be hungry but to be hungry and alone. The ration card could provide only so much accompaniment.

In the middle of the monsoon season, my regular home visits in Manuli with Mary for her social work took on an added urgency. The municipal government had shifted the ration shop for Manuli's residents even farther away from the neighborhood. This would force the elderly and infirm to travel an extra distance, which Mary assured me was unacceptable. Specifically, they would have to cross Hill Road—where vehicles and rickshaws careened toward the seafront road at high speeds. Mary wanted to have a meeting with Manuli's corporator (municipal ward representative) to discuss the issue. "If he won't budge on this," she said, "we'll threaten him with a *morcha* (protest march)." The ration shop foods were bad enough, she said—worms and stones littered the dal and rice was measured out from bulk containers. To make residents go farther from home for it was cause for protest. The problem was further complicated by the bureaucratic maze of the city's public distribution system (PDS) of ration foods. Even though some of Manuli's residents had faithfully gone to the "new," more distant ration shop for their food, according to Mary the shopkeeper refused to give them food because they were not on his list of recipients. They had ration cards and held them in their hands, but there was no record as far as he was concerned from his side of the counter. "We need to talk about why people are being harassed for the food that the government owes them," Mary said forcefully. She wanted to air her ideas at a meeting of the *mahila mandal* (community women's group) in order to get suggestions and feedback before she met with the corporator.

After a morning of household interviews, we headed to Trinity Hospital, just a few blocks away. In a satellite building opposite the main ward, the hospital had set up a community health center that shared meeting space with the *mahila mandal*. We were met at the door by a nun, Sister Eileen, who ran the community center. Mary explained to her the problem with the ration shops. "Ah, they're making us dance," Sister Eileen sighed. She led us into the main meeting room, where we joined a group of women already assembled into a circle. Health education materials were scattered on the room's tables, evidence of an earlier politics of health that morning. This current meeting had just begun. The guest speaker was a well-heeled woman named Paramita who ran a city-based NGO that worked on government accountability. She was visiting the group that day to educate them about the Right to Information Act (RTI), a 2005 law passed by the national government that gave citizens access to publicly available information. Paramita gave the group a general introduction to RTI. "Who is the government for?" she asked. "For us!" chanted the group. Paramita clapped her hands at what she seemed to read as enthusiasm. "Yes, the government is for everyone," she repeated, and the RTI "keeps government accountable."

She asked if any of the women wanted to share an appeal for information so she could help them streamline their complaints. A tall, thin woman in a purple sari stood up. "My husband is dead, but someone furnished a ration card with his name on it," she said. The ration card is a form of identification acceptable to many utility companies, and this faked card had been used to set up an account with the electricity company. The woman was now receiving electric bills for an account in her dead husband's name and had no idea how the forgery had happened or where the pilfering was happening. Mary, the next to share, explained to the group what had happened with the reassignment of Manuli's ration shop. "You should complain," Paramita said immediately, and launched into a mini-lecture on complaints. "Complaints are the way that things get done," she assured the group. But she cautioned the women against simply phoning the government office responsible for their specific problems, because there would be no paper trail. Instead, she explained, "you complain in writing to make a record."

With Mary's case as an example, she took out a piece of blank paper and showed the group step by step how Mary should approach the corporator about the issue. Mary had to write the address of the old ration shop and the address of the new one. She had to write the complaint like a formal government memo. The most important element of the complaint, Paramita said, was a deadline for action. "You set the date," she told Mary, "not them." From matters of hunger and government corruption sprang another world of paperwork and bureaucracy. While Mary had pondered a protest earlier that morning, after the afternoon's information session about RTI, she thought that Paramita had a good point. "We need to complain," Mary said to me as we walked home, "but we need to do it right." She asked me to type and print out the letter the *mahila mandal* drafted, and we would take it around the neighborhood for signatures:

> To: Ration Officer
> S. V. Road
> Bandra (W)
> Mumbai 400 050
> Sub: Complaint regarding transfer of ration shop from Ranwar to Perry Cross Road.
>
> Dear Sir,
>
> We wish to bring to your kind attention that about 25 to 30 people are not able to draw their ration from the new shop at Perry Cross Road. We would request you to allow them to draw their ration from the old shop at Ranwar. Please take action within the next 4 days and oblige.

Beginning early the next morning, we took the complaint letter from house to house, hoping for at least fifty households to sign in agreement. At each stop, Mary explained the situation and had to exert little effort to make her case: everyone was generally in agreement that their entitlements were moving farther away in terms of both real and imagined distances. This continued for over a week. We also went to both the old and "new" assigned ration shops for Manuli—small storefronts with samples of the different dal and rice varieties on display with their matching prices. The storefronts extended deep into miniwarehouses filled with sacks of goods. At each shop, Mary explained her plans to speak to the corporator and how she was filing a complaint. The men running both shops dismissed her. No comments. When the document had the requisite number of signatures, we headed to the area ration office, which sits in a heritage building on a main road. Next to the office, a makeshift warehouse had been set up to paint giant *murtis* of Ganesha in preparation for the upcoming *Ganesh Chaturthi* holiday. Inside the office, old wooden desks lined the perimeter of half the spacious one-roomed building, and the other half was packed floor to ceiling with record books. The desks were empty, except for one attendant, who politely accepted Mary's complaint but explained that he was too low in rank to handle it. She needed to come back again to find the proper person in charge. Ceiling fans blew flakes of weathered paper records from the books into our faces as we turned and walked out. Mary was too frustrated to speak. It would take multiple additional visits before someone formally accepted Mary's complaint about the ration system. Long after her meeting with the corporator, the issue remained unresolved around this measure of allotted eating: a paper booklet that evidenced diet and could disintegrate depending on how the winds blew.

In the June 2012 issue of *World Nutrition*, an editorial appeared that began with a simple Q&A:

Q. What drives global obesity?
A. This is obvious.

The editorial asserted that global obesity is already in front of our faces with bodies that have grown too fat and that we have overlooked the most obvious cause of mass metabolic disruption: food processing. The editorial quoted Brazilian obesity researcher Dr. Carlos Monteiro, who argued that food processing was a pivotal but as yet unexamined part of the global obesity story, especially in obesity's new hot spots, such as India. "The big issue is food processing," Monteiro said. "Or, to be more precise, the nature, extent and purpose of processing, and what happens to food and to us as a result of processing."[1]

Dr. Monteiro's quote struck me as an ethnographic challenge as much as a public health stance. It was an object analysis insofar as it isolated the object of processed foods as an agent of blame. His statement demanded an understanding of processing in everyday terms ("the obvious") and of the broader contexts governing food's ability to change as a result ("what happens to food"). The challenge was to do so in relational terms, because processing connected food and persons. It is common sense that one would never let a stranger into the kitchen, a space that is a place of purity in many Indian homes. But processed foods are the handiwork of many strangers: machines, marketers, corporate workers. The work of changing food entails work to make the food of strangers familiar.

"Food processing" calls forth an apparatus of industry focused on changing discernible ingredients and of distilling contaminants from a pure product. Processing also can be understood as a mode of value transformation, as raw elements become food through craft and industrial food sciences (Paxson 2013; Paxson and Helmreich 2014; Weiss 2012). I define "processing" in this light: it is a transformation that imparts value. In this chapter I examine such transformations as a powerful form of connective permeability. The power to tinker with food is the power to play with absorptive capacities on two fronts: first, in terms of what substances stay in and out of food; second, in terms of how people bring in or deter food in living spaces such as the market and the home. I open up Dr. Monteiro's statement into a question about metabolic living: What happens to food *and* what happens to us in the process of processing?

Quality Control

A food-processing story: Many of the *koli* (fisher) women who sold fish on Manuli's streets directly pursued possible customers with a hail.[2] There were several types, depending on the mode of selling. Some women moved through the neighborhood and its surrounds, singing their wares in the courtyard of apartment buildings and announcing the specific fish available that day. A housewife or a maid would come down the stairs and pay for fish for that day's lunch or dinner. Many of the *koli* women had regular customers in specific buildings, and so they themselves would climb the stairs and deliver the goods. They walk with baskets on their heads, and in the baskets there are often sharp knives. At vestibules of apartment buildings or in stairwells, they hack away at fish, turning whole fish into fillets or leaving the fish intact but scaling and gutting it so that it's ready to cook as a whole piece of food. This was the constant work of turning something into something eatable. It is very human and very taxing work. And it raises the question, prior to asking about what processing *does*, of how processing *fits* into ecologies of food supply.

Other *koli* women did less ambulatory work and situated their sales on the street. They anchored the several places on Manuli's main street where one could buy fish. This was where I sourced my fish, because I struck up a relationship with Surekha, one of the sellers. Surekha's supply wasn't particularly different from many of the others on the street; it was more the case that early on, I succumbed to her hails. Further, she was the first seller on the street when approached from the direction of my building, meaning that if I didn't buy from her, she'd know it because I had to walk past her. Surekha tolerated my questions about how to cook different fish. She also told me that she was diabetic when she learned about why I was in Mumbai and affirmed that many of the other *koli* women were diabetic. Surekha pointed out that Manuli's market women fulfilled the stereotype: they were supposed to be fat, jolly, and wear lots of gold. I could not easily parse this. Through Surekha I interviewed other fish sellers on the street and came up with the same diet: fish, vegetables, and rice. And they were climbing those stairs every day, and if not anymore, they had for years before. Weight and illness nonetheless appeared, despite what in many circumstances would be considered heavy physical activity.

I sat with Surekha on several occasions to observe the actual work it took for her to make a sale. Here, processing made for profit. The sale often started with the hail, best done as a targeted yell at a passerby. One morning evinced a typical interchange that began with Surekha's call: "Hey, *bhai* (brother)! Hey! *Arrey bhai!*" A man looked out of the corner of his eye, and Surekha caught him. He approached and examined the *surmai*—kingfish (which is "good for the brain," my research assistant, Mary, said). He asked for several fish; Surekha priced the group at 800 rupees. "It's 600 everywhere else," he said. I glanced around, noting that *everywhere else* was only meters away—there were at least five women on the street selling fish, all within line of sight. The man left. Five minutes later, he walked by again, glared; another ten minutes passed, and he walked by yet again. Surekha pointed at Mary and then at the man, who had stopped to buy bananas a hundred meters away. Mary pursued the indecisive customer but returned alone, shaking her head—he was uninterested. Surekha waved her hand— "If you're not serious about it, why bother?" she asked. She continued to gut fish, spilling entrails into a bucket. A yellow tabby cat popped its head out underneath the folds of her sari, licking its whiskers with the bucket in view. The *fayda* (payoff, point) of being serious was that someone got food to feed another person. And people were picky—about price, like the man who never sealed the deal, and about specific features of the fish, like a woman who arrived after him and fixed her gaze upon tuna fillets. "*Pink, pink, very good!*" Surekha announced to her in English, perhaps cued to it by the more formal businesslike dress the woman wore in contrast to a housecoat. The woman responded in Hindi. "I want a red one," she said softly (*lalwalla chahti hoon*). Surekha yelled at her that red fish are "not real" (*assal nahin*) and that the pink ones on the table were the right color. Vibrant red fillets meant that something extra had been added—a dye made from chili powder, perhaps. Surekha processed fish into fillets into money. One might question her prices but to question her quality meant the deal was not destined for completion.

Surekha's space in the market was located at the front of her house. She set up a large board on several upturned buckets and sat on the threshold of her front door. Many of the fish on her board came from the Colaba fish market, at the other end of the city. These had been previously frozen. Some, she would tell me, came from fishers in Manuli—from the men who push boats off the shore or a seawall into the water at specific tide-related times. They catch fish through trawlers or through purple nets, called "disco nets," that off the boat, men would darn in the afternoon lulls. After a morning catch, the beach transforms into another market, one that directs fish to several of the city's fish markets beyond the one in Manuli, including the major ones at Sassoon Docks and Khar Fish Market. Leftovers would go to the men to feed families or to give to wives to sell throughout the neighborhood or even to sell to other women—thus the "local" fish on Surekha's board.

A hollowed-out boat anchors the scene. There is a man with a scale who holds court. Men transfer the contents, baskets of lobsters or fish or prawns, into a main basket. The scale is counterbalanced to 100 grams. Seafood is added or subtracted to determine the gram weight. For a lobster, if it's more than 100 grams, the scale master tosses the basket to a sorter, who has three baskets of his own. Each corresponds to a category. For lobsters, this sorting is done for export purposes—and after the sorting here on the beach in Manuli, a truck loaded with lobsters will go to a company on the city's outskirts where they will be boiled and then weighed again, bound for an airplane. Most go to New Zealand or Singapore. Categories determine cash. Payment to the many men involved in this one operation is 500 rupees per kilogram for Category One, 300 rupees per kilogram for Category Two, and 200 rupees per kilogram for Category Three. What doesn't make it into the baskets for quality control, determined here by weight, makes its way into circulation in the neighborhood. "Process" here is an arc stretching from the sea to the hands of a fisher to the scale to an IOU-like receipt that a fisher can collect payment on at a later time.

Uninvited Guests

In Manuli, processed foods were indeed a common concern but not necessarily because of concerns about metabolic illness. In my interviews, the most common reason cited for using processed foods was to avoid food adulteration. "Health," in specifically biomedical terms, was rarely the reason given at first for buying packaged foods, which are necessarily more expensive than their bulk, "loose" counterparts. Certainly, despite the discursive intermingling of concerns about metabolic disease and acts of food adulteration, the two had little in the way of a close, causal relationship. Adulterated foods do not cause weight gain or insulin resistance any more or less than other foods, nor did anyone perceive them to do so. Processed foods did have ambivalent properties in the eyes of both public health authorities and those who bought them. Because many processed foods were snacks, they were often derided for being unhealthy and causing weight gain. Yet their aseptic packaging offered a "clean" alternative to potentially adulterated food. Concerns around metabolic disease generated an additional possibility: an opportunity for food companies to develop foods called "functional foods." Yogurts with "probiotic" enhancements for good digestion, breads with extra fiber, and cereals with antioxidants are all examples of functional foods gaining traction in Indian grocery stores.[3] These were foods specially engineered and fortified with nutrients with the explicit function of addressing weight gain, cholesterol levels, and blood sugars. Functional versions of staples such as rice and wheat could take on "extra" benefits and impart them to make the eater fuller, longer.

These two forms of foods, adulterated and functional, can both be understood as the result of processing. Both raise questions about what it means to be fed by a stranger. The two forms of processing share two features that I discuss throughout this chapter. The first is a bleeding of the boundary of food and drugs, a phenomenon discussed in depth by several medical anthropologists working on both Ayurveda and biomedicine in South Asia. The second is the porosity of the home, a permeable domesticity. These features operate in very mundane terms, but they also are highly productive about claims of metabolic disease. Absorptions between foods and drugs allow adulterated foods into the home but also enable food companies to create new foods to address metabolic illness. Here, the drug substantiates disease states, a phenomenon documented in depth in Joseph Dumit's work (2012) on pharmaceuticals. The permeability of the home allows adulterated foods inside, but this porosity also allows the cultural figure of the housewife to travel widely to food companies who must process her in order to create "healthy" foods that she will feed her family.

Through elemental and spatial traffic, the sciences and sites of processing are also sciences and sites of metabolic living, as people struggle and make do with a food supply that everyone knows is tainted and demands vigilance. Persons working in food companies that engineer "healthier" foods do the work of determination and discernment, too. They create moral visions of middle-class subjects who can address the risk of metabolic disease by eating processed foods with added benefits— much like following a drug prescription. Processing is a moral and material formation in this light and operates both within and outside the reaches of legality and medicalization. An anthropology of processing can contextualize the vectors of risk, harm, regulation, and benefit that permeate and animate such moral materials, and can elucidate their scope.

Empirically speaking, divisions between inside and outside the home structured nearly every conversation about food and eating I had during the course of my research. For instance, eating at home was often presented as natural and healthy in opposition to the dangers of eating "outside." This was so because of the possibility of food adulteration and because "outside" food couldn't match the nutritive qualities of home-cooked food. To situate these questions in an anthropological analytic concerned with the cultural logics of inside and outside, one approach might be to imagine food packaging as the fulcrum between the outside domain of the strange and unclean countered against the inside familiarity of kin and domestic order. There is certainly a vernacular rationale behind this line of thinking. Inside/outside oppositions have been fundamental to scholarship in South Asian studies, from Ravindra Khare's study (1976) of the Hindu home to E. Valentine Daniel's exploration (1984) of the fluid boundaries of the Tamil house to Partha Chatterjee's examination of the gendered spaces of the material, masculine, worldly *bahir* (outside) and the spiritual, feminine, familiar *ghar* (home, inside) in nineteenth-century Bengal. Works by Dipesh Chakrabarty (1991) on garbage and Jim Masselos (2000) on living spaces in Mumbai further explore how connections between the home and the street constitute a politics of habitation integral to South Asian expressions of belonging and citizenship. The transgressions of these spaces are as culturally productive as they are problematic. For example, Sara Dickey's study of relationships between middle-class housewives and their domestic servants in Madurai shows how the permeability of the home helps employers produce class boundaries.[4] Further, the spatial mapping of inside and outside relates directly to food production and consumption in India, in terms of a common semiotic opposition between "outside" food (*bahar ka khana*) and "home" food (*ghar ka khana*; see also Valentine 1999). Jonathan Shapiro Anjaria (2009) describes this dichotomy in his research on civic activism in Mumbai: "Where 'home food' signifies food that is pure and controlled, 'outside food' signifies danger and the possibility of ritual pollution" (396). Anjaria's work on hawking adds an additional analytic layer in terms of how consuming food outside the home raises questions about what it means to eat in public. Collectively, these studies also echo a long twentieth-century anthropological concern with commensality as a means to understand social tensions and compromises, especially regarding forms of kinship that constitute and transgress the space of the home in South Asia.

If a common concern in these studies has been about who is allowed in the kitchen and how kitchens and eating extend into other lived spaces, my interest is in how entities make their way into kitchens even when they are not invited—what they attach to and how. It strikes me that invitations are important to understanding metabolic living as a representational and material political formation in Mumbai (on the cultural politics and ethnographic history of hospitality, see Candea and da Col 2012). Because of the porosity of both homes and foods, controversies over processed food crystallized tenuous relations between the home and the market (however illicit). In this context, metabolic disease was as profitable as it was problematic. To address how processed foods scale up to a concrete metabolic threat, they must be taken seriously as open objects set in multiple, deeply gendered relations to the home and market. The claims that packaged food is bad for the body and that food companies are guilty of murder are both critiques about porosity in terms of food's constituent parts and the conditions under which those parts become embedded in homes and bodies. Adulteration entails putting the underworld inside. The entry of the corporation is at issue with functional foods.

The medical valences of food work unexpectedly in this context. As I have argued thus far, medicalization cannot be given all the credit here, as the realization of functional foods takes complex cultural work. Metabolic discourses overlay much of the earlier relations between processed food and sickness, whether in the case of more mundane cases of milk dilution or more exceptional cases of death by poisoning. Medicalization cannot fully explain the story of processed foods, because fatness is not uniformly medicalized in processed foods. Instead, what deserves attention are the critical dimensions of food generally overlooked in the causal jump from processed food to the effect of metabolic disease: the openness of food to the world, the thin lines between food and drugs, and how families, foods, and markets cross these lines.

The food-drug boundary blur is thoroughly gendered, because the primary point of intervention of processing is the home kitchen, a space crucial for the purity and health of the home and a space of women's household labor. There is much labor, done primarily by women, to filter out the worst parts of outside food, such as adulterated foods and to keep the family healthily fed. However, my aim is not to provide an ethnographic account of gendered domesticity that, in effect, confines women to the kitchen. Quite the contrary, I show how the kitchen and its key inhabitant—the cultural figure of the housewife—is relationally permeable. Women work through stances about specific food products in the market but also find themselves interrogated by food companies doing qualitative research inside the home to calibrate marketing techniques to a housewife's perceived wants and needs. Both real and imagined versions of the kitchen and housewife travel and influence decisions across the marketing boardroom, laboratories of new snack foods, and infrastructures of governmental regulation.[5] Neither kitchen nor housewife can be taken for granted as uniformly emplaced; both are multiply conjured and interrogated. My informants were primarily women who cooked for their own families and also had jobs cooking for others as domestic labor or as neighborhood caterers. The figure of the housewife extends to them, as well as to their employers (some who work in office jobs, some who do child care but not house cleaning or cooking). Channels of domestic relations build markets in several directions. Through these related spaces and persons, it becomes possible to better understand how the food-drug dynamic of processing makes the "obvious" site of metabolic disruption coterminous with gender- and class-specific modes of feeding.

Adulteration

Now a second story of processing: In April 2009, the advocacy organization Centre for Science and the Environment (CSE) tested multiple brands of *vanaspati* (vegetable shortening) for levels of trans fats.[6] CSE's lab results were "shocking," according to the *Navbharat Times* and other newspapers: several vanaspati brands had trans fat levels as high as 23 percent by volume, far above the 2 percent limit set by European standards. Because trans fats are cheap and shelf-stable, increasing their level in shortening allowed companies to "stretch" their products without visibly changing their taste or color. The *Navbharat Times* article (2009), headlined "Vanaspati ghee is the enemy of health," noted that setting precise Indian national standards for trans fats was locked up in the "red tape" (*lalfitashahi*) of Health Ministry bureaucratic machinations. At the time of the CSE study, the Indian government required companies only to acknowledge the presence of trans fats rather than to specify their exact levels. Sunita Narain, the director of CSE, explained that companies exploited this loophole. "If you consider what the Union Ministry of Health has issued in the name of labeling nutrition facts, you will know how our food is at risk," she said. "It literally allows companies to get away with anything—as long as it is on the label. This is just not acceptable. . . . This procrastination means that while there are no legal standards, companies are literally getting away with murder" (Sinha 2009). To acknowledge the porosity of food but not regulate it was the grounds of criminality.

I translated the *Navbharat Times* article about the trans fats controversy with my language tutor, Prof. Munir. After detailing how hydrogenation works, the article concluded that "the worst effect of trans fat is on the heart, because it reduces good cholesterol (HDL)." The effects of trans fat stretched beyond visceral body fat to influence risks of women's fertility, breast cancer, diabetes, circulatory system damage, and poor bodily development (*sharirik vikas*) for young people. Prof. Munir grew excited by Sunita Narain's accusations of companies "getting away with murder" by shirking regulations and infusing foods with unhealthy, unregulated ingredients that could be linked to metabolic disruption. Sitting on my couch, he tapped his fingers on the printout of the article. "We need this," he said of CSE's exposé. "We need people to be critical, because the poor are suffering at the hands of the multinationals." Prof. Munir acknowledged the dangers of trans fats in terms of health, but he also posed broader parameters of danger in which food absorbed harm and then passed it on to the absorptive body. He began a long lecture on the perils of food adulteration, beginning with loose foods like milk and dry goods measured out from a bulk batch. Loose food was the means and ends of everyday adulteration, he explained. Someone with just a little money can go to the store and ask for only five grams of ghee, which the store owner spoons into a small bag. Day-to-day living and spending matched perfectly with adulteration's logic. A store owner could stretch out his larger container of ghee with mashed potato but still keep the white color and soft texture. It was a more familiar form of the fleecing illustrated by the vanaspati scandal. From metabolic damage caused by one element (trans fat), he sketched out multiple possibilities for harm through absorption of food that was adulterated—*milawati*, "mixed, adulterated," or *naqli*, "fake."[7]

Tensions between real/fake and whole/mixed certainly governed what constituted adulterated food. But equally dynamic was the boundary between food and drug. Prof. Munir's use of the term "loose" for bulk food is an apt descriptor for this boundary's openness to elemental reconfiguration. In adulteration, processing rearranged the elements of foods to the eater's detriment by substituting dangerous elements for the expected. In the instance of functional food, processing adds to food's elemental ingredients in order to enhance the metabolism and impart health according to biomedical rationales.[8] Across these trajectories of processing, a tenuous boundary of materialities and morals makes food a site to experiment with and endure the limits of liveable permeability. How much can one be fed by another when the "other" in question is an assemblage like a food company? Processing governs matters of metabolic living, then, because it raises questions about what it takes and means to be fed by another in times of uncertain health. Processing puts emphasis on what a product can become and what it takes to get it there. This is in contrast to a focus on the product itself, on food already processed and "ready to eat"—a perspective that tilts too easily to claims of overconsumption for lack of attention to the work it takes to change and exchange food into something ready.

Prof. Munir loved stories of food adulteration, perhaps because they were vivid in ways that public health news stories (my usual homework assignments) simply were not. Many of the adulteration stories we read were horrifying but also sometimes comical, filled with cops and criminals fleeing the scene of the crime only to leave the evidence behind. It was the stuff of young city beat crime reporters, mixed with the narrative style of Hindi pulp fiction novels that fill the kiosks of Mumbai's train stations. Prof. Munir told me stories of fruits with added chemicals to speed their ripeness or milk that had soapy water added to it to make it whiter. The passive voice governed these claims: Prof. Munir never quite pinned blame on one agent. Instead, he narrated the soiling of foods as the handiwork of a shadowy network of perpetrators he called "the nexus," using the English word. The nexus, he explained, involved relations between corporations, the government, and local crime syndicates. The nexus was behind food adulteration, through and through, as well as nearly every other form of everyday corruption. Lawrence Cohen (2007), in writing about "the nexus" as it manifests as a publicly perceived link between homosexuality and India's urban crime syndicates, notes that "this figure of a nexus, ubiquitous in political reportage, suggests an affinity or attachment in which a civil institution is deformed by an underlying relation to criminalized interest" (106). For Prof. Munir, food adulteration scandals evidenced intensifying attachments between the home and the "criminalized interest" of the market, to deforming and disastrous ends. "Remember that everything is part of the nexus in this city," he warned me. "It's destroying the people of India."

Like Prof. Munir, public media also built links between concerns about metabolic disease and food adulteration. For instance, one newspaper article, "The Perils of Packaging," began with a declaration: "Due to our lifestyles, India has become a hub for many of the world's deadliest diseases, such as heart disease, hypertension and diabetes. To a large extent, the management or cure of these diseases depends on what we eat." The author of the article, a diabetic himself, decided to study the nutrition labels of several processed foods and contacted the manufacturers to discuss their labeling policies. He was largely ignored. "My take is that [food companies] aren't prepared or have chosen to ignore the health of their consumers until the law forces them to publish complete nutrition information," he concluded. A commenter on the online version of the article put this squarely in legal terms, opining that laws were weak, policymakers were corruptible, and the adulteration of foods should be punishable as a crime under the Indian Penal Code's section 307—Attempt to Murder. This was because adulteration "can finish or cripple the generations." The perils of packaging had generational effects, in this vision, and the generations needed protection from what was in their food.

In discussions about food adulteration in Manuli, my neighbors were insistent that the nexus reached into the home through adulteration's pernicious effects. This meant that someone inside the home needed to be responsible for managing the threats of adulteration—and that someone was most often the housewife. "I've just stopped eating grapes," my neighbor Sarita told me, because "the skins absorb pesticides." She told me this as the fruit wallah shouted his daily offerings from the main road into the alleyway, where we could hear him from her kitchen window. I found myself asking more and more frequently about food adulteration in household interviews as my time in the neighborhood passed, but sometimes without any prompting the topic pressed its way to the surface as the most concrete food-body connection. This was as true for food staples as it was for indulgences. Milk was at the center of many household discussions about how the nexus had tainted the building blocks of the Indian diet. For some individuals, packaged milk was doctor's orders, as I learned from interviews with nutritionists who often used milk to increase their clients' intake of protein so that they might feel fuller longer. One nutritionist admitted that branded, boxed milk might have more preservatives than fresh, loose, bagged milk, but she still "prescribed" it to patients. "You have a choice between the devil and the deep blue sea," she said in reference to the choice between adulteration and preservatives, but preservatives won out in her view. This illustrated an additional dimension to adulterated milk; namely, that there was a certain expectation that milk would be adulterated if you didn't buy it in boxes. One neighbor told me simply, "You should *expect* your *dudhwala* (milkman) to water the milk."[9]

There was loyalty involved at many scales. A friend from the neighborhood yoga club, Jyoti, told me that for years she had bought bagged milk but recently observed that it was "too watery." "Those men put the water in the milk," said Jyoti—the nexus again. Her sister, bedridden with cancer, had doctor's orders to drink milk every morning to restore her strength. Jyoti told her sister, "Don't drink that milk, it won't do anything for you." She and her sister asked their servant, Manu, to find a new milkman. Manu managed the daily food purchases and cooking. Jyoti often had me over for meals, and I had a decent relationship with Manu because Jyoti often left me in the kitchen with him under the pretense of me learning to cook "traditional" food by watching him carefully.[10] I spoke with Manu about the change. His and Jyoti's accounts converged: Manu protested the idea of a new milkman because he and the current milkman were friends ("They have adventures together," Jyoti would say). To change the house's milk supply was tantamount to a betrayal of the relationship and the company they kept. Jyoti acknowledged the personal relationship but pleaded with Manu to take the business element out of it: "The milkman is *cheating* us," she begged him. She reminded Manu of the details of processing that everyone knew: how the milkman took the old milk bags, cut a slit at the top, and put in contaminated water. As the milkman stretched his product and profit, he shortened her sister's life—not the kind of drugging her sick sister needed. Manu ultimately carried out Jyoti's wishes and began buying Amul brand boxed milk for the home, something I noticed during a subsequent cooking lesson. Manu and the old milkman let business be business and, according to Jyoti, still ran about the neighborhood together.

## Readiness

Hydraulics of loyalty and betrayal, like those Jyoti detailed, structured most of my discussions about adulteration. It took work to manage adulterated food as one of many streams of food coming into the home. One morning, Mary led me down Manuli's waterfront to a row of concrete, seafacing hutments. The pathway was dirt but later that year would be paved with concrete because of Mary's protests to the municipal government. At the time, though, it had just rained, and puddles crowded out dry spots for the neighborhood dogs to rest. I waited in a clearing on the beach by the communal latrine. She walked down an alley, and a few minutes later returned with Almas, who in her midtwenties was pursuing a career in fashion that she hoped would take her abroad. Her mother didn't approve of her choice of "lifestyle," and so Almas preferred that we conduct the interview in the open rather than inside her home. Almas said she was used to speaking to foreigners given her work in the fashion industry, but since Almas and I were similar in age, Mary thought it prudent to "chaperone" us lest rumors arise from anyone who saw us on the beach. Almas had enough trouble at home, Mary said, and being seen alone with a foreign man in a public place wouldn't help things.

Almas grew up in Manuli, in the same home she lives in now. Her family of Gujarati Muslims was one of the only Muslim families in the neighborhood in her youth, although that changed with the influx of more Muslims into Manuli during the 1990s. Growing up, she was "addicted" to *Baywatch*, which she watched on a neighbor's television. She was convinced she wanted to be a professional diver. She quickly learned "there's none of that in India," and so she set her mind on fashion. She moved to Delhi after high school, stayed with friends, and worked at small jobs in fashion design that exposed her to the fashion industry. She garnered enough experience to return to Mumbai to work as a fashion director tasked with recruiting models for fashion shoots. She spoke earnestly about the group of eastern European models she was in charge of that week but was frustrated with the challenge of feeding them. It wasn't because they didn't want to eat, and it wasn't even that they were wary of "heavier"

Indian food. It was because they were afraid of "getting poisoned," in their words. Almas explained to them that food poisoning could be avoided by refraining from eating on the street but added another caveat that surprised the models: They also had to be careful about accepting foods from people's homes. *Ghar ka khana* (home food) was usually the cleanest food possible, but one could never be too sure because of food adulteration.

Hearing the direction of the conversation, Mary interrupted Almas's story and offered her own insights: "My aunty told me that, when we were small, we used to love to drink *lassi* from a place in Dadar. And *lassi* has to be thick. She told me that to make it thick, in the middle of the night the men used to add toilet tissues in the milk. They would grind up the tissues and put it in the *lassi* and sell it to people. When people started becoming sick, they checked into the cause. When they went to the doctor, there was a layer of paper tissue in their stomachs. The cops went after the men who did this. But what about the people who suffered with the tissue in their bodies? So now I'm buying boxed milk. It's safe." Mary felt that if *lassi* vendors put tissue in their milk, vendors of loose milk in the local stores could do the same, and so switching to boxed milk made by Nestlé made the most sense.

Almas confirmed this sense of packaged milk as the locus of safety, but Mary continued her condemnation of "the nexus" and its work of food adulteration: "And they do other things, too. I heard about them injecting things . . . they're injecting fruits with color, so that when you cut the fruit, like the watermelon, it's pink. I think only in India we have that— not in your country? Let's be frank, OK? It's too much here. It's because of the politicians. They get poor people to do these bad things. If [the middlemen] stop injecting foods, [the politicians] won't get their money. Everybody wants to grow, to become rich. But how? And who lets them get rich?" In Mary's view, the get-rich potential of adulterated foods was understandable, if contemptible. It was simply a way for low-income middlemen to make a little extra money at the hands of greedy politicians who would inevitably siphon off most of the profits. But everyone suffered. "Why should we die slowly when we're paying for food?" she asked.

She and Almas continued the conversation together by laundry-listing several possibilities for adulterated foods:

*Watermelons*: Injected with dirty sugar water to make them sweeter
*Bananas and mangoes*: Dipped in powdered lime solution to ripen them quickly ("Oh so perfect on the outside when you feel it," Mary said, "but inside it's garbage")

*Milk*: Soap, chalk, paint, talc, and lime added for whiteness
*Radishes*: Scrubbed with dirty runoff groundwater to make them whiter
*Chili powder*: Mixed with ground-up red brick mortar to enhance red color
*Black pepper powder*: Mixed with ground-up papaya seeds to enhance black color

The list was endless, the possibilities of deception and reconfiguration seemingly infinite. This was food science carried out on a mass scale, using mass objects like water and chilies. The guilty party was always in the third person plural: "they," "them." I came to understand their explication of this science as an explanation of what it means for others to feed you and how these entities might be treated as relations. Paying for food only to die slowly was an expression of kinship's betrayal through shared substance. But it was not precisely food sharing that enacted relations here, so much as it was elemental processing that created this perverse connection. Well and good that buying food was like a drug deal—but the product needed to be the real thing.

The exchange between Mary and Almas surfaced a repeated act of commensuration I came to understand as "readiness." In literary scholar Richard Ohmann's study (1988) of the formation of mass culture in nineteenth-century America, he pays close attention to an advertisement for Quaker Oats. The marketing behind Quaker Oats, he writes, "did not so much create a need (the common charge against advertising) as show housewives how a generalized and very real historical need . . . might be narrowed and met through purchase and use of a particular kind of commodity" (363–64). In other words, Quaker Oats advertising made homes *ready* for the product by "instruct[ing] the housewife in creative and caring use of the new product," which ensured, Ohmann continues, that "the new bond between corporation and home was secure." Harnessing attention rather than simply peddling products became the means for moving packaged foods into homes *and* the rationale for intensified relations between homes and corporations. Packaged foods are not merely food but food with invitational qualities. Put differently, food packaging invites a sense of filtering: filtering out public scandals of adulterated, open-market foods while retaining the nutritional, healthy goodness connecting bodies to companies. The pervasiveness of packaged foods in urban India made readiness—an assemblage of economies of attention, loyalty, and reputation—the apparatus of the filter.

Unlike Ohmann's example, however, the food supply that Mary and Almas sketch out shows readiness to be an expansive act, managing food for oneself and one's family, that requires attention to all sorts of invitations—not just to the "buy me!" quality of packaged foods but also to the allure of extra-red watermelons or chili powder *which everyone already knows is adulterated*. Adulteration here is not simply a crisis of knowing. Knowing difference is only one part of this story. If knowledge was all that mattered, the story would end with confirmation: one *knows* that one is being poisoned. Mystery solved, certainty attained, and on to the next threat. Readiness in an ecology of adulterated food is a crisis of knowing good and well that what you can rely on for food is most certainly uncertain. To feed others, one must filter all sorts of persons and investments in the food one buys, many of them less than savory. "Choice" is a politics of pursuing or avoiding substances to absorb that overlaps and even overtakes a politics of individuated consumer preference.

Mary and Almas's narrative register of the list also surfaced a historical formation of listing complaints about adulteration pegged to constituent parts. Twentieth-century news articles combined the wonder by foreign journalists amazed at the corruption of the food supply with the anger of Indians who demanded that the government simply *do* something about systematic poisoning. For instance, a 1964 Associated Press article found "the slowness of justice" in India remarkable considering the extent of the danger: "Ever eat spices with coal tar in them, or salt adulterated with chalk dust, or milk diluted with water? A lot of Indians have—unwittingly. Food adulteration is a big racket in India, so big that one is never quite sure that he is eating what he thinks he is. Not even sealed containers, ostensibly imported from abroad, are always safe." The article noted that finding the persons responsible for adulteration was an exercise in moving targets: "if an adulterator is caught, he usually is a small fish. Retailers caught with adulterated food blame wholesalers who blame importers who point enigmatically across the seas," it explained (Associated Press 1964).

Some reporters positioned food adulteration in counterpoint to widespread malnutrition. A special article for the *New York Times* in 1974 reported from New Delhi that "ironically, in a country where it is commonplace for many to become sick for lack of food, many are now suffering because of it." Its report on food adulteration scandals could easily have been lifted from newspapers thirty years later: "Lentils that cause paralysis. Used tea leaves collected from garbage dumps and mixed with fresh tea for resale. Soft drinks colored with dyes that produce cancer. Within the last six months the problem of adulterated foods—some crippling and even fatal—has gripped the attention of Indians in such urban centers as New Delhi, Bombay, and Calcutta" (Weintraub 1974).

The article quoted then Prime Minister Indira Gandhi, who called adulteration a "serious problem" and who "urged that guilty traders and merchants should have their names displayed in markets and railway stations." This approach made public shaming the instrument of accountability and state-sanctioned food-supply purification. This was all the stuff of crime and punishment, a historical antecedent of Prof. Munir's assertions. Food adulteration had an arc that historicized the deprivation of the city.

This form of elemental relationality formed connections within the community as much as it did between the community and the nexus. Back on the beach, as Mary stepped away for a minute to take a phone call, Almas spoke quietly: "Mary is taking good care of her family. I've seen it since childhood. She's feeding her daughter well. But others, I don't know. Others drink Coke, but I don't. The day I realized it was harmful, I stopped. I was fifteen, and a friend of mine told me that Coke was harmful." Almas was speaking of another food scandal, when the Centre for Science and the Environment accused Pepsi and Coke of producing products with high levels of pesticides (see Vedwan 2007). Almas was clear, however, that it wasn't only the rich who bought packaged foods that inflicted harm. She pointed to a door a few homes down the lane, which marked the house of one of the poorest families in Manuli. Almas said that the mother who lived there was disliked by most of the neighbors because she didn't take good care of her children. According to Almas, this had to do in part with the woman's junk food indulgences: "She spends her money on rubbish for herself—Coke, Mirinda [an orange-flavored soda]. If she just spent it on rice, chapati, and dal, her kids would be healthy, not short and skinny and undernourished." Not only did the woman's love of sugary sodas damage her own body, but her money was "wasted" on that damage at the expense of nourishing her children. In this register of health-inflected neighborhood gossip, anyone could work processed food into an insult to the familial body. Almas's portrait of the bad mother down the lane was one of a woman patently *unready* to handle certain foods.

There was, of course, the monetary cost to reckon with. Paying for packaged food involved an initially greater outlay of money compared to cheaper, loose food, but it also insured against expensive doctor's payments. Seema, a middle-aged housewife with two small children, said she strictly followed her doctor's dictum: "5 rupees for bad food means 500 rupees for medicines," meaning that cheap food was risky because of the chance of adulteration and subsequent sickness. Little outside food found its way into her home unless it carried a familiar brand name. Such brand loyalty was another form of affinity between persons and packages. Mary was quite friendly with Seema, but she expressed doubts about Seema's comfortability with branded foods. She freely discussed this with her on another occasion, when the three of us had tea. Mary shared a story about her daughter's discovery of yet another corporate conspiracy channeled through a crunchy corn chip snack called Kurkure:

MARY: My daughter loves Kurkure, you know—that snack? But she learned in school from a teacher that it has nylon in it.

HARRIS: Nylon? As in [*pointing to pants*] nylon?

MARY: Yes! Nylon threads. They put nylon threads in Kurkure for some reason. I didn't believe her, but she told me to burn a piece of it on the stove, over the flame, and we did and saw a nylon thread. So she totally avoids that brand now.

Hearing this, Seema vowed to never give her kids Kurkure anymore, albeit in half jest to acknowledge how difficult it was to find cheap snacks they could buy at the *kirana* shop (small, local provision shop) across the lane. While adulteration could strike familiar elements of the home kitchen, trusted packaged foods could also be targets of adulteration. This was a point made clear to me by Father Matthew, one of the priests in Manuli's church, who once pulled out a small packet of *aloo bhujia sev*, a *namkeen* (snack) of fried vermicelli noodles made from gram flour and mashed potato, during one of our conversations. Father Matthew had been a diabetic for the past five years and paid very close attention to his diet, but he still liked to snack in moments between seeing parishioners. "What do you think is in this?" he asked me. I looked at the packet closely. He turned it on its side and peered at the nutritional label. "You can see what's in it here," he said, but that was merely an assertion by the company that manufactured the food. If we sent the packet of food to a lab, he said, the *real* components would be revealed. He didn't even want to think about what might be inside in terms of adulterated ingredients. Even the label, backed by science, told only half-truths at best.

Whether through Mary's loyalty forged to boxed milk, Almas's loyalty disconnected from Coke, or Seema's turn away from Kurkure snacks in hearing Mary describe their danger, food adulteration scandals produced relations of loyalty to some foods even as they tarnished ties to others.

When Seema vowed to never buy Kurkure snacks again after hearing Mary's accusation that they were really made of nylon, she aimed to protect her family's health against corporate interests that offered some solutions to life's problems but could never be fully trusted. The cultural figure set in relation to the nexus and its acts of processing, then, was the housewife charged with protecting the home against pollution and harm. Domesticity was the site for crafting relationships with corporations in both the protective and proactive sense. A good housewife needed to protect herself and her family against adulteration, and like many women in Manuli who worked as domestic maids and cooks, she was responsible for the health of her second "family" as well. To care for the home was to master the sciences of danger. The path to protection entailed being at the ready in order to keep loose foods at the margins of the kitchen.

## From Punishment to Prevention

Daily expressions of frustration with food adulteration drove sentiments about foods in Manuli, but readiness was a policy refrain, too. While the responsibility for everyday safety fell within the scope of the home, the state also formulated protective measures against adulteration to make the nation ready for safer foods. The threats to the home posed by adulteration aggregated to a national problem, according to public media. Along with public pressure to regulate how the nexus tampered with the food supply came equally pressing requirements for the national government to adhere to international food standards. If India wanted to export its food products as a member of the "developed" world, it had to be prepared to tackle food safety through other means than busting food adulteration rackets. Instead, it would need to transform its approach to food safety completely, by using "risk analysis" to identify the most expedient and cost-efficient means of regulating the food supply. One of the most promising solutions would be to strictly regulate nutritional labeling by requiring food companies to detail every ingredient in their products as a matter of law, turning processing into a matter of state-mandated nutritional regulation and a form of governmental "preparedness." This framing of processing addressed public demands for accountability but also opened the door for food companies to exploit the hypervalued virtues of nutritional qualities and quantities. Food packaging could seal in food that was unadulterated *and* hypernutritive. Readiness for adulterated foods could produce a readiness for functional foods through policy infrastructures. Once there was a consensus that metabolic diseases were large-scale threats, specially formulated packaged foods could offer one solution to the problem, even though their relations to food adulteration scandals remained muted.

Coverage of food adulteration scandals by Indian media outlets often directed outrage on the government and called for public sector action. For instance, an editorial reminded its presumably middle-class readers of the omnipresence of adulteration and the need for policy solutions to bring adulterators to justice:

> "Give it up, buddy. You can't eat your way to health in our country. And your attempt at giving your child healthy nutrition is doomed. No, I am not talking about the underprivileged who go hungry. Nor about the protein- and vegetable-free diet of those who barely get to fill their bellies in this spiraling price rise. I am talking about you, my privileged, aware reader, you who know all about health food and fancy diets and have access to it all. Or so you think. Let me break it gently. You are probably poisoning your family. . . . The only way to protect yourself and your child is by getting proper safety regulations for food and beverages in place. If we can stick to international quality for export, we could jolly well do it for ourselves as well. Let's take ourselves as seriously as we take the foreigner." (Sen 2010)

In the absence of an immediately tangible policy solution, individual consumer choice circulated in public media as the best form of protection. An article entitled "Be a kitchen detective" cautioned the reader that "Danger lurks in the packaged food we find on the kitchen shelves. Profiteers routinely adulterate food items like milk, dal, ghee, honey and so on. In recent years, food adulteration has evolved into a very profitable business, causing serious health hazards." The best way to handle this, according to the article, is to "Get to work, Sherlock Holmes," and to individually check all items on the kitchen shelf (Sujata 2010).[11] These accounts followed processing as it worked its way into the family's moral underpinnings. A common form of reportage on food adulteration involved coverage of "busts" of adulteration "rackets," whereby food adulteration becomes a criminal event policed by cooperative arrangements between state Food and Drug Administration officials and local police. Rackets and busts move adulteration into the realm of public justice discourse and operationally loop Mumbai's police into protecting the food supply (see Natu 2009 and Siddhaye 2010 for just a few examples of coverage on food adulteration "busts"). Popular forms of urban heroism also converge on saving the food supply, such as the 1987 film *Mr. India*, in which Anil Kapoor plays an invisible superhero. With the help of undercover reporter Seema, played by Sridevi, Mr. India force-feeds an underworld henchman named Teja a bowl of dal with stones in it to punish him for doing the same to orphaned children. (In this scene, before Mr. India's force-feeding intervention to right a wrong, Teja and Seema have a lavish dinner. The waitress asks if they need anything else. "You know I'm on a diet," Seema responds coyly, as she inhales tandoori chicken with two hands.)

The workings of criminalization point out the complex institutional moves required to keep adulteration in check.[12] Given the large amount of trade between states, the national government moved toward a central legislative instrument beginning in the late 1930s. Following independence, the issue took shape as the Prevention of Food Adulteration Act (PFA) was ratified in 1954 and became effective on June 15, 1955. The PFA emerged as an effort to coordinate what had until that time been a state-by-state effort to craft and regulate food laws. It later underwent several revisions, beginning in 1955 when the government elaborated technical specifics on matters ranging from infant formula labeling to packaged (bottled) drinking water regulations. The actual enforcement of the laws, however, was left to individual states and Union Territories and was further decentralized to subregions and cities. In Mumbai, for example, the city's Food and Drug Authority (FDA) would enforce food safety rules, largely in the form of adulteration racket busts and raids on warehouses containing illegal imports. This responsibility was further complicated by the fact that certain foodstuffs, such as edible oils and fats, were regulated under an entirely different legal apparatus concerned with weights and measures. For decades following independence, food adulteration was highly regulated but in a somewhat haphazard manner due to the diverse regulatory mechanisms in place, each with its own line of accountability and administration.

This overlapping approach was completely centralized at the national level in 2006. Following economic liberalization and accession to the World Trade Organization (WTO) in 1995, India instituted WTO-mandated changes to the regulation of food safety. These standards and rules are set out by the Codex Alimentarius, a set of international norms that regulates additives, colors, packaging, handling, "safe" cooking temperatures, and a host of other metrics whose adherence is required as part of WTO participation. More generally, codex compliance is the operational standard for food exports. Any food or food-related product in India intended for export must be certified as adhering to codex standards. The codex sets standards for food packaging in terms of its material components, and these standards are required as part of "good manufacturing practices" (GMP) that allow Indian-produced products to circulate in domestic and international markets. But the codex also regulates what appears on the package: logos, brand names, and crucially, a list of the food's ingredients.[13] Despite critiques from several scholars that the codex is essentially a handmaiden to transnational food and agricultural conglomerates, it remains the fundamental regulatory mechanism for food safety.

To adhere to the codex regulations and to centralize national policing of food safety, India created the Food Safety and Standards Act of 2006 (FSSA), which effectively replaced the Prevention of Food Adulteration Act of 1954 and its subsequent revisions. The FSSA created a statutory regulator for the food sector as a whole, the Food Safety and Standards Authority of India (FSSAI). According to its charter, FSSAI was created "for laying down science-based standards for articles of food and to regulate their manufacture, storage, distribution, sale and import to ensure availability of safe and wholesome food for human consumption" (FSSAI 2006). Administratively, the FSSAI falls under the jurisdiction of the Ministry of Health and Family Welfare, meaning that it has cabinet-level bureaucratic influence. As much as its creation has involved bureaucratic shuffles, FSSAI has not ceased its criminalization of food adulteration and even proposed in 2009 to create "food safety courts" dedicated to prosecuting adulterators with punishments as severe as life imprisonment (Chandra 2009).

In 2009, Union Health Minister Anbumani Ramadoss mandated that all nutrition information should be listed clearly on food packages, one of several health-related shifts designed to bring India "in line with the developed world," according to one report (Sharma 2009). Among the required elements of labeling would be the precise amount of trans fats. While one high-ranking civil servant in the Health Ministry explained the impulse for mandating labels as a matter of fulfilling WTO requirements, the Health Minister had a different explanation: "Changing lifestyles have led to a spurt in the number of people suffering from diabetes and heart-related problems," he said. "It is essential for an individual to know what he is eating." Regulating nutrition labels would enable the government to simultaneously work on "preventing" diabetes, obesity, and other cardiovascular diseases while also "preventing" food adulteration and instances of noncompliance with WTO regulations. Packaged foods thus joined concerns about metabolic disease to concerns about food adulteration and made precise declarations of nutritional values a useful solution on several fronts. More generally, this process signaled a change in the governance of processing from "reaction" to "risk prevention."

Food company workers found the new regulations somewhat irksome. When I interviewed Satish and Tejas, two members of the quality control department of a snack company called Enjoy Foods, they expressed frustration at the labeling requirements. Both Satish and Tejas thought the regulations were simply an import from the US Food and Drug Administration. "Especially trans fats—it's so ridiculous," Satish said. "It's clear that Americans eat lots of trans fats—they love animal fats. But here in India we don't. We eat vegetables. We eat rice. We're a milk-rich country, but we're not dependent on milk. We have a vegetarian, grain-based diet. We eat fiber and vegetables. You won't find heart disease in villages, where people eat simple diets. The US is full of obesity, but not here."

Tejas thought the requirements to measure nutrition levels by portion sizes was another American import: "My full plate is the American quarter plate!" he exclaimed. Indians ate too little and too simply to be subject to standards that were clearly intended for overconsuming Americans. As the two men traded other reasons why Americans were obese while Indians were not (e.g., "Americans sit inside air conditioning all day, while Indians sweat out their fat"), they eventually settled on the "real" problem of the new nutrition regulations. While they found it more convenient to report to one authority—FSSAI—instead of seven different authorities as before, they felt the nutritional regulations were a convenient means for the government to limit the potential for private industry. "We [private industry] are freebirds," Satish said emphatically. "We don't want regulations. We're part of the democracy. Everyone is spending their time and energy complying with these regulations, but they're ignoring the overall quality of the product." For Satish, government nutrition regulations threatened both the taste of the product and the profit potential of the company. "Quality" here had a link to the ideals of an incorrupt, democratic India.

I was curious to know what the person in charge of enforcing the act in the city thought of these connections. When I spoke with Mumbai's FDA Commissioner, Mahesh Zagade, I first asked what he thought were the challenges and opportunities of taking a law from the 1950s and putting it into renewed motion in 2012. He characterized the 1954 PFA as having a "single focus" such that offenders were "raided, caught, and punished." The new FSSA was completely different. It took a "360-degree approach" to food safety, as opposed to the multiple separate laws under the PFA umbrella. Through federal, state, and municipal hierarchies of food safety regulators, the work of the new act hinged on audit. When I asked for a specific example, Mr. Zagade opened the thick book of the complete FSSA that sat on his desk, feathered with colored Post-it notes. "I will just read it out to you," he said, and recited chapter 3, section 18, "General principles to be followed in Administration of Act." These included pursuing "an appropriate level of protection of human life and health" and "carrying out risk management."[14] After his recitation, he looked up. "For me," he said, "this section is really beautifully worded. It's about the protection of human life." I mentioned invocations of "freebirds" and industry concerns. Mr. Zagade was quite straightforward that his work as a government regulator made him "quite unpopular" with the industries and restaurants that had to comply with a new set of rules. But he felt it to be essential work—even "on a personal level." He was committed. He was ready. The city needed to be, too. He made it clear that he was the drug regulator and was refreshing his role as the food regulator. Regulating the world of processing was about which elements did and did not belong in a material. For him, these differences connected ingredients, the state, and the protection of human life.

The creation of FSSAI and its main policy, FSSA, enlivened private contractors who worked as intermediaries between the government and the targets of the act. One company, Meridian, began as a lab testing company that would test for chemicals in water samples. It also tested for chemicals in foods, and with the advent of FSSA, it saw an opportunity to grow from just testing into "awareness building" and publicity. I learned this from Adil, who began as an auditor at the company and worked his way up to head marketing and PR. He wanted Meridian to be the public face of the FSSA, even as it was the machinery behind testing for "noncompliance" with the law. I asked what a typical "compliance audit" looked like. Meridian takes food samples, collects swabs of the machinery and other parts of the operation, and works through a detailed checklist according to the details required by FSSAI. "We help them get better," he said of those parties under investigation, from street food carts, to restaurants, to large-scale food companies. He told a story of a restaurant that seemed fine during initial investigation despite rumors of infractions. The workers even wore gloves. Meridian's auditors watched a man who was cutting vegetables while wearing gloves. He went to the toilet wearing gloves and emerged wearing gloves. They asked the man why he did what he did. The man replied that his boss instructed him that he would be punished if he ever took off the gloves, no matter the circumstance. These were some of the contingencies Meridian had to work with, according to Adil.

Meridian sought to build a complex surveillance system to monitor adulteration incidents. Adil proudly described the company's sources of "intelligence" on outbreaks of sickness from adulterated food, such as a recent case in a university cafeteria that sickened six hundred people. The company was launching a campaign to turn the city's residents into what he called "citizen journalists." "Everyone has a phone that can take pictures," he explained. Meridian was planning to launch a contest that challenged people to take a photo every time they witnessed a food safety infraction—a man washing vegetables with gutter water or a street vendor not using gloves. The citizen journalists would post the photo to Facebook, sparking outrage and awareness. The most compelling picture would net an award of 50,000 rupees. I asked what would happen to the person caught in the action. Adil assured me that there was no "enforcement" involved, really. "It's about making awareness go viral," he said. People needed to be ready for the new laws. While FDA Commissioner Zagade celebrated a move away from the punitive toward the protection of human life, Adil seemed to suggest it was only through punishment—popularized through social media and given monetary compensation for that reward—that people would take FSSA seriously.

## The Family's Healthy Heart

Just as Meridian took an instrument of governance and regulation and turned it into an opportunity for profit, food companies themselves saw opportunity, too. As one industry representative told me, "Lifestyle may be the problem behind obesity, but foods can be used to combat that problem." Borne out of the impulse to regulate, label, legalize, make honest, and infuse health into India's food system, packaged foods also productively blurred the boundary between food and drug and brought the home and the corporation into more intimate relations.

One afternoon, in the crowded aisles of my small neighborhood food market, a gray-haired man struggled to balance a shopping basket and a fussy toddler. The girl brushed up against a bright yellow display case of cooking oils that towered over the neighboring shelves of toothpaste, spices, and cookies. The man took this as an opportunity to grab her interest by pointing out the display case by its brand name: "Look sweetie, Saffola!" As they hurried toward the cashier, they missed the woman three steps away wearing clothes that perfectly matched the yellow of the display: a hired in-store marketer for Saffola foods. She was passing out pamphlets about their new "functional" rice to anyone who managed to squeeze by in the narrow aisle. I asked her casually about the rice: What made it different? She gave a well-rehearsed explanation. "It helps you lose weight by making you feel full longer," she said. "Scientific research shows that obese people benefit from it." Gently pressing, I asked how that worked. She shrugged. "I'm just here to sell it," she said pleasantly, turning to dole out a pamphlet to the next potential customer.

Between the issues of science and the home, what happens to food in the name of healthy domesticity? Here I take a cue from Geeta Patel's reflections on "homeliness." Patel (2004) notes, "Homeliness does not necessarily render women into commodities. Women might become commodities whose value is given through homeliness, but in each instance described in this essay, the women themselves are not exactly nominalized into a commodity form. The possibility of their homely domesticity is held out as probability (as a portion of the contracts or promises I articulate in my examples) precisely because women are not merely reified into commodities. Through the intimacy invested in homeliness, women become intrinsic to circulations of capital that are also not reified" (154). This sense of homely domesticity has particular importance for the formulation of new foods geared specifically to address health. The domestic woman becomes crucial to food companies, as she is the arbiter of invitation, the filter of foods that feed the family.

I had seen Saffola products advertised in billboards around town before and knew that the company's mainstay product line involved cooking oils. Saffola is one in a line of products produced by an Indian company called OilCo, which got its start selling cooking oils but in the last decade expanded to hair oils, functional foods such as "healthy" snacks, blended cooking oils with "heart healthy" fatty acid balances, and the weight-loss rice I saw in the market. When I arrived at the OilCo headquarters in Mumbai via a friend's introduction, the OilCo CEO, Mr. Chanda, was pressed for time; he simply wanted to learn more about anthropology and offer me a taste of some of the company's newest snack products. More in-depth conversations about the marketing and science of the foods could be arranged, and he gave me some names to contact. One of the individuals on the list was Dr. Laxman, OilCo's head of research and development. Months after meeting Mr. Chanda, I attended a medical conference on obesity and was surprised to see Dr. Laxman's name on the list of speakers. After his presentation on how OilCo's line of functional foods could treat obesity and diabetes, I introduced myself, and he invited me to visit OilCo's R&D office.

Dr. Laxman, a biochemist by training, explained that "if you take the entire business of food production, 5 percent is branded products, and 95 percent of the market is unbranded, loose commodities." This offered an unprecedented opportunity for a company like OilCo. Dr. Laxman hoped to intervene in what he called "the gap" between biology and modernity, whereby "the gut is traditional but the lifestyle is modern." This gap, embodied as diabetes and obesity, had immense potential for both profits and losses. "Ultimately, how the government acts doesn't matter if you end up with a country of sick people. Sick people means lost productivity," he said. It was private industry that could remedy that sickness, as well as the awareness of brands that could accelerate the supposed lag time of the Indian gut. For Dr. Laxman, consumer "awareness" fit into the rubric of enlightenment through science. He acknowledged the many types of "experiments" people do every day with functional foods: adding *methi* (fenugreek) seeds to rotis to help regulate blood sugar or grating carrots into *idlis* to add nutrients to what otherwise is simply fermented rice batter. But putting functional foods in packaging gave them an added credibility and a sense of safety that these home remedies couldn't sustain. I admitted to him that when I first heard the term "functional food," I thought, "what's a *dysfunctional* food"? He laughed:

> "I agree, all foods are functional foods. If I eat bread, it's functional. It's providing calories, fiber, gluten, it has protein. So that way, I really don't see a difference between foods and functional foods. I'm just redesigning your food. I'm giving it functionality. So functional food is a food, and food is a functional food. See, it's the concept. Functional food doesn't mean going to a lab and making some funny thing and saying it's now a magic thing. It is a lifestyle adaptation, it's an adaptation of your cooking style. The realization is coming about what happens if you don't have a healthy nation. You don't want to have young diabetics and young obese people . . . it's lost productivity. And there's nothing better than preventing all of these things in the first place, and food and lifestyle are the two most critical factors for making that happen."

OilCo avoided a strategy of directly releasing a line of products into the food supply. Instead, it carefully conducted a dynamic research process of market research, on one hand, and lab research on taste, texture, and nutrition on the other. Initial market research on functional foods concluded it would not be strategic to offer products such as meal-replacement bars or protein powders.[15] OilCo was known for its cooking oils, and this was its market advantage: its products were already considered inside foods by women willing to pay extra for health benefits. The company wanted to build on that loyalty as it launched new products.

Additionally, its market research revealed that rice was highest in the list of foods that overweight and diabetic persons missed the most on their diets. OilCo's solution was to alter the staple foods themselves. By sorting through over twelve thousand varieties of rice in a food lab, testing the glycemic index (GI) of each one, it finally found one variety with a low GI, meaning that it elicited a more dampened insulin response after eating and would be suitable to market to diabetics. The variety grew in the hilly regions of the southern state of Karnataka, so it was a domestic product and would not involve foreign import taxes and logistics. Dr. Laxman's lab tested the rice for texture and taste after confirming its nutritional virtues; it seemed to be an ideal candidate. The crux of this blockbuster was its formulation of domesticity: it was domestic in its Indian origin, and its corporate pedigree gave it the quality of inside food.[16]

I was curious about the production of messages behind the rice advertisements, and so I returned to Mr. Chanda's list of OilCo employees and met with Sudhir, a marketing manager. He led me to his glass-enclosed cubicle, stuffed with boxed snacks. Sudhir explained that consumers see OilCo as a company that transformed itself from merely a company selling edible oils to "a company concerned with the national problem of heart disease." When it launched its "healthy" oil products line, it sponsored roadside health checkups, where passersby could have their blood pressure and cholesterol tested. He reminded me that four Indians die every minute from a heart-related problem and that OilCo formulated products with that statistic in mind. The ideal medium of product positioning emerged from the market research, which as an aside Sudhir noted involved a form of "consumer ethnography." OilCo hired social science students to go into homes and conduct consumer research. The interviewers asked the housewife to imagine a situation where she had run out of food but suddenly learned that extended family members were on their way. "You get the consumer to imagine situations, moments, and events that tie in with food, and then you construct the product in response to those attachments," he said. These sentiments formed the basis for a product's "message." He called this research process "insighting." Even before the product was finalized, the corporation had entered the home on the pretense of perfecting a safe offering and with the expectation of attachments. Just as Dr. Laxman focused on positioning OilCo's functional foods as natural, "inside" foods, Sudhir described them as "unintrusive" to the rhythms of everyday life.

While OilCo's marketers emphasized the health threats to men, they focused on women as the ones who "notice" new products. They also recognized that in some families, a woman might be unwilling to reveal to her husband that she had bought a new food and was trying it out. OilCo's flour and grain extra-fiber mixes were the perfect vehicle, then, for surreptitious preventive health. A woman could simply mix it in to the flour and make rotis, and her husband would be none the wiser. Sudhir said OilCo gave housewives products to "intervene" in their husbands' well-being; he called this alliance a matter of "making women partners in the management of the risks of their husbands' lifestyle." Thus the primary means for garnering public attention about Saffola's products emerged through domesticity's gendered axes of care. The company's design and marketing team combined advances in food science with highly gendered marketing campaigns to pose packaged foods as the solution to metabolic disease and tied the brand loyalty of housewives to emotional investments in the home. This affective appeal, they hoped, would help surpass any preconceptions that functional foods were elite indulgences and instead would make foods a "natural" element that belonged in homes across Mumbai's socioeconomic ranks. Specifically, OilCo marketed the rice as a way for women to "manage" their husband's excess weight. The ads, which appeared on bus stops, billboards, and other public signs, featured a picture of a young woman who had picked up her husband and slung him over her shoulder (see figure 3.1). Headlined with the message "Saffola Rice to Manage His Weight," the subheading that "Keeping an eye on weight means keeping an eye on the heart" (*Weight pe nazar yaane dil pe nazar*). The ads marked the gendered stakes of obesity: for men, it was mortality, but for women, it was marital obligation.

OilCo's products were suffused with the hope that they would mediate domestic forms of care. This was all a question of loyalty, at the end of the day: a question Sudhir posed as brand loyalty but one deeply gendered through demands for subversive feeding and care. "Brands don't exist to sell," Sudhir explained. "They exist to improve customers' lives. Once you recruit an OilCo customer, you have her for life."

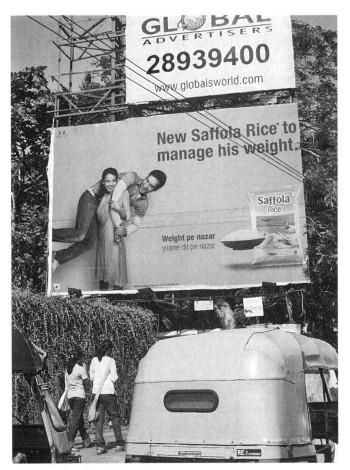

**FIG. 3.1** Saffola Rice billboard

## Processing the Housewife

Sudhir had repeatedly mentioned that Saffola products were born out of necessity—not only in terms of health writ large but also out of the specific needs of the Indian housewife vocalized to market researchers who entered their homes. In this sense, "insighting" in food marketing research was a complex "para-site" of knowledge production, to use George Marcus's term, because it is a place where the ethnographer can observe other ethnographies in action. In other words, the home and the home kitchen in particular were spaces not only of my own interest but also of corporate researchers whose work would be used to craft new kinds of foods. And like my own engagements, the figure of the housewife was utterly central to the speaking, writing, and doing of this kind of work. Most at stake was the question of what she—and by extension, her home—could handle. What kinds of new foods was the housewife ready for? What could she bear? How did readiness translate into novelty and market niche?

I secured an invitation through a friend to a market research focus group. This group was the intermediary between the preliminary data the in-home researchers collected and the report the market research firm would send back to the food company. The group I participated in was a sounding board and an instrument of finesse of sorts. It also had a specific task: to funnel its qualitative data toward ideas for possible products. The experimental space of the home moved into the space our group occupied and would be transmuted into concrete foods.[17] The focus group was an intense two-day workshop whose participants were all food "experts" in some way or another: food writers, restaurateurs, bloggers, and caterers. Almost all were women, and almost all identified as upper middle class. Some were involved in producing and distributing organic foods. This seemed a bit odd to me, given that our task for the two days was to ultimately produce preliminary sketches of a new processed food to help a multinational food company cement its reach into the urban Indian prepared foods market. The entirety of the workshop was videotaped, and the market research firm had note takers, audio techs recording every word, and "visualizers" to draw our thoughts into pictures. The leader of the workshop, Himanshu, explained that its mission was to "bring the city home": tastefully but safely, for housewives who live in smaller cities and are lower middle class. Our task was to embody and think like that housewife. Glossy, plastic-wrapped boxes of packaged foods were circulated among the participants as a cue to think about the kind of goodness and appeal that could be sealed inside a package.

The key variables a housewife works with, according to preliminary interviews, included variety, religious mandates, "quick and tasty," comfort food, and wholesome. Her specific concerns included experimentation ("trying to replicate restaurant food at home"), appreciation ("her biggest joy"), and being a magician ("she has a planned life but has to be ready for surprises, sudden guests, and her kids' demands"). We learn that the housewife has to be the "Masterchef" of the house—named after the popular Australian reality television show—for several reasons. She learns from watching *Masterchef* (and specifically, Himanshu said, the version dubbed in vernacular languages rather than the English-only version). But she also must possess the versatility of a Masterchef, because as their research shows, "the kitchen is her battleground." Her children want pizza, not dal. Her husband wants conventional food but nothing too mundane. Her in-laws who live with her want *sadha khana* (simple, plain food like dal, a vegetable, and rice—especially appealing to older generations with digestive problems) but also demand snacks throughout the day. A clash of culinary interests crystallize in the kitchen, often prompting the housewife to prepare three different meals/dishes all at the same time. Excerpts from interviews delineated the stakes of these obstacles, including "Inconsistency in taste makes my husband angry"; "Guests will gossip if my food is too bland"; "My dignity is at stake in my cooking"; and "I am under constant scrutiny—I can't afford to make mistakes." Himanshu aptly summarized this part of the research, categorized by the firm as "woes of the newly married bride." "This sounds like a TV serial," he said, "but it's true." Although our task was to take these insights and brainstorm a packaged food, there were also concerns about processed foods to consider. These included potential protest from the in-laws and the question of food's religious functions, given that only fresh food can be used for *prasad* (offering) to deities. Cost of course was an issue, as was a patent worry about preservatives.

Throughout the exercise, the housewife was processed as a specific subject who can go to the market, be vigilant, and maintain the right balance between the porosity of the home and the foods she invites inside for both eating and ritual offering. Himanshu gave us parameters for our brainstorming. Our food had to help the housewife multitask, to make her happy without being cumbersome (*jhanjhat*), and to eliminate the repetitive vegetable cutting and spice grinding characteristic of food preparation (*katne pisne ke jhanjhat se chut kara*). One of the organic food producers sighed about the task: "Ugh, we're being used to make *them* a whole range of products"—*them* here meaning the corporation. Nonetheless, she carried out the task. She, too, thought it had some purchase. Some of the ideas that percolated in our group included diabetic-specific functional foods and foods with less salt or sugar. In reviewing these ideas, the group split. Some thought that a product advertised as healthy would seem out of price point for our targeted tier of housewives. Health, in other words, seemed too middle-class-y. Another person agreed: our housewives would identify the food with a disease, and that would spell doom for marketing. Other team members felt differently: "You can charge more for it because it's healthy," one said. "And after all, India has the most number of people with diabetes in the world, so it will sell." My own silence during this whole process reached a breaking point when one of the team members said with exasperation, "*you have to contribute something*." I had grown a bit weary of instructions to imagine the newlywed girl serving fiber-rich cake to her mother-in-law. "Can we propose something that *doesn't* involve the daughter-in-law being subservient?" I asked. The intersectionality of gender and class was well taken but also deemed a fait accompli. "You're looking at those women at this table," one of my team members said. "*We're* not like that." Another woman responded with a joke that itself was a marker of privilege, given its sheer utterability: "You just have to wait for the bitch mother-in-law to die," and then the poor housewife would be free to experiment culinarily.

The urban upper-middle-class makeup of the group posed challenges. As the "visualizers" sketched our ideas on paper, Himanshu walked over and deemed our fledgling product "too Western." "It should have a *kaḍai* (wok) or roti in the background. Not all white and modern. Maybe some warmer colors, like red, yellow, and brown. It needs traditionalizing, localizing. Maybe sari borders on the side of the package."[18] The workshop continued on like this: iterations of products and constant questioning by Himanshu and his team as to how we thought the housewife would handle them. Were they ready? Was their family ready? Not being ready was always front and center, and as such, the housewife was as much a technology as she was a person: the domestic cyborg. In the focus group, there was a constant reminder to think like someone of a different class, to grapple with her struggles by generating a packaged food product that could be a solution for her. Each time someone proposed a gadget or something fancy, like bottled pasta sauces, we were reminded of the constraints of the lower-middle-class tier. Readiness had technological moorings sometimes, criminal/corrupt ones other times, intimate ones in even other times. To issue calls for nutritious food was one thing, but to appreciate who would be making it was another. At the interface of the inside and outside of food, the question of readiness was in motion. Readiness arranges the metabolic across homes and foods. As problems of bodily well-being, domestic life, and public disorder are recast as problems for food companies to solve, readiness emerges through the science of nutrition, headlined by the cultural figure of the housewife who triangulates the home and the corporation.

## "You Can't Listen to Them All"

On a later visit with Sudhir at the OilCo office, he mentioned that the rice was selling well but that OilCo had decided to "reposition" the marketing message, which he couldn't yet share because the revamped product hadn't launched. The company didn't want to continue to associate the product with obesity and diabetes, even peripherally. To link a product to a disease limits its sales. It was good for an introductory strategy, but expansion was necessary. Medicalization helped create channels into the home, but constantly shifting messages were needed to keep those channels open. The ultimate goal was a woman's loyalty to the brand, which took on the form of a lifelong contract that promised her safety in return for her continued investment. With Sudhir's hints at change, I kept an eye on the rice and asked my neighborhood grocer if he might let me know when the "repositioned" product arrived. When the new product came, it wasn't in the same yellow packaging. Instead, it was green and white and in a large plastic container quite different from the yellow plastic kilogram bag in which the "weight-loss" rice had been packaged. The new product was called "Saffola Arise." It was priced at sixty-nine rupees for a one-kilogram pack, in comparison to "regular" varieties of basmati rice priced between twenty and forty rupees loose per kilogram at the same grocer. The rationale behind the new product—which was the same rice as before—was not that it would help you lose weight but that it would keep you "active" and not sleepy.

Television commercials and nutritionist testimonials posted to the product's website emphasized this point. One commercial showed a man in an office looking longingly at a coworker who was eating heaps of rice for lunch; when the coworker offered to share, the man declined—"I have a meeting, I can't eat rice," he explained. The rice would make him too sleepy. Similarly, another commercial pictured a woman at a lunch party who confessed to the camera that she wished she could eat as much rice as she *really* desired but instead settled for just a spoonful. The coworker in the office in the first commercial and the party host in the second both presented the solution in the problematic moment of self-denial for fear of poor productivity or sociality: Saffola Arise would satisfy your hunger, keep you full, and—most importantly—not make you sleepy. The product's new tagline captured this magical, superadded property: *Active Rice, Active Zindagi*—"Active Rice, Active Life." Rebalancing the inner energy of the body, so closely linked to the thinking and productivity of the man in the office and the woman in the home, now had another solution in the form of a processed food that spurred metabolic efficiency of a person's body-brain.

I rarely saw Saffola rice used in households in Manuli, because of its comparatively high cost. But OilCo's other products made appearances in many homes. During another visit to Seema's house, I noticed that she had a bottle of Saffola cooking oil on her kitchen counter and asked her about it. Seema ducked into the kitchen and returned with the yellow plastic jug. "It's good for your heart," she explained. "See? It says 'The Heart of a Healthy Family' on the label." Reluctant to let the product's tagline have the last word, I pressed on the issue: "But why do you buy it?" I asked. Seema explained that she was simply too busy to be bothered with the media craze around obesity and chronic disease: "There are all these threats, but you can't listen to them all—how would you live?" The "heart-healthy" cooking oil was a convenience because it dampened worry about her husband or her children needing active interventions to prevent disease. Whatever "function" it served in terms of public health prevention efforts, Seema easily integrated the oil into her daily repertoire at home. Public threats faded into the background, as the more private aspects of processing came to the fore.

Seema's use of functional foods was not so much a matter of meeting concrete needs or being fooled by ads as it was distracting her attention from chronic disease so she could focus on more pressing daily matters of family relations. Readiness, more than feminized foolhardiness of instrumental consumerism, structured relations between persons, objects, and the qualities of excess added to packaged foods. I have suggested that the affective formation of readiness was at the heart of framing what belonged in the home and what belonged outside it. In contrast to the vision of OilCo, however, readiness for packaged foods emerged not as a sentiment of a choosy housewife who ventures into the market. Instead, it cohered as the echo of the market's approach to the home, a metabolic footprint rather than housewifely choosiness. The echo came as a calm shrug, as Seema pointed out: "You can't listen to them all." Hypervigilance over invitations had its limits. The permeability of homes, foods, and housewives featured prominently as processing became part of the arbitration of inside and outside, of familiar and strange. To be fed by another in this circumstance had uncertain qualities, illustrated by Seema's shrug. This highlights the tenuous nature of a politics of processing, despite its connective powers across home kitchens, commercial snack markets, global import/export policy arrangements, and the gray markets of adulterated foods.[19]

Not food itself, nor what is added to it, nor who adds to it are independently sufficient to explain how metabolic disorder and food adulteration link to processed foods. Processed food was not home food, but neither was it quite outside food. Packaging defied easy categorization and allowed individuals to formulate loyalties that helped processed foods move easily inside the home. Selectively porous processed foods allowed the filtering out of public scandals of adulterated, open-market foods while retaining the nutritional, healthy goodness of connections between bodies and private food companies. These objects complicate clear differences between feeding and drugging and elicit different moral appeals and appellants who converge on the issue of accessing the metabolic body. Food processing indeed constitutes the obvious, but it does so in ways that trouble the idea that metabolisms and bodies map precisely onto each other. What meaning, then, can this haziness between food and drugs absorb in moments of medical therapy?

It is said in Bandra that you can't throw a stone without hitting a pig, a priest, or a Pereira. This longtime saying imprints urban adage with the neighborhood's density of Portuguese derivations: pork, Catholicism, and family surnames. The saying's degrees of truth signal the times. I lived down the street from a five-hundred-year-old Catholic church surrounded by families named Gomes, Alves, Fernandes, and yes, Pereira. Pigs were few in number in their live form, but pork products abounded. If I wanted to purchase meat, I could walk in any direction and arrive at a shop called a "cold storage store" that connects the slaughterhouse to the neighborhood to the eater. Many of Bandra's cold storage stores have been in business for decades. I interviewed several of the owners. A store might have begun with one freezer in the early 1960s, and through the years family members would have procured the things that made meat sellable, like a slicer, a grinder, and a cash register. During one interview, a shop owner invoked the pig/priest/Pereira aphorism unprompted but then exposed its fragility when situated in Mumbai's contemporary real estate economies. He explained that the neighborhood was gradually becoming less Catholic. Longtime resident Catholic families were selling their bungalows and moving to the city's outer suburbs. His store's sales volume had not changed with this demographic shift, because he did not sell pork or pork products like sausages. His chicken, beef, and mutton were halal. Thus his Muslim customers kept the business as brisk as when the neighborhood was primarily Catholic. I asked after the provenance of the meats; each cold storage owner responded that chicken came from various distributors but that all beef products were sourced from Mumbai's central, government-controlled abattoir in the area of Deonar.

One owner introduced me to a veterinarian, Dr. Pillai, who had been the chief animal inspector at the facility. Dr. Pillai invited me to tour the facility to observe slaughter and meat processing. Arriving at Deonar, his car was inspected, and I was reminded that no photography would be allowed. Dr. Pillai led me into an open grazing area that functioned as the market for farmers and wholesale buyers. A shepherd (*gvala*) kept goats in line. Most of the meat processed at Deonar is exported to the Gulf. We passed a large sign declaring, "Cruelty to animals is a serious offense." The air smelled like a petting zoo, conveying the scent of the abattoir's sixty-four acres of animal processing facilities, often regarded as Asia's largest in terms of facility size. Animal caretakers approached Dr. Pillai as we walked through sheds for bulls, buffalo, and goats. They held up hooves and ears and other areas of concern: possibilities of infection or jaundice or wounds from tussles with other animals. A caretaker pointed out a bull who had a bloody, gouged-out eye from getting into a fight with another. Dr. Pillai advised him on wound care and antibiotics. Doses were relative to the animal's size and weight. The caretaker put his hands around the goat's flank to assess relative proportions of bone, flesh, and fat: sixteen kilos total, he announced. I noticed that each animal had a label. Some had yellow numbered tags on their ears, but all were marked via a brand, called a *garam chhaap* (hot stamp), burnt into their hides. Before moving from market to slaughter, an animal's skin receives a mark, "VD," for "Veterinary Department," a stamp of approval attesting that it has no cancer, no walking deformities, and is at least three years old (the required minimum age for slaughter).

Dr. Pillai drove us to the slaughter area. Two types of slaughter occur at Deonar. The first is called "ground" slaughter, where all processes are done by hand in the open, from the slitting of arteries to the dressing of the animal. The second type, "line" slaughter, is mechanized and carried out in a concrete building next door. Ground slaughter was in high gear when we arrived. It takes place in a covered but open-walled structure paved with slabs of concrete spaced apart at certain points for water channels. Concrete and stone bathing areas line the structure's inside perimeter. There, butchers scrub in and out of their work. Beams with dangling hooks hang carcasses in the air. From these hooks, shirtless and barefoot men flay animal quarters. They strip off hides with long knives and divide a carcass into quarters. I noticed some movement out of the bottom of my visual field and looked down to my shoes. I nearly stepped on a pile of bull hides, furry and bloody. The movement came from the topmost hide, still quivering: rigor mortis.

I asked about the hides as a young man trucked them away on a hand-cart. Dr. Pillai explained that they are sold to leatherworkers in Dharavi. While he explained this to me, something brushed the back of my leg. I turned around and saw hooves. Men were wheeling in a three-hundred-kilogram bull on a wagon. It appeared dead to me, but I was mistaken. Dr. Pillai said it was not dead but somewhere between life and death. It was trampled by other bulls. It arrived at the open area for what he calls "emergency slaughter." Deonar produces halal meat, and thus a mullah must perform the actual act in the open slaughter area (on the automated line, the mullah stands at the very beginning when animals are brought in and performs the required invocation of God's name and the required slitting of the throat to ensure that the animal can be hung upside down to freely bleed). Meat produced here in the open area, by ground slaughter, will be immediately taken to cold storage shops in the city; line slaughter begins later in the evening, and meat is then packed overnight and shipped out the next morning. The butchers, mostly in their late teens and early twenties, tucked sharp knives into the back of their shorts. Once they suspended quarters of an animal carcass on hooks, the men sluiced buckets of water over the meat and then on themselves to wash away droplets of blood even as they waded through blood with bare feet. It is as if we were at a *dhobi ghat*, a place to wash clothes, red instead of white. Life seemed miscible between species and skins: water and blood, all the way down.

My own blood reacted. "You are scared," Dr. Pillai said, observing the color drain from my face. Yes. He led me to the bathing area; blood water splashed me as butchers finished with a shift clean up in the concrete tubs. One of the mullahs I observed hand-slitting the throat of a bull told me that he has done this work for twenty-five years. Many of the men working with bulls are from the Qureshi community of Muslims, whose members have extensive and complex historical links to animal slaughter and trade. He beat his wet work clothes on the concrete walls of the tub to get the blood out. He and the others changed into fresh clothes from plastic bags tucked in corners, and a man appeared with a set of fresh knives. Another round began. Ground slaughter processes roughly forty-five animals per hour. With the line slaughter added in, the Deonar abattoir as a whole processes approximately ten thousand animals each day. A junior veterinarian approached and consulted with Dr. Pillai on some inspection-related questions. He took me to the carcasses and narrated what his eyes sought out: evidence of hemorrhagic disease. If the carcass passes this inspection, it receives a new mark, a purple stamp indicating veterinary approval. I peered at the mark, making out the imprint that reads "Deonar." The vet noticed my own inspection of the ink on the carcasses. Like a slap, he stamped an open page of my field notebook. First blood, then water, and now ink. My notes soaked them all in.

A tour of the line slaughter facility required dodging fast-moving carcasses of goats, thorns from their fur, and their entrails spilling into buckets after line workers slit their bodies open to the world outside. Dr. Pillai narrated each step. He offered to take me to lunch immediately after our visit; I was less than hungry. We opted for tea at his nearby home instead. There, Dr. Pillai spoke of the complexities of labor unions at the facility, of the changes over the years brought by automation, and of his desire to visit slaughterhouses in the United States, which he understood to be an impossible request because of the ways that meat-processing facilities there are hermetically sealed to curious outsiders. I asked if he ate meat. "I use to be a pigger when it came to food," he said, and he loved meat. "But now I eat mostly salads, and cook only in olive oil." He showed me a scar on his chest. A triple-bypass surgery, several years back. A fleshy stamp of his own.

Patients queued in long lines in the mornings before Trinity Hospital opened. From emergencies to routine clinic visits, many of Manuli's residents wound up at this hospital on the neighborhood's outer edges. During outpatient hours, each person who wanted to pass from outside to inside received a number that determined place in line and appointment time. The line snaked to the road. A set of guards flanked the main door, admitting only a few patients at a time into the hospital in order to manage crowd capacity. The endocrinology ward was on Trinity's second floor, past another number checker at the stairs and elevator. Patients met lines upon arrival in the ward, too, this time managed by a charge nurse. Like the crosses along Carter Road, these lines were signs of the times: a community and city bearing the load of metabolic disease. How much of this load could Mumbai (and by epidemiological extension, India) absorb? The lines sketched out a landscape of metabolic living's therapeutic features.

I devoted much of my time to observations in the hospital's second-floor hallway and in the rooms it connected to. On one side of the hallway, doors opened to the exam room for the hospital's head of endocrinology, Dr. Chitre. Trinity's diabetes foot clinic was on the other side of the hallway, across from Dr. Chitre. This clinic, led by Dr. Samant, is where patients would see a specialist to care for complications with diabetic neuropathy, a condition that arises when feeling is lost in the extremities and that puts persons at high risk for infections from undetected wounds. Left untreated, those wounds could lead to amputation of toes, a foot, even a leg. No matter how "successful" a person might be in following Dr. Chitre's treatment regimen, it seemed that there was the specter of loss in that room across the hall, as one could lose flesh and blood walking on the streets or go about daily routines but accidentally hit a carnal snag. I began to see the hallway as a line. It directed bodies and diagnostic categories toward drugs on one side and toward amputation on the other.

Built through interviews with dietitians, clinical observations, and discussions in Manuli, this chapter considers the making and unmaking of metabolisms as a multisite for clinical therapy. Persons appearing at Trinity for clinically applied metabolic science had often mounted other attempts to alleviate metabolic disorder. From diets to homeopathy, individuals in Manuli and elsewhere appealed to many sciences that took the metabolism as their centerpiece. Lines around and in Trinity Hospital formed one of many convergent lines that presume and remake the metabolism as a site of clinical science. Close attention to this set of lines shows how clinical care makes sense and nonsense of the metabolism as both resource and target for bodily betterment.

Clinics, hospitals, and their cadre of nutritionists and physicians had a strong hold over treatment for metabolic disease. Care for metabolic illness also reached outside clinical spaces into everyday life, as persons monitored the ups and downs of their bodies in concert with adherence to medication and diet. As a therapeutic site, the metabolism can be understood as absorptive in the ways that it extends beyond the walls of a clear-cut biomedical space. As a site of uncertain knowledge—of not knowing if a treatment would stick—it was porous in that it had selectively empty spaces. This allowed for multiple disease categories to bubble up in the same person and for several types of therapies to be applied to one body (sometimes additively, sometimes synergistically, sometimes in tension). My aim is to elaborate the morals, somatic experiences, and techniques of healing that absorb each other as the domain of the metabolism grounds clinical practice.

Collateral Care, Collateral Damage

How might absorption as a set of lines of relation between persons and objects matter for therapy? To address this question, I first take a closer look at clinics as spaces of relation. Some of these relations are interpersonal, as persons arrive to therapy on their own accord or, reluctantly, at the insistence of (and often accompanied by) family members. Caregivers would diagnose and treat a patient; this person might disappear but often cycled back into the clinic for follow-up and recalibration of orders. Relations of time also defined the clinic. For a person with diabetes, somatic schedules matter. Beta cells in the pancreas are diminishing, and therapy must accommodate that dynamic. Quotidian schedules matter, too: patients have work and study, and so any diets or pills or insulin injections must be integrated with time in mind. Time matters as therapy passes in and out of the day and of the body.

Absorption is never a simple matter of moving one substance or action into another without collateral effect (see Carsten 2001 on the many ways that "substance" can be deployed in anthropology). Insulin goes into the body, but the blood that comes out for sugar testing has mostly likely already interacted with added insulin. Pills are swallowed, but they also garnish the table between the doctor and patient, even as pharmaceuticals course through the body of the person holding the blister pack. In the foot clinic, toes fall off. Feet and even whole limbs are scheduled for amputation. Here the body stops its actions of absorbing things from the world outside the skin. In a frame of gross exchange, the body alone or the amputating surgeon sends the body part back into the world outside. None of these exchanges are equal or evenly hydraulic. The question about metabolic living that can be addressed at the site of this bind is how much collateral damage and repair is ultimately bearable.

My thinking about lines derives from Julie Livingston's concept of a "therapeutic pipeline," which she describes as the often cyclical, resource-constrained, and deeply personal therapeutic trajectory entailed in chronic illness. Livingston's ethnography of cancer in Botswana shows how empathy, understanding, indifference, and impatience charge clinical spaces. A focus on the different therapies people do and do not receive offers a more precise account of patients and care providers than too simple accounts of patients as medicalized subjects and caregivers as biomedical automatons. Therapeutic pipelines allow us to follow the work it takes for people and their ailments to traverse clinical care. In the clinics I observed in my own research, such pipelines were overloaded with both substances and solutions, and the work of therapy was the work of getting things to sluice through. It seemed that each person—patient, dietitian, accompanying family member, physician, even administrative staff members—was invested in directing the traffic between the material world, full of harms and healing, and a state of better metabolic balance. Whether through diets, counseling, or drugs, there were deep investments in keeping fat out or sugars low. It was differing visions of the metabolism—how it worked in a healthy person, how it might "get sick," how it might be repaired through dieting—that cemented the hope and discipline of experts and the bodies they sought to repair. These visions were prescriptively linear, even though everyone understood well the complexity of digestive and circulatory systems (that is, that guts and blood vessels were anything but straight lines). Nonetheless, linearity was the best way to make sense of a short, intensive clinical consult: what could the doctor and patient do in those ten minutes? They could follow an algorithm. A line offered some help and hope. Where it led was a question to be dealt with downstream.

With so many lines crisscrossing the hallway, the room of the clinic, the courtyard of the hospital outside, and the trajectories of drugs, I began to see therapy as a bundle of lines; more specifically, as a matter of *collateral*. "Collateral" as an adjective may be defined as something on the same side; something parallel. As a noun, it is something pledged, such as money. It is a term in anthropology about kinship, referring to the siblings and descendants of siblings in relation to a given person ("collateral kin" is here different from "lineal kin"). "Collateral" is also a term in the science of anatomy that describes supplementary support structures. Blood vessels or ligaments can be defined as collateral to a given anatomical structure because they support it subordinately. A clogged main blood vessel, for instance, may have collateral circulation develop around it because smaller, often adjacent vessels circulate blood to circumvent the passage in something like a backup loop. "Collateral" is a term I use to make sense of the multiple lines and knots that open up bodies to therapy. I take lines of therapy quite literally, because for my interlocutors, a line down the hallway as an entry to receive drug prescriptions from Dr. Chitre or a line down the leg toward a thickened spot in an artery in Dr. Samant's clinic ultimately led to different conditions of living with metabolic illness.

This chapter has its own line, a narrative one that arcs from food (through a discussion of nutrition and dietetics) to drugs (through a discussion of Trinity Hospital's diabetes clinic, with Dr. Chitre prescribing pharmaceuticals) to amputation (through a discussion of the other side of the hallway in Trinity, in Dr. Samant's foot clinic). The concept of collateral inflects my narrative approach to this chapter. As an observer sitting next to dietitians and physicians in clinical settings, I watched patients enter the room, undergo a time-delimited consult, and then exit, only to be replaced by the next case. I relay the work that providers did to manage the heaped load of patients and the interloping anthropologist. I saw lines outside clinic doors, and once inside a formal clinical space, I watched the coming and going of patients in lines. These sessions produced field notes with cases linked by malady or complaint. Gathering together observations on clinical cases is a common data collection method and subsequent narrative trope in medical anthropological studies centered in clinic settings. I follow that tradition here, in part, but I also want to highlight its limitations and strengths in an attempt to narrate the power of therapies that take absorbing bodies as rationale and relation.

## Lose Weight, Gain Life

*A forty-year-old man, Mr. Bala, comes in to the diet counseling room with his wife. He explains to Usha, the dietitian, that his hypertension, obesity, and diabetes were the result of a too busy work schedule that didn't allow regularly timed meals and thus made him feel "slow." "Your sugars and your cholesterol are out of control," Usha explained. "You have to eat something, you can't starve yourself. If you increase your veg intake, your hunger will go away [apka bhuk khatam ho jaega] and you'll get back to normal." As she wrote an updated diet regimen, Mr. Bala's wife interrupted to ask, "A family doctor told us about some syndrome? A syndrome that he has?" Without looking up, Usha answered, "Metabolic syndrome. That's what he's got." "Metabolic syndrome," Mrs. Bala repeated to herself softly. "That's it." Mr. Bala came into the clinic already convinced that his meal timings were the root of his "slowness." He left with instructions that it was his own responsibility to normalize his metabolism by eating more regularly. In the clinic, his malady and his metabolism were nudged inward, as Usha instructed his wife on the possibilities of possessing a metabolism just as much as he possessed disease or food itself: That's what he's got.*

As with much of my clinical fieldwork, my opportunity to undertake long-term observations in Dr. Bhatt's clinic emerged after meeting him at a national medical conference. His clinic was very close to Manuli, and I asked Dr. Bhatt if I could interview him and his staff of on-site dietitians. He offered even more: the opportunity to regularly conduct observations in the clinic during evening consults because he also worked at several hospitals during the day. Dr. Bhatt was a metabolic disease specialist, so his patients were diagnosed with metabolic disorders such as diabetes, hypothyroidism, iodine deficiency, and polycystic ovarian disorder (PCOD). Sometimes, though, a patient would receive a diagnosis simply of "obesity." In addition to a waiting room that was eternally jam-packed, the clinic had two main consultation rooms, one for the dietitian and one for Dr. Bhatt. It was customary to remove one's shoes at the door, and often the door could barely open because of the mountain of shoes lined up inside it. I learned to estimate the evening's patient load by how easily the door would open. It took work to pass through the door. The door offered a steady material testament to the unresolved question of how many patients a clinic can take on in a city suffused with persons under their own internal metabolic duress.

A patient first saw a dietitian who would solicit a dietary recall and suggest possible changes based on both the recall and the patient's recorded diagnosis (either by Dr. Bhatt on a previous visit or by another a physician the patient had previously visited). The patient would then return to the waiting room until it was his or her turn to see Dr. Bhatt. The doctor would signal his readiness for the next patient by pressing a button that triggered a loud buzzer in the waiting room. The buzz was a sign for Ram, the man at the front desk, to wave the next patient in. Ram was always on the phone scheduling appointments and listening to patients explain complex itineraries of lab work and other physician consults. With the phone handle always appended to his ear and cradled in a shoulder, Ram communicated deftly with people in the room around him via hand waves: "Go!" and "Doctor's not ready for you yet!" and "Don't leave yet—you need to pay." (I believe that in the half year I spent in the clinic, the only times we actually spoke were when I phoned in to ask a logistical question; in person, we simply gestured to each other.)

Given my interest in diet and nutrition, Dr. Bhatt first assigned me to sit alongside the dietitians. Over the course of six months in his clinic I shadowed two, Usha and Rashmi.[1] The rhythm of the clinic ultimately came down to cases: short interactions, then the buzzer that signaled that Dr. Bhatt was ready for the patient. What was compelling to me about Dr. Bhatt's clinic was how nutritional therapy came first, a prototherapy before the pharmaceutical and clinical consult he would give. In this way, the care of nutrition held the metabolic clinic together through a blending of food and drugs—a person-object arrangement invested with the hope of long-term, lasting effects on illness. Connecting someone's weight gain to a specific disease opened up the possibility for the "best" therapy, according to the dietitians. Personalizing treatment was key. The dietitian would begin with a subset of possible foods for therapy based on diagnostic categories; then through individual consults would further tinker with the regimen. On the side of the dietitian's desk was a paper organizer for photocopies of different diets, each tailored to a different condition: Obesity Diet, Insulin Sensitivity Diet, No-Salt Diet, Thyroid Diet. In addition to the elements of these individual diets, dietitians often would "prescribe" corporate food products, thus integrating packaged foods into the diet sciences they asserted. Even when food company products were in plain sight, however, they were always secondary to what dietitians considered the most pressing problem at hand: a noncompliant patient whose injured metabolism was no excuse for "bad" dietary decisions.

The nutrition counseling room was cramped, with just enough space for two chairs on the consultation side, separated from chairs for patients and their accompanying family members by a small table. One side of the room was crammed with medical and dietetics journals. The only other available space was taken up by a life-sized cutout of an obese man. The cutout had a built-in height measurement ruler, and at its base was an outlined area for a bathroom scale (figure 4.1). Ostensibly, someone could step on a scale to learn his weight and simultaneously have his height measured to yield the two components of a BMI calculation. While staring at the smiling fat man, the person saw a sign at the top of the measurement stick suggesting "Lose Weight. Gain Life." The cutout also had a clock, in the shape of a heart, where the man's heart belonged. "Time is ticking" was printed above the clock, and there was a small container for pamphlets describing the sponsor of the cutout: Xenical, a weight-loss drug. The cutout was a technology of measurement, an advertisement for pharmaceutical approaches to weight loss, and perhaps most intensely, a visual connector between fatness and a bodily timeline at risk of stopping too early.

Despite the life-sized interactive drug ad that dominated the room, I quickly learned that prescriptions and proscriptions in this room centered on eating food. A patient would enter the room, sit down, and hand over a folder of laboratory reports, referral papers from other doctors, and past dietary recalls and food regimens if the patient had come before. Lab reports were compulsory, meaning that patients arrived having already spent money and blood and urine to produce baseline information. Often these lab reports came from the diagnostics company ScanTech (see chapter 1). If there was no lab report, there was no consult. "I can't do anything for you without reports," was the standard line the dietitian would deliver to the unfortunate few who showed up empty-handed. Sometimes patients would bring their medications and slide them across the table: insulin

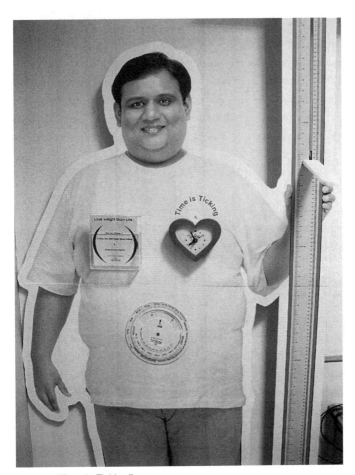

**FIG. 4.1** "Time is Ticking"

pens or metformin tablets for diabetics, thyroid medication for patients
with hypothyroidism. A ceremonious dump of *things* on the table began
the counseling encounter. Usha and Rashmi would proceed to scrutinize
the paper records and looked first at key indicators: serum glucose levels
from the last fasting blood sugar test, levels of indicative hormones, and
past diets they or their colleagues might have prescribed. This quick look
bridged multiple sciences, such as biochemistry and pharmacology, with
something to say about the metabolism, and landed them in the domain of
medical nutrition therapy.[2] Usually patients had been diagnosed by their
family doctor, so there was a diagnostic category to work with, such as
"diabetic" or "thyroid patient," and the diet recall helped the dietitian fill
in the specifics. In circumstances in which no prior clinical diagnosis was

apparent, the dietitians would do their best to diagnose by reading the lab report's assessments of HbA1c (a measurement of blood glucose over the three months prior to a test on a blood sample, used to give a more generalized picture of glucose levels than a measurement of a single day) or levels of creatinine (used to measure kidney function).

An integral part of the counseling was the initial diagnostic diet recall, a personalized and historical line of ingestion. The dietitian would instruct the patient, "Tell me everything you eat, from morning until night." Depending on the patient's "problem," the dietitian would pull out a specific diet sheet and fill it in for the patient, both questioning and explaining directives for every meal of the day. Some patients did this with no problem; others were slower and less clear on the recall part. The dietitian would prod: "Breakfast? Lunch? Tea? Dinner? Snack before bed?" The rhythms of the day pegged the rhythms of eating and made the temporality of the metabolism legible in terms of meals eaten or skipped.

The diet recall spoke volumes about social class. Who packed whose *dabba* (lunch box), who ate only on the street, what kinds of vegetables or meats were regular parts of the diet, the distance and time commuting between home and work, and the kind of labor at home that structured mealtimes all were key elements of these alimentary chronicles. Many patients explained that their primary obstacle to weight loss was a lack of time to think about what they ate. Diya, a twenty-five-year-old who worked at a public relations firm, came in one evening and laid out the problems immediately: "My hours at the office are damned crazy. I like my tea sweet. I drink lots of Tang during the day—that's wrong, I think? I'm pure veg, so no eggs or anything. I eat a huge dinner in the evening; I'm Gujarati, it's what we do." Rashmi patiently asked Diya about her "lifestyle": Did she ever walk anywhere? (No, she went to work in a rickshaw). Could she pack and carry a lunch to work? ("Listen, I don't have the time. Most people in my office call out for Subway sandwiches.") In spite of her protests, Diya confessed that she was willing to change, to do whatever it took. "Anything, whatever you say, I can give up anything . . . even rice," she said. Her only condition for change was that it fit her work schedule, a condition expressed in similar terms by the patient who followed Diya: "If I have the time, I eat; if I don't, I don't," she said.

Portion sizes were as important as the substantive contents they measured. The dietitian would refer to different-sized cups or spoons lying on the desk and ask patients to point to the size that corresponded to the amount of rice they ate in a meal or how much oil they cooked with.

Rashmi often used laminated cutouts of drawings of different sized chapatis for this purpose; Usha asked patients to draw with their finger on the table the size of chapatis in a typical meal. They made regular use of a set of *katoras* (small bowls) on the table and asked patients to show how many servings of rice they ate. Thus, along with laboratory measurements and predetermined diagnoses, food measurements played a central role in ascertaining basic information about patients.

Patient complaints rarely centered on their biomedical diagnosis but instead concerned matters of balance and metabolic speed. Balance was a concern at the scale of meals as much as it was a sense of inner bodily pace. For example, Sundays were an important day for "indulgence," when "rich" (*charbi*, "oily") foods like meat curries or creamy, buttery vegetarian dishes would be eaten. Many Hindus identified as semivegetarian but avoided labeling themselves "non-veg," which to them was too closely identified with meat eating and, by extension for some, too constitutionally similar to Muslims or Catholics. They broke their vegetarianism frequently on Saturdays during meals eaten outside the home, often at local Indian-Chinese or Punjabi outlets. For Hindus, different days counted as fasting days when non-veg food was prohibited—Tuesday, Thursday, and Saturday were all possibilities, depending on the lineage of Hinduism an individual or family followed at the time. Matters of speed also delineated the relationship between meals and their digestion. Patients continually complained of body systems that were too fast or too slow, mostly too slow for the patients who were overweight and/or diabetic. "Metabolism" was mentioned less often than the English word "slowness." A frequent refrain was "It feels like things have really been slowing down inside" (*Andar se, lagta hai ki bahut slowness ho gaya hai*). *Andar se*, "from the inside," located the problem inside the skin but also gave it directionality. These concerns with balance were compelling for me to observe because they were possibilities to see the overlap of multiple medical systems and the overlap of physiology with directions of body-environment force.[3]

Sometimes a quality of foods, such as fattiness, mattered most. Other consults revealed the importance of "hot" and "cold" foods, general markers of Indian medical systems premised on the humors (see, e.g., Leslie 1976; Alter 2014; Langford 2002; Ecks 2014; Nichter 2001).[4] As described in this book's introduction, my path to metabolism did not extensively cover the grounds of Ayurveda, Unani, or other nonallopathic medical systems as thoroughly as it did systems of biomedicine. Occasionally, though, patients in an allopathic (biomedical) setting like Dr. Bhatt's had concurrent or previous homeopathic treatments on hand. This could possibly be understood instrumentally, as a matter of medical pluralism. But in cases of these patients and others who had no explicit "traditional" medical engagement to speak of, there still seemed to be an Ayurvedic understanding of the body's sensitivity to environments reverberating in a biomedical space. For example, the matter of bodily constitution often came up in discussions with dietitians, a matter that grounds Ayurvedic assessments of body type. Patients would express self-diagnosed feelings of difficulty or ease in digesting certain foods—again, an Ayurvedic resonance at work. Due to the structure of my own research methods, I could not corroborate the lines of healing systems that stretched across a given patient-nutritionist encounter. This was especially tough given that the nutritional diagnosis was a prerequisite for a pharmaceutical one. Patients did not leave after seeing the nutritionist, and indeed they often seemed annoyed that they had to pass through the nutritional pipeline before they saw the "real" expert, Dr. Bhatt. Nonetheless, in these moments, one could appreciate different kinds of lines of healing systems shooting through the nutritional counseling room. If the "time is ticking" sign made manifest the presence of pharmaceutical companies, the dietary recall and attendant commentary made it possible to trace the imprint of other healing systems that converged on the metabolism.

Conversationally, I never heard the terms *sthul* or *atisthula*, the Sanskrit-derived Ayurvedic terms for "obesity," in clinical observations. However, I did have two key Ayurvedic encounters. The first involved a presentation I observed on Ayurvedic approaches to obesity at a major medical conference on obesity in Mumbai. The presenter, an Ayurvedic physician, laid out modes of knowing and treating obesity according to Ayurveda. He said obesity could be caused by excess intake of food (*atisampurnaad*), especially of foods that were heavy (such as red meat), sweet (such as milk), cold (such as ice cream), or oily. Certain bodily states could factor in, too, including lack of exercise (*avyayamaad*), lack of sexual activity (*avyavayaad*), sleeping during the day (*divaswapnaad*), or genetic predisposition (*bijaswabhavaat*). The presenter reminded the audience that according to his practice, a thin person is easier to treat than an obese person (*karsham eva varam sthaulyat*).

The second encounter was with an Ayurvedic doctor who was quite active in an Indian association of doctors (mostly biomedical) researching diabetes and obesity. Dr. Vishali had the unique perspective in this case of being trained in Ayurveda but now holding a leadership position in an organization that included India's leading biomedical and public health specialists (including surgeons). I often asked her to parse the exchanges between Ayurveda and biomedicine that might be occurring in clinical practice or in the minds of her patients (she ran her own Ayurvedic clinic in the Mumbai suburbs). She found allopathic and homeopathic/naturopathic modes of healing consonant and fluid. Her best gloss was that in matters of diagnosis, Ayurveda was excellent; in matters of treatment, biomedicine and Ayurveda could together effect a positive change. For example, she reminded me that according to certain principles laid out in the *Charaka Samhita* and *Sushruta Samhita* texts (the two key texts for contemporary Ayurvedic practice), a body can be understood in some senses to be like a watch that one winds each day by following certain repetitive processes of self-care. One must wind the watch, or it won't reset, she explained. "Time is ticking" here took on a different-than-drugs but still urgent sense, as the lack of reset could result in several symptoms that could add up to the collateral category of obesity in an Ayurvedic diagnostic account: pendulous abdomen, fatigue, difficulties in sex, weakness, bad body odor, oversweating, excessive appetite, breathlessness, lethargy, and sleep apnea.

As a key member of the Indian association concerned with obesity, Dr. Vishali was also part of nationwide clinical studies of obesity and diabetes treatment programs. One of these programs was multipronged, meaning that patients in the program first saw a biomedical physician for basic diagnostics (BMI, waist-hip ratio, body fat percentage), then a physiotherapist, who assessed and prescribed possible postural and exercise changes, then a nutritionist, then to Dr. Vishali for yoga and Ayurveda treatment. Patients would stay in the program for two to three months. Dr. Vishali was pleased with the results: significant loss in weight among patients, and better blood glucose profiles. Thus, while Ayurveda informed her work and thinking, her professional practice could never be isolated to a particular modality of practice and knowing. She called her approach "multidisciplinary," with the "multi" here signaling several systems of healing as well as Ayurveda's encounters with a global public health concern.[5]

Instead of specific healing systems, organs often surfaced out of the conversations around bodily constitution in Dr. Bhatt's nutritional counseling room. For instance, a fifty-seven-year-old woman in a bright green *salwar kameez* came into the consult room with her daughter and husband. Her eyes were very bulgy, which indicated to Usha (along with the doctor's diagnosis in the folder) that she was "a thyroid patient." "My only problem is my eyes. . . . I get headaches," she said. Usha parsed her diet with her and suggested that she take some protein powder. "But I don't want to put on weight," the woman protested. "But we're pure vegetarians." "But I already put almond and *pista* [pistachio] and *elaichi* [cardamom] in my milk." Protest after protest. She then asked about the temperature effects of fruits as they would affect her body and thus her systemic response in terms of the thyroid condition. "What about citrus?" she asked. "What about *thandai* [a cold, sweet, milk-based drink]?" "*Chalega* [fine]," Usha said. Usha wanted to emphasize protein; the woman wanted to emphasize temperature. Usha's compromise was to suggest low-fat milk. The woman wrinkled her face: "I don't like the smell." In her household, they drank Amul Gold, a packaged full-fat milk. The woman's daughter took this impasse as an opportunity to add some of her mother's offenses for Usha's adjudication: "She eats chocolates, you know." Usha mentioned the importance of physical activity. The daughter wanted to know if her mom needed to join a gym. Her mother and Usha settled on something less hot: some basic yoga. "I did it once, yoga," the mother said quietly. She could do it again. The balance of substances mattered, temperature-wise and otherwise. This balance could be undone and reconstituted in environments of stress, indulgence, and exercise. The line of therapy here moved from thyroid to metabolism to mother-daughter cross-talk to the feminized aesthetics of body size and would have a temporary stop in Usha's prescription sheet as a set of foods to pursue or avoid taking in.

Even as it allowed a "big tent" for multiple understandings of bodily operations, the metabolism's distributional possibilities also could strengthen biomedical authority. One evening, a thirty-one-year-old woman named Mrs. Qadeer sat quietly across from Usha, who clicked her tongue as she looked over the woman's records. Mrs. Qadeer was deemed "obese" by Dr. Bhatt according to her records, and her weight gain stemmed from PCOD. Usha solicited a meal-by-meal food intake recall from Mrs. Qadeer and concluded afterward that she didn't seem to be eating very much. "Don't skip meals," Usha told her. "You're torturing your body. The torture is lowering your basal metabolic rate." Mrs. Qadeer expressed surprise at this conclusion. "Actually, my body is yo-yoing [*mera body yo-yo ho gaya hai*]," she said. For Mrs. Qadeer, body weight was an elastic line. "It goes down, and it goes up. I'm afraid if I eat [my weight] will go up the next day. I'm losing patience. After three months, I lost three kilos, which the doctor said was good, but I didn't think it was enough, so I quit." Usha scolded her for her impatience and ignorance: "You don't know what's going on from

the inside, right?" (*Andar se aapko nahi pata hai ki kya ho raha rai, right?*)
"You should listen to *me*." From Usha's perspective, Mrs. Qadeer simply
couldn't understand the metabolism's complexities and should leave it
to medical (specifically, nutritional) authority to guide that understanding from the interior outward. First and foremost on the list was to understand that the metabolism was inside the body. Its workings may be
mysterious and may be realized in terms of hydraulics and humors, but
Usha reinforced the point that as a dietitian she was the one who would
handle Mrs. Qadeer's yo-yo. The metabolism could be highly individuated
in terms of its problems and potential therapies, but its collateral dramas
also invited in experts to help navigate porosity.

The expert could be the nutritionist, but patients had plenty to say
about their own condition, too. This was apparent when a patient would
come to the clinic to specifically discuss metabolism in terms of a unique,
possessive bodily system. For example, a woman in her early forties named
Anjali arrived one evening and announced that her weight was steadily increasing. She also had taken Obimet, an antidiabetic medication. Obimet
is one of the trade names in India of metformin, one of the most widely
used first-line drugs for diabetics, which inhibits glucose production. Anjali understood that she was taking a medicine that targeted one substance
(sugar) but discussed it in terms of another substance: fat. After relaying
her complaint about weight gain, she implicated the Obimet as a thus-
far-ineffective treatment: she called the drug "her fat loss pill that didn't
work." On her own, she stopped the medication. She did this because, as
she put it, "I have really strenuous workouts" at the gym and during seaside walks on Carter Road in the evenings. Anjali continued to sketch a
constellation of promising therapies that had no effect in her body, inasmuch as effect was measurable by weight gained and lost. "I'm doing all
the right things," she said. "I'm not eating egg yolks, I eat *jowar* and *bajra*
[sorghum and pearl millet], I take protein shakes. I'm a vegetarian. I'm
losing motivation, because I'm the only one gaining weight at my gym,
but I work my ass off. It's not like I'm lazing around, eating pizza. People
keep telling me that it's good to speed up my metabolism, but I'm gaining
weight, so to hell with it. When your jeans are getting tighter, and button-
ing them is a major achievement . . . it's just that losing weight was easier
for me years ago."

Usha suggested that she eat more foods with antioxidants to speed up
her metabolism. After all, Dr. Bhatt would be in charge of discussing the
ins and outs of metformin; it was Usha's job to take all problems, includ-

ing pharmacokinetic ones, and translate them into food. So Usha detailed for Anjali all the foods high in antioxidants, especially leafy greens. "But will I lose weight?" Anjali pressed. Usha tried to explain that the increased speed of the metabolism was a "goal," if there was any, rather than weight loss. Anjali repeated that nothing she did seemed to attain that goal. Nothing in her hands could "speed up" her body. "I'm still gaining weight. It's the weight," she insisted. She mentioned a therapy she heard about from friends that involved wearing an oxygen mask for short "oxygen treatments" rumored to burn fat. Usha promptly told her this was *bhakwas* (nonsense) and wrote out a diet for her.

While the "complaints" from patients centered on problems with balance and internal speed, the clinical setting allowed the dietitians to engage the fuzziness of the metabolism by emphasizing specific comorbid conditions that accompanied weight gain. My observations were certainly partial, but I was struck by the number of women who came into the clinic needing to lose excess weight gained through polycystic ovarian disorder (PCOD) and thyroid disorders. Rashmi told me once that PCOD has no real cure, and so the easiest way to treat it is to encourage women to lose weight. The weight loss would metabolically "rebalance" the system and decrease the severity of related symptoms. The challenge, Rashmi said, was to convince women to change eating habits (not, as one might observe from a different vantage point, to take their medicine—these patients were also often on Obimet). Compliance was an uphill struggle for nearly every patient I observed, and thus while I wondered if Rashmi was critiquing a perceived stubbornness of women's bodies, in truth she held *all* persons and bodies as already stubborn upon entry into the room.

As with the example of Mrs. Qadeer, sometimes prescribing a diet required direct explanation of responsibility and medical authority. With a twenty-one-year-old patient with PCOD, for example, Rashmi simply told her, "Nothing will change for you as long as you're not eating healthy. So just do what I say—it's because you're not eating well that you're like this." The young woman, who came in with her mother, expressed disdain at the prospect of eating more vegetables. When Rashmi emphasized that the woman needed more fiber in her diet to feel full, the young woman's mother wrung her hands and asked if chicken had fiber in it. This question precipitated a series of volleys across the table. "Salad!" Rashmi declared. "She needs to eat salad!" "Can I put mayonnaise on it, at least?" the young woman asked Rashmi sweetly. "And can I have Chinese food? I love pizza and burgers, but I can resist those. But not Chinese food." Rashmi scratched out more prescriptions on the diet sheet and suggested that if she absolutely *had* to eat Chinese, that she try and get something stir-fried or steamed. Rashmi didn't bother negotiating with the next patient. When the woman gently confessed, "Everything's gone haywire, hasn't it? My reports must be bad," Rashmi looked her in the eyes with a calm intensity and said plainly, "That's because you're not following the diet. When you follow, you lose weight and get back to normal." The metabolically meek would inherit the diet.

A key element of prescribing diets was to suggest specific branded foods. Usha and Rashmi each had their favorite, I learned. Usha preferred Saffola rice, a brand of low-glycemic-index rice (see chapter 3). Usually pitching it as a "new" rice, she suggested that patients try it out. Sometimes, spare pamphlets from Saffola were on the desk in the room, offering patients information on Saffola rice and other products in the "healthy heart" line such as "healthy" safflower cooking oils. Rashmi was a little more suspicious of Saffola rice. A patient asked her specifically about it one night: "I'm taking [Saffola rice] now, can I still take it? It's better than regular rice, yes?" Rashmi thought it might be worth exploring brown rice for this patient. But the woman pressed her on the Saffola product, claiming that she already had bought it and felt "lighter" when she ate it. "It's been tested by the drug people, right?" she asked Rashmi. Rashmi had to agree: "Yes, the FDA tested it; they say it has a low glycemic index. You might as well just use it." For this patient, Saffola was not merely a food but a drug to "take." The absorptive language of "taking" and food's pharmaceutical definition emerged from an institutional backing (via the FDA) and from personalized, expert approval (via Rashmi's nod). Rashmi herself preferred to "prescribe" Treptin biscuits, which were protein-enhanced, artificially sweetened cookies appropriate for diabetics. She told me that she liked them because patients always wanted something to snack on, and they grew tired of the oil-free, somewhat tasteless snacks that she generally suggested. The special biscuits were like treats, with added nutritional benefits. In the language and action of prescription, Usha and Rashmi could observe and manage absorption in the clients, although never quite as fully as they wanted to.

These counseling visits illustrate the power of diets to coordinate the uncertainties of the metabolism. Diets patched up the cracks between dietitians and patients who couldn't be trusted to eat right (*sahi*) and to relay eating truthfully in a context of bodily operations no one precisely understood. Diets worked as a way to keep patients answerable to an authority that cut through ambiguity: nutritional expertise penned in every handwritten diet prescription that Usha and Rashmi slid across the table. In this sense, diets were something to be taken as a therapy, much as one would consume a pill. Taken properly, they could bring a patient "back to normal"—but taken lazily or partially, they had little effect, if any. But all the correct consumption in the world could not predict the moves the inner force called "the metabolism" might make. Absorption did not follow a checklist.

In a strict sense, dietitians operated much like Margaret Mead's "nutritional gatekeepers," the housewives who dutifully regulate meals that Mead (1943) describes in her extensive studies of eating habits in post–World War II families in the United States. But even more than regulation, dietitians worked to pass food through patients' bodies in specific combinations, in hopes of metabolic repair. Put differently, dietitians stepped into the ring of the illness environment in order to change the terms of absorption and to distribute the terms of metabolism as clinical science from the singular form of instrumental, individuated consumption. The implementation of the diet had to originate with the patient, but her knowledge was linked intimately to the dietitian's expertise and to the hope that the metabolism would "take" to a dietary prescription. The moral force of the diet, along with its science, were matters of concern in these rooms. Willpower may have been the ingénue, but the metabolism was behind the scenes. Where the metabolism overdetermined the possible reasons for weight gain, diets could channel some authoritative clarity and slim the body in the process. The metabolism and the mouth were partial filters, and nutritional gatekeeping was a constant negotiation with what the body could possibly absorb.

Simultaneously, nutrition worked as an expert science of the metabolism. I understood this most clearly when a young man, about thirty, came in during Usha's shift, accompanied by his wife. The diet recall evinced that he never ate outside food: "*sab ghar pe*" (everything at home), he said. Food at home, with the metabolisms affected therein, became the site of investigation. Usha asked him to cut out his morning toast. "But it's brown bread," his wife said. Brown bread, with the promise of whole wheat, was always an appeal in the clinic. Here was a place where patients knew a thing or two about nutrition and its bodily effects. Usha and other nutritionists had a scripted response, understanding but direct: brown bread was a sugary trick. Like many diet foods, it put persons into a comfort zone where a single food anchored hopes for metabolic balance. That comfort unraveled once one sat across from Usha. "Brown bread is 20 percent whole wheat flour, but the rest is *maida* [white flour]," Usha said. "But the doctor recommended it," the wife said, frustrated. She was referring not to Dr. Bhatt but to a neighborhood doctor she had taken her husband to see before. Again I saw the plurality of care, the ways that one troubled metabolism became the task of others in the household. The wife and the husband both thought that starting the day with brown bread rather than white toast put him on a better path. They were not unknowing; they were following a doctor's orders. Usha was unsurprised and sympathetic. "I know," she said of the incongruity that a doctor would err in matters as simple as toast. "I know. But nutritionists know better than doctors."

### "We're not sick, we're addicted"

Usha's claim that "nutritionists know better than doctors" emphasized that metabolic science as a clinical science required specialists in nutrition. Admittedly, I did not find dietitians and their operating science to always be held in terribly high regard by those under their care. For instance, on the train one morning, three high schoolers climbed into the carriage I was sitting in and took seats opposite me. There was a girl accompanied by two boys, one of them short and a bit chubby, the other tall and lanky. Settling into their seats, they compared lunches. From his shirt pocket the tall boy took out a packet of black candy pebbles, called *fatafat* (quick, on-the-go) candy according to the label. The girl took out a small packet of Good Day Biscuits and reached over to take one of the little black pearls of candy. The lanky boy jokingly warned her: "It's rat shit!" They read the ingredients together out loud: rock salt, common salt, glucose, *jeera* (cumin) powder. "It *tastes* like rat shit," she replied. The chubby boy rummaged through his backpack and took out his lunch tiffin. With disgust, the girl pointed to the contents of the lunch box: "What's *that*?" I glanced over as the boy dissected it in front of the two others. It was a sandwich of white bread with tomatoes and paneer inside, spread with green chutney on the bread. "They want me to eat this for *breakfast!*" he said ruefully. "This is what it's like to be a fat kid, *yaar*. My mom took me to a *dietitian*." This was expert punishment, planned and executed. To be *mota* (fat) was to be forced into the domain of nutritional science.

Dietitians were quite familiar with this disdain. When I recounted the episode on the train to dietitians I interviewed, they recognized how they were often the first stop on the train of expert consults (prior to biomedical physicians). This roughly consigned nutritionists, along with homeopaths and Ayurvedic doctors, to a group that collectively produced knowledge and advice that, compared with doctors, cost less to seek out and usually less to fulfill, given that foods were the target of complaint and intervention. Further, nutritionists were the first to attest that the equation of weight loss was far more complex than simply recommending a diet and waiting for the kilos to disappear due to a sluice of willful compliance. They disputed the sober linearity of this kind of diet thinking. Lines were part of their work, but they knew that it took finesse to understand and apply trajectory.

Watching Usha and Rashmi opened up many questions for me about the kind of training they received and how they came to be placed in Dr. Bhatt's clinic. I was curious about the kinds and content of knowledge areas they drew on in order to assert that a metabolism was not right and required intervention to effect bodily change. The relation between prescription and nutritional knowledge seemed tied to occupational history. Rashmi, for instance, had worked previously at a slimming center, where no doctor was present. Usha's previous jobs had all been similar to the one she had with Dr. Bhatt: as the consulting nutritionist alongside an endocrinologist, diabetologist, or general medical practitioner. They kept in contact with former classmates from their college and graduate program; some worked with Ayurvedic doctors, some worked in hospitals, and some had branched out on their own to operate home-based consultation services. Usha and Rashmi had both graduated from one of Mumbai's most established nutrition education programs at a women's university not far from Dr. Bhatt's office. I sought out the chair of the Nutrition Department, Dr. Srinivasan, to better understand the forms of knowledge I saw deployed in the small consult room. Dr. Srinivasan did her undergraduate studies in India and received her PhD from a prominent nutrition science program in the United States. She had conducted research on clinical nutrition in both settings and knew the ins and outs of the attendant politics of university research. Further, she had type 2 diabetes herself. She was in a unique position to reflect on the passages of food and knowledge that made the metabolism into a clinical construct.

I first asked Dr. Srinivasan to sketch the differences between the fields of nutrition and dietetics in India, because I heard the terms used so often and so interchangeably. Nutritionists, she explained, "deal with all aspects of food related to nutrients." This includes matters of food processing, what happens to nutrients during cooking, their individual and related functions, and importantly, "how they are metabolized in the body." Thus *nutritionists* would be the ones to think through the problems and opportunities posed by the interface of food and genomics that conditioned a conundrum like the thin-fat Indian (see chapter 1). Nutritionists in her definition had a more population-scale view of food science, thus the field of "public nutrition" was a coherent one. Persons in this field studied large-scale issues of, as she put it, "metabolism and toxicity" and did so with the aim of alleviating malnutrition at all levels of severity.

*Dietitians*, by contrast, "are more into applying" nutritional science and specifically do so by counseling patients. If nutrition was the science, dietetics was the art, she suggested. Her department has a separate trajectory for each field. The focus on training dietitians is a focus on how to work with patients—a clinical, one-on-one, practical science of counseling. Dietitians draw on nutritional knowledge, but they and nutritionists do so in different occupational spaces. Dietitians would be placed in clinics (like Usha and Rashmi), or put in charge of kitchens at a hospital to make sure that there were food options for patients with a range of needs (e.g., low-salt, high-fiber, low-fat). Where the metabolism was concerned, "dietetics focuses on the diet of the patient," she explained. As a therapeutic art, it required study of basic sciences, specialized applications (e.g., diets in pediatric, geriatric, oncological, or intensive-care units), and internships to understand the organizational structures of clinics and hospitals and how nutritional knowledge can be embedded. This was all with the understanding that while many of the graduates from the dietetics program would work in health care institutions, many would also go on to work individually as private consultants (often later in their career).

Dr. Srinivasan clarified that the "knowing" part of nutritional knowing must be parsed according to the gendered and classed ways in which the practice of "nutrition" and "dietetics" split in India. She entered the field in the early 1980s, a time when "the dividing line between dietitians and nutritionists was not so fine." This related also to the health care landscape of India, particularly in urban settings. In Mumbai at the time, for instance, there were private and charity hospitals, but primarily it was public hospitals that hired experts in diet. Corporate hospitals were few in number. Later, after her return from the United States, she "began to observe this trend of having all these upper income hospitals increase." The knowledge about rising rates of diabetes was still fractured, but the interest in how nutritionists and dietitians might help doctors was on the rise. Through different trajectories of employment—with nutritionists increasing in university/college settings and dietitians fanning out to work with a single doctor or hospital department—the sciences of dietetics and clinical nutrition took on different shades of purpose. From the research end, Dr. Srinivasan witnessed a split in publication patterns, too. This split was furthered by the ways that the field of nutrition science and its relative of dietetics stratified across gendered, classed lines. Dr. Srinivasan teaches at a women's university with what she called "first-generation learners"—women who are the first in their families to go to college. These women, along with a section of the student body who came from "fairly well off homes," collectively wanted to work in business/corporate settings. This left a vacuum in the jobs in rural areas and urban slums that also needed their expertise, she explained: "I felt that [these students] needed to learn to communicate with every subgroup in society, not just go to this five-star and seven-star hospital or sit in air-conditioned offices in industry, you know? That's not India. India is a huge mix of things, and at the risk of sounding passionate, if you don't do something for the 70 percent [below the poverty line], that section is going to collapse very soon."

Dr. Srinivasan addressed this issue by introducing a required internship component in the curriculum and strongly encouraging the students to split their internship between time in hospitals and time in communities. As lower-class and middle-class women aspired to higher-paying and more prestigious jobs in companies, she wanted to even the field by making practical work among the poorest communities of Mumbai a common ground. Dr. Srinivasan's explanation of the dynamic field of nutrition science in India ended on the note of a lingering element of willpower that she herself explained was difficult to resolve:

*As a diabetic I've analyzed myself. I respond to stress by eating. It takes a lot of effort to analyze yourself—not everybody's willing to think. That's why in the first class [of the nutrition course for first-year students] I ask them "What's the first thing you do when you get inside your home," and they said, "We tell our moms that we are hungry." And then I asked, "Suppose you're going to have some friends or relatives over. What's your mom's first reaction?" They said, "What are we going to give them to eat?" So you see, we're a food-centered society and I told the students that when you tell a patient, "Don't eat this!" the "no" becomes a big attraction. I found that in myself when I knew I couldn't have sweets. I never loved sweets before—but they became like a forbidden fruit—like the apple in the Garden of Eden. And here I am, I know everything about diabetes, at least enough to know the pitfalls of not controlling your blood sugar—yet I violate all the rules. How do you expect a common man to do it?*

Dr. Srinivasan had the vantage point of someone who produced nutrition science, applied it to others, and was subject to it herself. She made it clear that the lines of therapy themselves tangled food and willpower.

I observed such power relations as the centerpiece of metabolism as therapy in the work of one of Mumbai's well-known dietitians, Poorvi. I first encountered Poorvi's therapeutic approach after reading a magazine article she wrote entitled "I looked as though I had walked out of a Nazi concentration camp." The article was a tell-all of her own journey through weight gain and loss and an explanation of her approach to counseling clients based on the concept of food addiction. In the article, Poorvi described her transformation from a healthy child to a food addict, beginning in her early teens when she "had gone from skinny to plump to fat to obese." After trying a host of solutions—naturopathy, massages, laxatives, health farms, high-protein diets—she finally arrived at a doctor's office and stuck to a "sensible" diet that helped her lose weight. However, her rapid weight loss also was accompanied by anorexia and a body that evoked the concentration camp imagery for her. She "became obsessed with the effect food has on our bodies and minds," studied naturopathy, and opened her own independent nutritional counseling practice. In the article, she clearly stated her vision for India, writing, "I want India to wake up, to not follow America in its eating habits—its epidemic of obesity, psychological disorders and preventable life-threatening diseases. We are not the dustbins of the West. Let us rid ourselves of packaged foods and return to real food."

I was compelled by Poorvi's descriptions of addiction and condemnations of packaged foods, particularly in her postcolonial critique of India as the West's "dustbin" for unhealthy, packaged foods. I contacted her to request an interview, and after an initial brief meeting at a restaurant (where she ordered a fruit platter for us), she invited me to visit her home in South Mumbai, where she also runs her nutrition counseling service. I told her that her magazine article had introduced me to her story, and she offered to elaborate on her childhood in the late 1960s, growing up in an upper-middle-class vegetarian Gujarati family. "Nothing was wrong with me as a child; I was born normal, not overweight," she said. But she was "a fussy eater." It would take her an hour to finish a meal, because she ate slowly and carefully. She was also skinny, which became a source of concern for her family. "All mothers have a thing where they need to just nurture more and more, especially when their child is thin, because the sign of health is a child with a big build, not a skinny child," she explained. Pressured by her family to eat more, she took up the habit of eating cheese, drinking milk, and consuming considerable amounts of sugar via powdered flavors added to milk, such as Ovaltine and Horlicks. This had the effect of adding weight, to her family's delight, but it also cultivated a deep attachment to these foods that she was unable to sever. She identified with this mind-set—it was the one that guided her life as an overweight person for nearly twenty years until she had a revelation about what she was putting in her body: "I had absolutely no idea until 2001. Then I thought: Oh my god, the sugar. The sugar. *This* is why I can't concentrate. This is why my brain is a mess. Imagine the calories of it. Imagine the addiction of it."

She saw this addiction to junk food all around her, across all social divisions. Her vegetable seller, a relatively poor man, asked her recently which flavor of Kellogg's Corn Flakes was best to purchase for his finicky daughter. She described a mother from a lower-class family who brought in her twelve-year-old daughter for diet counseling the previous day. The daughter was so obsessed with Maggi brand instant noodles that she refused to eat anything else. "I don't know how to handle her; she throws a tantrum if there's no Maggi," Poorvi recalled the mother saying. Poorvi asked the daughter directly, "Why Maggi? What is it about that food?" The daughter responded simply: "I just need it." To Poorvi, that "need"— an addiction—underlies the rise of diabetes and obesity across social classes in India. She felt that the importance of addiction remained unacknowledged among the medical community. Instead, doctors focused on prescribing drugs or engaging dietitians to promote weight loss through specific foods. Doctors missed the point by using an exclusively biomedical approach. "We're not sick," Poorvi said. "We're addicted. And the drug is food."

Poorvi was correct in her assessment that addiction remained relatively invisible in clinical settings.[6] In all of my observations and interviews, she would be the only person ever to mention addiction, much less focus on it as the fundamental cause of obesity. To Poorvi, food addiction was one of the fundamental causes behind the weight gain in her clients. She posed the food-drug relationship as the problem rather than the solution (as was the case with functional foods). As such, she mapped out a different moral trajectory for her clients, whereby they required a certain kind of responsibility to know the systems of production and marketing that led to desire in the first place. Therapeutic success was measured not just in pounds lost but in knowledge gained, but this was not solely knowledge tightly tied to a doctor's prescriptions or the "nutricentric" knowledge of ingredients. Rather, success required knowledge of the dangers of food companies and their influence over individual willpower. For Poorvi, addiction was another layer to the forces of the metabolism, whereby desire and attachment had morphological consequences. Poorvi prescribed reattachments. She distanced her patients from what she viewed as poisonous substances, such as sugar and fat, "pushed" by food company "dealers." In doing so, she distanced them from the institutions that pushed those substances. Risk was as much about corporate harm as it was a matter of biomedical, nutritional self-knowledge. Persons were answerable to themselves and to food, with no doctor in the equation.[7] Poorvi urged a total rethinking of the attachments that constituted dieting in the first place. To do so required understanding the fluidity between what counts as food and what counts as drug and how the mind and its requisite clinical expertise could be a first-order connector between these domains.[8]

This was not a clean split wherein addiction belonged to the realm of the psychological, on one hand, and weight gain and loss were matters of the material world on the other. Poorvi complicated easy divides between persons and foods, because the question of who nourished whom was her work's target rather than its assumed condition. She encouraged her clients to locate their desire for food in a field of corporatized temptations and inner bodily machinations. Dispassionate responsibility was certainly a moral language for weight loss and gain in her practice. But it had its limits. This was so because overweight patients also sought diagnosis for the dimensions of their weight gain that they deemed to be medical. There was a porous overlap between the attachments of food-drug and person-medicine.

## Trinity Hospital Hallway, Side 1: Getting Control

*A nun in a blue sari, aged sixty-two. "You'll have to take insulin," Dr. Chitre tells her, because her sugars keep rising. The nun came in with a quiet smile but is not happy about this news. "I'll bring it down," she says, pleading. But her sugars are high. "Are you seeing well?" Dr. Chitre asks. "I think so." "You think so? Tell me accurately. When you cross the road, can you see from side to side?" Yes, she can. Dr. Chitre is assertive about insulin: "Your sugars won't come down only with diet, so I'm giving you insulin." She's supposed to check her sugars and if they're greater than 130, then she should take the insulin.*

The distributions of care and of clinical space in the stories I heard in Manuli eventually brought me to Trinity Hospital. Founded in the 1940s, the hospital now has nearly 250 beds and is administered by a public charitable trust. The management structure of the hospital includes a strong component of leadership by an order of Ursuline Catholic nuns dedicated to several other health care missions in India. The hospital serves the surrounding community in Bandra, including Manuli, and tends to have a lower-middle-class to poor clientele because of its low, sliding-fee structure. As in the case of the nun, many of Bandra's Catholic clergy, social workers, schoolteachers, and convent residents are patients as well, although admission to the hospital is not restricted to Catholics. Indeed, many of the patients were Muslim because of the socioeconomic profile of many Muslims living in this area of Bandra. A dietitian in the hospital explained to me that there were culinary factors that stratified the patient profiles, too: Trinity was one of the only major hospitals in Mumbai to have a full "non-veg" menu, meaning that chicken and beef were served. She felt that this deterred some Hindus who might otherwise come to the hospital and attracted Catholics and Muslims who wanted meat in their hospital meals.

I had obtained permission from the medical director of Trinity to conduct long-term observations in the hospital's endocrinology ward, starting with Dr. Chitre, who did much of the diabetes care. I saw it as a potential contrast to Dr. Bhatt's clinic, both in terms of patient population and also because with Dr. Bhatt's setup, I was often sitting with the dietitian. In Trinity Hospital, however, I observed the clinical and pharmacological dimensions of metabolic care because I shadowed Dr. Chitre, the endocrinologist in charge. At Dr. Bhatt's, I witnessed nutritionists attempting to pass food through persons. With Dr. Chitre at Trinity, the matter of concern was passing drugs through persons. As historian Robert Tattersall (2009) notes, pharmaceutical treatments for diabetes remained largely constant between 1960 and 1980. In the period that followed, which he calls "the pharmaceutical era" (159), the rise in the number of diabetics in the United States prompted drug companies to invest resources in new and reformulated medications. Dr. Chitre's room sat squarely in this era, as it did in a history of pharmaceutical company intensification in India around diabetes.[9]

The rhythm of Dr. Chitre's exam room was fast paced. She sat at a desk, with a chair next to it for the patient. There were two extra chairs on the other side: one for me, and one for a retired physician named Dr. Rita, who wanted to keep up with "the latest" in metabolic care, as she explained to me. Because there was nowhere else to sit, I often volunteered to excuse myself if several family members came in with a patient. Dr. Chitre and the family members both hushed me and told me to stay. My notebooks filled up with paragraph-sized records of entries and exits of persons and disorders, a set of cues about who patients were, their diversity, and the clusters of similarity and difference the clinic would take in.

*A first-time patient, a man aged sixty-five. Dr. Chitre checks his throat and feet. "He's borderline, with sugars at 159/135. It's debatable whether or not he's diabetic," she says. There's disagreement among clinicians about which is more important, the pre- or postprandial (i.e., fasting or not) blood glucose measurement. She says that he doesn't need a special diet now, but he does need to have a full blood lab assay, including sugars and HbA1c. He assures her about his eating: "I don't eat potatoes or sugar [main batata aur sugar nahin khata hoon]," but she says, "Doesn't matter!"*

*A patient with polycystic ovarian disorder, aged thirty-one. "Before I got married, I wasn't fat," she says. [Shaadi se pehle, main moti nahin thi.] After marriage, "there was a lot of food, and the obesity intensified [bahut khana aata hai; motapa baḍa raha hai]." Dr. Chitre tells her: "You need to lose weight. Lose weight, and your period will get regular." There's also a genetic reckoning. Dr. Chitre tells her that obesity runs in the family, and she says, "My father's dead." Dr. Chitre responds: "It comes through your genes [tumhara genes me aata hai]." Dr. C instructs her to see a dietitian to help her lose the weight. Her insulin level is high right now at 210. This is because of the obesity, Dr. Chitre tells me. It's causing her skin to darken. Around her throat there are discolored circles that a high-collared blouse mostly covers.*

*A sixty-five-year-old woman. Diabetic, but also her kidney profile is not good, because her serum creatinine is at 60. She needs dialysis, Dr. Chitre says. "Can I take pills for it," the woman asks? "No," Dr. Chitre says. The woman protests: "There isn't any medicine for it?" [Koi dawa nahin?] The woman also says that she has two kidneys. Won't the other one take care of things? "They're both bad [donon kharab hain]," Dr. C tells her, and explains that she's given her pills for high BP, for her sugars, but she can't give her pills for her kidneys. "You'll need dialysis, period," she says. It's her last chance.*

*A wife accompanies her husband, the patient, who is fifty-eight. His sug-*
*ars are 343/411—exceedingly high. "How can this be?" Dr. Chitre asks. The*
*wife assures Dr. C that they keep a very strict diet. He's not yet on insu-*
*lin. But no more. Dr. C issues her decision: "He'll have to have injections of*
*insulin"* [Injection lena parega, insulin.] *The going rate for human insulin*
*is about 160 rupees for 40 units (a little over $3). On his list of current medi-*
*cations, "Diabecon" appears. "What's that?" asks Rita, the retired physician*
*sitting next to me. "It's Ayurvedic," Dr. C says. Rita wonders if it has any*
*side effects or interactions with insulin. "I follow their faith," Dr. C says. "It*
*doesn't harm anything." She bids them farewell with this: "You must take*
*control"* [Control kar ke denge.]

In these field note passages and their representations of human/drug/food passages, commonalities emerged in terms of key cultural figures whose very existence had to make room for a relation between alimentation and clinical concern. One was the figure of the office worker, stressed and unable to line up "correct" eating with labor rhythms. In contrast to the dominant public representations of the office worker as a man, however, the clinic showed the ways that the office became a place of health risk for women as well. Gender and sexuality came to the fore in other moments, too. One patient who entered was a twenty-three-year-old woman whose listed complaint was "throat pain." Her thyroid levels seemed OK, but Dr. Chitre told her they would monitor it. The woman needed to walk and watch her weight. "Why is it happening?" the woman asked. Dr. Chitre: "It's hereditary." This seemed unsatisfactory. The woman requested an alternative treatment. "I read that this can be caused by an autoimmune disorder? Can you give me something for that?" Dr. Chitre was stern: "You can only treat the end damage—you can't change the genes. Look at my nose: Why is it like this? It's genetic! Only maybe in the next birth can you change your genes!" The woman still seemed unsatisfied with this, but Dr. Chitre closed her folder, marking the end of the discussion.

After the woman left, we had our sidebar. Dr. Chitre explained to me and Rita that "the Internet is the worst enemy of patients. They go reading something and get freaked out. Especially women with thyroid issues. Girls look on the Internet and get worried, because their in-laws will cause problems if their pregnancy isn't OK." Here Dr. Chitre traced anxiety around metabolic disorder to marriageability and to the pressure of a woman's in-laws. As patients worked through different moves of therapeutic negotiation with Dr. Chitre, the sideline discussions she would have with me revealed that the question of tolerability—how much of a metabolic trigger or treatment was viable—was a question that stretched across families in the making, along with current and possible contributions of labor. Losing weight here marked the absorption of women into the marital home.[10]

In between these shuffles—each case striking a chord with an anthropological domain—I learned more about Dr. Chitre, who was the daughter of two doctors and grew up in Mumbai. She was used to seeing patients around her house from an early age and ultimately decided to enter medicine. "I would never have been a capable surgeon, to be frank. I'm a hyper personality," she said. "You've observed this, right?" I demurred, telling her that she was hyperattentive if there was any hyper in the mix—not a bad thing for a physician. She decided to specialize in endocrinology because it was a medicine of systems, with many organs involved. She liked the complexity. While she treated patients with all types of hormonal disorders, she spends most of her time treating diabetic and obese patients. "It's the sedentary lifestyle and the food habits," she said. "You just see so many bakeries on the road now; in my childhood, we never used to go out to eat."

To illustrate this, she brought up the case of a thirteen-year-old patient who came into the clinic earlier that morning. His parents accompanied him. "He weighs too much," his mother had said (*uska weight bahut zyada*). Behind the examination curtain, Dr. Chitre kindly asked the boy a series of questions while his parents sat next to me by the desk. "Do you exercise?" "What do you eat?" The boy replied that he exercises plenty at school. She pulled back the curtain and reported that she wanted a check on his testosterone levels to see about his hormone balance. I was in the clinic the next week when the boy returned with his parents, lab report in hand noting that his testosterone levels were normal. His mother was anxious. She pressed her hand on the boy's stomach: "Look! There's so much fat!" Dr. Chitre issued her diagnosis: "It's obesity, so it's important that he loses weight. Go to the dietitian. He'll get better then."

In recalling the boy's case in the interview with me later, Dr. Chitre said that it wasn't only obesity that was the concern. "That boy, you remember him, right? He's only thirteen and he has diabetes." I assumed she meant type 1, "juvenile," diabetes. I was incorrect. "No, his reports are suggestive of type 2," she explained. "But it's actually good that we know this now; he can control things even without medicine if he follows a good diet and exercise." That was an open question, though. She described the boy as a typical teenager who got sick from too much computer time: "They use those Nintendos for playing . . . they just don't go outside to play." Sedentarism was a curse throughout life, too. Like many people I spoke with, she pointed to call centers as a bastion of metabolic provocation: desk work, night shifts, odd times for meals, poor sleep, no exercise.

Dr. Chitre clarified that therapy and disease rarely shared a starting point. As had nearly every other physician I spoke with, she reminded me that by the time she diagnoses a person with diabetes, the pancreas has already lost 50 percent of its working capacity in terms of its ability to produce insulin. There was a long time lag between the onset of diabetes and the time of diagnosis because few patients notice any manifest changes. There often was little to no pain associated with diabetes. A patient may have noticed increased urination or dizziness, but not in all cases. If the person was considered overweight, she screened for diabetes because of the risk factors associated with excess weight. "So what we do is try and move ahead with what remains of the patient," she said: half a working pancreas. A person less than whole, perhaps a metabolism less than whole. Collateral self-work could do something piecemeal. A patient who took tablets and controlled diet and exercise could extend pancreatic runtime. Dr. Chitre did her best to anticipate the line that a patient's body would follow. In most cases, at some point she would need to move a patient off tablets and on to insulin.[11] When insulin failed, then dialysis. But then the line led across the hallway, where what remained of the body might diminish even further with the possibility of amputation. This was the end of the line for Dr. Chitre's side of the hallway; the patient would leave, directed to other possible branches of therapy.

*A forty-five-year-old man, diabetic for fifteen years. He dumps his tabs, his insulin vials, and his syringes on the table. He's been on dialysis before. He has a question about how the forty-milliliter dose of insulin measures up and how he should administer the dose. Dr. Chitre checks his foot and sees that he has an abscess bandaged up. He complains that his "belly is getting bigger" and that he's feeling* kamzori (weak). *All matters treatable in her room, but she is most concerned about the foot. She instructs him to make the soonest appointment he can to see Dr. Samant, the foot specialist across the hall.*

Dose/Response

What happened when persons left the clinic, pills and instructions for insulin in hand? They did not easily move from one room on the side of Trinity's hallways to the other; after all, these were separate sides of a line with separate physicians running separate appointment schedules. And after waiting for quite a while just to see Dr. Chitre, for example, patients were under no false impression that upon referral to another specialist, they could simply move across the hall and get their next consultation. They knew that their trajectories were punctuated by pauses and that the wait outside the hospital would have to happen again the next time they returned. Dr. Chitre and Dr. Samant were separated spatially by just ten feet, but they were in a hospital running their own outpatient clinics, and so regular bureaucratic protocols of appointments, preparatory paperwork, and required lab tests all applied.

So people often went home, sometimes for a significant length of time, between consultations. Pills went with them. Moving between clinics and homes in Manuli, I found myself in a world of tablets (pills): from pills moved across counters at the chemist to pills tossed onto kitchen tables in household interviews. Pills could be multivalent: "These are my sugar-pressure pills," someone would say. Or "tablets for my diabetes," more specifically. As in the earlier vignette about Anjali's nutritional consult, a tablet could be intended for one mechanism of action (in Anjali's case, metformin for blood glucose management) but rendered as something else ("my fat loss pills.") Given the explanatory investment in the clinic, patients were often quite clear as to what tablets were intended to do physiologically. To think through the contingencies of medicines, then, this section focuses on how tablets were a steadying force in otherwise turbulent times.

Mary's elderly uncle was content with his need to take pills to manage hypertension. As long as he had two pieces of bread with breakfast, he was "under control," he explained. Uncle Salman spent his working life as an elevator operator; for decades, he had pushed the buttons to take people up and down the floors of the nearby building, where film superstar Salman Khan lived—thus his nickname, Uncle Salman. Even after the elevator was replaced by an automatic one ("a Japan-wallah elevator," Uncle Salman called it), he still sat on a stool in the elevator car's corner, pushing the buttons for directors, producers, reporters, socialites, and Khan family members. His wife, Aunty Noelle, kept the house in meticulous order. She also kept Uncle Salman's medical records: a notebook that had various entries with his blood pressure and the date he got the reading from a visit to the clinic. During a visit in 2012, I noticed that the entries never carried past 2010. I asked how his pills were going: "God is great," he said, and opened a canister of chewing tobacco to both Mary's and Noelle's dismay.

Noelle brought out a cluster of pills for me to examine. She bought pills at ten rupees per packet at Manuli's chemist—the generic version instead of the "brand" version, which cost forty rupees. "Same drug," Uncle Salman said. Tablets, branded or otherwise, were a steadying force (when they were available).

As I interviewed persons with diabetes in Manuli, I attempted to avoid replicating the "tell me what you eat, from morning until night" approach that I witnessed in Dr. Bhatt's clinic. It seemed a bit too behaviorally inter- rogative for neighborly discussion. Yet it also seemed inescapable: food lent itself to laundry-listing, however confessional or dispassionate. In the process, these questions and their answers enacted ontological cuts be- tween body and food, with the metabolism often presumed as the canvas upon which their interrelations would act. The inquiry itself could not pass through the stickiness of the metabolism. I returned to the original deal I struck with the church archivist, Mr. Gomes, to first ask after the food. I spoke with several of the church's priests, most of whom had diabetes. If I was not out on visits for Mary's social work, the church's main office and social spaces hosted these interviews. The older women who recorded births, baptisms, and burials would clear out a walled-off corner of the room with a ceiling fan for me for my "food chats" with parishioners, as they called my research. It was in these discussions outside a biomedical setting that I attempted to understand what kind of illness environment a person faced in more everyday terms. For example, Paul was a retired computer technician who regularly volunteered at the church; he was the first person everyone told me to speak with, because he had "amazing con- trol" of his adult-onset diabetes. Paul was from Mumbai but spent much of his adult life overseas in the Gulf working for IBM. He returned to Mumbai to tend to his brother, who was on dialysis for kidney failure stemming from diabetes. Both of his parents had diabetes: "It goes from generation to generation," he said. He learned he had diabetes when he was fifty. Paul was walking to the bank on Manuli's main road and felt dizzy (chakar). He paused, thinking it was just an aberration, and went on with his business. He did go to the doctor to check his blood pressure, given his family history of cardiovascular disease. The doctor checked his blood sugars, confirming Paul's diabetes.

Paul devotes an extensive amount of time to self-monitoring: "I check my sugars all the time," he explained. He self-imposes a strict diet if his sugars are high: dal, chapati, and vegetables for a week, with no excep- tions. If his sugars are low, he'll eat a sweet. He doses himself, blurring

possible differences between eating and drugging. He walks thirty minutes each day on Carter Road; again, no exceptions. He takes metformin
tablets for his diabetes but also tries to regulate his blood sugar through
herbal means. He eats raw *karela* (bitter melon), a vegetable with insulin-
regulating properties, and makes and drinks an herbal tonic from *karu*, a
long, bitter bark from a tree in Goa that some vendors in the local market
carried. I asked if he ate much *methi* (fenugreek), a common herbal remedy
for high blood sugar. He didn't, he said; it caused too precipitous a drop
in his blood sugars. I asked if he took any Ayurvedic medicines, and he
scoffed: "That stuff takes too long. I'm already fifty-seven. Who knows how
long I'll last? I want something that works immediately." Paul dosed himself, blurring the lines between eating and medicating even in instances
when the medication in question was homeopathic, or more simply, a
home remedy.

Almas, the young fashion director, had a seventy-year-old father,
named Muffazal, who worked as a driver for a family in Bandra. He also
experienced several brushes with death due to diabetes, a series of close
calls he elaborated one evening as he sat in the car parked in the church's
back alley. Mary raised one of the more recent episodes. Months before,
Almas had called her, saying, "My dad's passed out on the bed—I think
he's dead." Ever the calm one, Mary responded: "I don't think you can die
from diabetes like that. I'm coming over." They found someone to drive
Muffazal to Trinity Hospital, two blocks away. In the car on the ride over,
they gave him water with honey. As Mary put it, "We did the glucose drip
before the doctors did." Muffazal remained mostly silent as Mary narrated
his medical history, which passed him through beds, cars, and emergency
rooms. As she finished what became known as "the glucose drip story," he
extended his hand through the window, with a packet of sugar in his palm.
He shook the packet, like ringing a bell. "If I'm feeling dizzy (*chakar*),
I make tea and put this in it," he explained, shaking the sugar packet
again. It was the very substance that made balance precarious for many
diabetics; in the clinic, there was so much talk of sugar (Hindi: *chini*;
Marathi: *saakar*, colloq. *shaakar*). Usually this was in terms of a substance
one needed to block from entering the body. In this instance, *shaakar* was
restorative.

I asked Muffazal if he took tablets for his diabetes.

"Sometimes." He didn't recall the drug's name.

Do you feel anything else, I asked?

"My legs feel weak [*kamzor*]. It goes into my feet."

Weakness (*kamzori*) spread through his limbs. Metabolic disorder came down to a distributed discomfort beset with drop-offs and recoveries. But wherever he wound up for therapeutic intervention, Mufazzal had the sugar packet accompany him. This *shaakar* was a little substance with large reaches of power. But as was true for many other persons I encountered, Muffazal might hold on to food or drugs in the hand, but there was no ignoring the feeling—or slowly, the lack thereof—in the feet.

## Trinity Hospital Hallway, Side 2: Demarcation

*A man in his sixties. His scalp is all black, but only some of it is hair. I can't figure out what the rest is: Dye? Fungus? His foot is mangled, with open, pus-filled wounds. His big toe has already fallen off, and his second toe is in the process of dying. In this room, persons might die, but first on death row are the appendages. Dr. Samant tells me, "It's very simple arithmetic. Below the knee, there's 5 percent of the body's blood. If it doesn't reach the wound, the wound won't heal." Dr. Samant says they won't amputate this man's leg. It's better to let the body kill off the toes, one by one, through a process called demarcation. The body marks out which parts of itself will die. The nurses put a sterile bandage on. I ask the man how he's feeling. "It burns," he says. Very simple arithmetic.*

One afternoon I sat in Manuli's church office, waiting for Mary to finish her work before we took off for neighborhood rounds. It was always tough to figure an exact end time to her office work, because even as she would pack up to leave, someone would come by the window. The window was open, lined with bars, and faced one of the courtyards off Manuli's main road. Parishioners often would come up to the window to ask questions and neighbors would stop by with news instead of walking around inside to the office. That day was no exception. Mary's cousin Genevie came to the window, and Mary beckoned me over. The news was not good. Aunty Cecilia, an elderly woman who had given me cooking lessons, had died from a heart attack during the time I had been back in the United States. Mary said it was diabetes that really killed her. Aunty Cecilia was survived by her husband, Joseph, who was diabetic as well. Genevie took on cleaning duties in Joseph's house to help him out. Right after Aunty Cecilia died, he cut his foot and the wound became gangrenous. It was because of diabetic neuropathy—he couldn't feel stepping on a nail, and the wound became infected. Genevie described her morning routine of cleaning the floor and then hours later seeing bloody footprints all over the tile: "I thought someone had been killed in the house, there was so much blood!" Joseph denied being injured. Then Genevie checked his feet, saw the gangrene, and immediately hauled him the three blocks to Trinity Hospital, injuring her shoulder while propping him up as he limped. The doctor at Trinity stitched up Joseph's foot and prescribed a strict diet. Genevie took on cooking duties for Joseph and thus enforced the diet, too: No rice, only chapatis, no sweets. Joseph resented her deeply for this. "He yells and screams at me, and sometimes stops talking to me, but the next morning he's OK again," she said. "It's because he's depressed from losing his wife," Mary added. For a while, things seemed to be fine with Joseph's foot, but then "somehow he went out and injured it again," Genevie said. This time, the toes became black. He had to have two toes and a part of his foot amputated soon after.

Lost feet, lost feelings: these were the limits of drugs and diet and came under the purview of the diabetes foot clinic on the other side of the hallway from Dr. Chitre's room in Trinity Hospital. Dr. Samant, a diabetologist for thirty years, was in charge of the exams in this room. He told me that roughly 15 percent of India's 62 million diabetics experience foot problems. When neuropathy progresses in the leg and foot, the person experiences loss of sensation. "If a person walks to the temple barefoot and there's hot marble, he'll get blisters, he'll keep walking on the wound." This leads to infection. Moreover, because of nerve dysfunction, the elasticity of the skin changes. Sweat glands don't function as usual, and the skin becomes dry and itchy; patients scratch and further induce injury. Blood vessels are also prone to thickening in diabetics, and so as vessels in the leg and foot lose their elasticity, "it's like a water pipe getting rusted, and the flow slows to a trickle," he explained. There can be clots and increased risk of gangrene. All that is needed to prevent these problems is a simple annual foot examination costing two hundred rupees. "This is a national problem," Dr. Samant said of diabetes, "but the government hasn't understood it." Despite the intensification of media coverage around metabolic disease, there was little mention of foot issues. Mumbai had only two sites where doctors could train in care for the diabetic foot. Dr. Samant taught at both.

Dr. Samant made it clear that the younger age of diagnosis for metabolic disease in India has profound implications for patients who will eventually require amputation. One percent of the 15 percent with diabetic foot issues will lose a limb, he explained, and with younger and younger diabetics, the limb loss is occurring "in a very productive age group." "It's a loss to the family, to the nation, to the economy," he said. The only saving grace thus far has been that in comparison to other countries, young smokers in India are fewer in number. This means a lower incidence of vascular damage, such that the onset of vessel damage because of diabetes is a bit more damped than in places where rates of smoking are much higher. Nonetheless, he estimated that of all the amputations he performs, 85 percent are completely avoidable by annual foot checkups, patient education, and simple footwear.

Dr. Samant's work occurred in the context of Indian and global histories of pain connected to the loss of limbs, particularly those concerned with leprosy (see Staples 2003, 2004). Specific historical figurations around the foot circulated in this field of medical science: missionary doctors carving out wooden feet, suggestions by early twentieth-century British physicians on which Indian shoe companies produced the best sandals for persons with foot injuries at the risk of amputation, and colonial and contemporary public health efforts to destigmatize diseased feet. Related objects also circulated in this milieu: poorly fitted sandals, indoor shoes that signaled how feet crossed barriers between the worlds outside and inside domestic space, and movements of the body during the hajj. The foot taught Dr. Samant, his patients, and their families about environments and signaled other parts of the body in turn. At some point, those signals slowed down in the course of their circuit. Feet withered, slowly.

Amputations were costly affairs. A basic prosthetic leg for a below-the-knee amputation cost between 25,000 and 150,000 rupees. The body bore the cost as well. The remaining leg's muscles put in extra work to lift the prosthetic leg ("it's like a patient carrying a dumbbell with every step," Dr. Samant said.) The heart had to pump 15 percent more blood, too, as a result of this extra work. Consequently, more than three-quarters of persons who have below-the-knee amputations die within five years of the procedure because of the strain on the heart. Thus the guiding principle of his clinical work was that early intervention and good footwear were more lifesaving than amputation and a prosthesis.[12] Absent those possibilities, he tended to let the body take care of things. This meant allowing for "demarcation," wherein the body would eventually stop the flow of blood at the line between dead and living tissue. He could then remove an extremity with fewer complications than an active amputation. In his room, parts of the body really did become things. Dead skin, dead toes, absent feelings—parts of the body disconnected themselves and lost their animation. In Dr. Samant's clinic, load bearing played out viscerally. One could point a living finger at a dead toe whose line between living and dead showed where passing through was no longer possible.

His exam room, across the hallway from Dr. Chitre's, presented a clear contrast to my seated, notebooked station in the dietitian clinics, where I was more or less a silent observer. Dr. Samant wanted me to understand pathology firsthand. The first time I observed his clinic, I sat in one of the chairs across the table from him, scooted back into the corner in a cloak of false invisibility. He would have none of this. He positioned me by the examining table, moving me deftly out of the area if it was a female patient or closing the curtain around himself and the patient if there was something he didn't want me to hear or see. He was my gatekeeper. Nonetheless, he wanted me to take a close look. "How could you possibly write about this?" he would ask, given that I did not possess a medicovisual vocabulary. I did not understand the differences between ulcers or between stumps; all I knew was the location (on the leg or where thick black skin was where once a toe had been) and the circumstance the patient reported ("I stepped on a nail"; "I clipped my nails too close"; "I don't know"). I needed to see to understand. Nor was there ever much mention of diet. Instead, it was a visual exchange: "Show me," he'd say to the patient or the patient's caregiver. The patient would sometimes walk in on her own but often would enter in a wheelchair, pushed by either a nurse or a family member. With Dr. Samant, the position of my sightline was also quite different. In the nutrition counseling room at Dr. Bhatt's office, the line of sight bounced between the dietitian and the patient, both staring at the diet sheet on the table. I could witness this from my perch in the corner. In Dr. Samant's office, however, I stood by him as the line of sight bounced off a supine patient's foot or leg and the patient's face, often staring out of the open window or at the portrait of Christ on the Cross above it. The paperwork that would otherwise clue me in to some details was quite secondary to the flesh. It was the foot that mattered in these cases.

How the foot mattered varied widely. For instance, one afternoon a man in his sixties entered the room, pushed in a wheelchair by his son and also accompanied by his wife and the son's wife. Another man came in: the caretaker (or perhaps the household servant), who shook all kinds of pills on the table, backed away and stood in the door frame watching the consultation while scrunching plastic bags that carried the meds back into a leather case. Dr. Samant sat in his chair to be laterally positioned to the patient. He explained that while the man's foot was healing well after a toe amputation, he needed special diabetic shoes and sandals. Pressure must be taken off the scar. With too much pressure on it, it will break and may not heal properly. The wife should allow the man to walk to the toilet, and that's it until the next visit, when Dr. Samant can clear him for more activity. The entire conversation centered on the toilet and the scar—that was the line that mattered.

Other times, the foot would be the line connecting a body part to holistic well-being. A woman in her sixties who came for a consult following the demarcation of her toes began by saying that her legs were in pain. Dr. Samant examined her. He declared her feet to be healing well. She asked: "Doctor, will you look at me?" I was confused hearing this, because Dr. Samant had indeed just looked at her feet. She asked about putting creams and medication on the feet and then asked about any possible tablets she might need to take. "All of these things, you're doing fine," he said. She pressed: Would he look at her? Is he sure everything is OK? He reassured her that it was. In the foot clinic, "me" did not always mean "my foot." Patients appealed for systemic care, as they too understood that lines connected the locus of pathology to a greater somatic complex that could be vulnerable and resilient.

The cases continued; my notes would start and stop as I moved the chair or as Dr. Samant had me drop the writing to watch his technique.

*An older woman in a wheelchair, pushed in by her son and daughter-in-law. The old woman wails: "Lai lai lai lai lai." She doesn't stop; she only changes the pitch of the wail to express deep pain when they put her feet on a stool for Dr. Samant to examine and when they remove the bandages. "Lai lai lai!" The son and his wife try and soothe her, kindly, softly. Her toe is dying. So is her brain. Dr. Samant tells me: "This is what happens with diabetes. Dementia. Age is part of it, but age itself isn't the only cause. The circulation stops in the feet but also in the brain. There's neuropathy in the brain. For younger patients, we might propose amputation. But she's already getting round-the-clock care from her family. For her, what can we do? We wait till the toes turn black, and the body will demarcate it and it'll fall off."*

*A man in his fifties. He gets up on the table, and Dr. Samant looks at the bottom of his feet, filled with ulcers. He got them during hajj, Dr. Samant explains to me. "Mecca is so hot, and they have to walk barefoot, it's fifty degrees centigrade sometimes [122°F], and the paths are uneven." It really hurts the feet, even though the man may not have felt it.*

*A man in his fifties. Dr Samant calls me over: he's shaving away dead skin around a wound with a scalpel. The dead skin bits fall off the table onto the floor. I wonder who will clean it up. "See here," he says, "the toe hasn't been moving properly so he's developed these dry bits, and this is how the ulcer develops. In the US, a podiatrist will charge a hundred dollars for this scraping, but here we do it for free." A global leader in diabetes-related surgery, barbering the feet.*

*A man, thirty-six. The toe is yellow. "It's gone," Dr. Samant says to me and to the nurse. "Gangrene." Dr. S turns to the nurse: "Admit him. Amputation." (In other cases like this, he might simply say to all of us or to no one in particular: "There is no other alternative.")*

*A woman in her sixties. Another case where Dr. S calls me over to watch how he scrapes necrotic tissue. I disobey, and take my eyes off the foot to look at her. "Does it hurt?" I ask her. "No, beta [child]," she says. "I can't feel anything."*

The differences in cases showed the wide variability in feeling and pain. For some, it was like the woman just described: "I can't feel anything." For others, pain came in many flavors and intensities. The chance to see Dr. Samant was the chance to narrate a history of selective feeling. His clinic was a place where "metabolism" entailed vascular function and the gradual degradation of atherosclerotic tissue. By the time a patient came in, sent by Dr. Chitre across the hall or otherwise, the body's vital lines—its blood vessels—were often blocked or in varying states of decay. Pain was a sign of "intermittent claudication," or the obstruction of circulation in lower extremities. The metabolism that mattered to Dr. Samant and to his patients was the set of signals in the connection between the extremities and the heart. Little blockages turned into lost limbs and, later, lost life.

We were in a different clinical setting than Dr. Bhatt's setup, inside a hospital rather than a private clinic. No advertisements for pharmaceuticals were to be found; the signs of hope were crucifixes. Across the hall, Dr. Chitre was up against the clock of the pancreas, whose beta cells were diminishing in absolute numbers and in their collective tolerance for drugs over time. In the foot clinic, Dr. Samant either waited for the body to do the cutoff or, in the worst cases, to do it himself. On his side of Trinity's hallway, time had taken its toll, and he had to create new therapeutic paths. Ulcers had already developed, nails already had been stepped on, tight-fitting sandals were already worn. Diagnosis with a specific condition, where a person passes through uncertain, ticklish, or dizzying symptoms to categorical, biomedical knowing, had a different set of temporal parameters. In the hallways of Trinity Hospital, things were lost and gained across the lines of therapeutic contrivance. Limbs were collateral in their own right—the price paid.

## Passing through Therapy

How does the metabolism come to be a multisite for therapy? As discussed in chapter 3, the blur of food and drugs, one of metabolic living's key features, plays out through the home's permeability and the domestic science of food processing. This chapter has offered a look at the permeability of the body under states of metabolic duress. I have focused on an additional kind of food-drug blur, one in and around the space of the clinic, to show how it emerges in clinical care practices involving the diets and pharmaceuticals that underlie clinical care. These practices are key to mapping illness environments; they illustrate how neither the body nor medicine is absolute. Amid dietitians and doctors, I observed a great amount of therapeutic approximation, from the guesswork of diets to the more intensive fine-tuning of drug therapies to the final stop in the line: limb amputation for diabetics. Consistencies and instabilities of different expert fields of knowledge such as clinical nutrition, dietetics, Ayurveda, diabetology, and surgery take the metabolism as their rationale and target. Clinicians may task their patients to change "risk behaviors" (generally around eating and exercise), but simultaneously, the clinical interactions I observed introduced the risk that something *will* work as a desirable gamble. This double bind of risk was clearly frustrating for many patients; "Will it work?" and similar questions made me wonder what precisely "it" was: The prescribed diet? The medicines? One's insulin sensitivity? Body weight? The metabolism itself? The combinatorial symptoms and therapies surrounding metabolic disorders allowed for such ambiguity. The lines that divide and connect clinical therapies offer clues as to what is in and out of order in body and in mind; what a nutritionist and a doctor can and cannot accomplish; and the complex movements that add up to therapy. We see this occur as measuring bowls, pills, scalpels, and skin shuttle across the lines between persons and clinical spaces.

Scholars of food studies have pointed to the ubiquity of diets as evidence of the centrality of nutritional thinking to self-perception and, specifically, perceptions of responsibility. Termed "nutritionism," this ideology produces what Jane Dixon calls "nutricentric citizens" and Gyorgy Scrinis calls "nutricentric persons": individuals who craft a sense of well-being and control through nutritional rationales.[13] This definition means that every time someone eats under the rubric of nutrition, he or she makes truth with each bite. There is thus a Foucauldian dimension to this process, suggest Guthman and DuPuis (2006b), meaning that nutrition is as much an avenue for domination and discursive production as it is self-definition. The authors compare the American war on obesity and its concomitant emphasis on dieting to Foucault's analysis of masturbation and explain that "just as proscriptions on masturbation were designed not to curtail a practice but to create new centers of power and knowledge in the surveillance of children . . . the point of the war on obesity may not be to curtail it—to have people eat less—but actually to imbue eating with a greater kind of power" (Guthman and DuPuis 2006b: 436). In this analysis, dieting channels biopower because it makes nutritional knowledge a site of moral reckoning backed by an imperative of good health.[14] To diet well, then, is to be in charge of the body. Yet this scholarship prompts questions of how and under what circumstances distant biomedical rationales gain intimate moral traction. If a strong focus on diet imbues eating with "a greater kind of power," what solidifies that power in the first place? Who and what is really "in charge" of the outcome of diet? How much passing through between food and the body can one bear, if passing through therapy means movement between repair and damage?

One conclusion might be that this greater power emerges from individuals. Diets certainly work as an effective technology of the self, whereby individuals incorporate moralized expertise from doctors, dietitians, and public media to craft new, improved, thin selves. The good dieter can be the person whose nutritional savvy and responsiveness puts her in more control of a seemingly uncontrollable system like the metabolism. The good dieter can also be the good patient, when goodness emerges as a matter of medical commensurability. As historian Sander Gilman (2008) notes, dieting "becomes the means of self-liberation, self-control, or self-limitation. It is a process by which the individual claims control over his or her body and thus shows their ability to fulfill their role in society" (1499). However, as I repeatedly posed this question to doctors, dietitians, and their patients—what kind of power does food have when used as medicine?—their responses suggested that the metabolic body opened itself to interventions in ways that developed outside of singular, self-oriented frames and involved specific arrangements between persons and objects.

In this rendering, metabolic science crystallized as collateral—a gradient of damage and repair. Passing through this gradient reveals lines to be environments in their own right. Diets worked through object relational fields of the senses, according to a certain set of rules, and made evident connections between food and pathology. This had implications for the question of the authority of medicine as well, because the charge of therapy worked as a multiway street. To be sure, declarations of responsibility and failure were forms of address to patients deemed noncompliant by care providers. But I observed that persons did not so much resist biomedicine as they asserted that they were doing *everything* right—everything in their available arsenal, that is, only to be stymied by the metabolism. Persons moved objects in and out of the clinic, sometimes plopping them down on the table to announce the start of the rhythm of therapy. Lab reports, insulin vials, pills, sugar, chapati cutouts, paperwork, notebooks: the thing-y-ness of the clinical encounter was central. So too were people's spatial relations, as they emerged in hallways, waiting rooms, and even in the body itself as certain body parts shut off as a result of overload or depletion. Here, biomoral substances were in play: blood, fat, even limbs. This condition brings us back to the deeply human dimensions of these stories, filled with sincere performances of patients being (or trying to be) good and thus filled with relations to medicalization more lateral than vertical, more about a passage of bioscientific authority than a strict adherence or resistance to it.

Across lines of therapy, the "greater power" involved in weight loss was the power to link persons and food as much as it was a means of self-definition. It is certainly possible to take this intensified focus on nutrition as evidence of "nutritionism," whereby diet becomes an ever more salient moral language of subjective self-fashioning. This move would place India alongside the United States as an ideological exemplar of a country filled with "nutricentric citizens." It also positions diets as techniques that fulfill the overweight consumer's need for change and self-redefinition. But this analysis would be inadequate, because it glosses over the co-occurring vulnerabilities at stake in weight gain, such as embodied stress or gendered double binds of home and office labor. An overemphasis on diet as a moral prescription for subject making cannot account for the ways in which the metabolism unites the sites of inquiry described here. No amount of responsibility and compliance can help patients if their metabolism doesn't respond favorably to dietary treatment.

The chapter has described collateral resources and damages in therapeutic environments that occur as biomoral substances spark bodily dramas. By "biomoral," I mean the ways that substances such as blood sugars, insulin, rice, and a foot's splintering skin are semio-material. This means that they are symbolic and visceral signs that make metabolic disorder intelligible as a clinical target and a sign of the need for intervention in everyday conversation. Patients and their caregivers constantly engaged in gatekeeping work that determined what stayed in or out of the body. Foods and drugs did not pass through the body like a silent wind; they could catch if a patient over- or underate or took too much or too little of a prescribed drug. I found that the rhythm of substances like fat and sugars—bodily and culinarily—were most at the center of therapeutic work and talk. Temporality articulated the absorption and emission of therapy.

The intake of, encounter with, and aversion to substances had a hefty relationship to the kinds of morals deployed in the back-and-forth between patients and caregivers. For example, prescriptions for diets and drugs came with appeals for responsibility and control: take this pill, eat this food, and do it right and regularly. While seemingly ham-fisted at first glance, the power of such therapeutic directives was quite diffuse, because patients were as creative as they were "compliant."[15] What matters when the dangers and the resources of the contemporary world are or are not successfully metabolized? Therapeutic environments centralize this question, because from simple diets to complex drug regimens, how much a person can take on and tolerate is of ultimate concern. The bundle of lines and all their side branching opens up several analytic standpoints for thinking about therapy. One is about the load-bearing limits of care, wherein the weight of individual knowledge cannot ultimately anchor the performative and promissory relations to dieting. Instead, the tether of this charge was the passage between objects and the metabolism. The compliance of the metabolism was as crucial as the compliance of the determined patient herself. In this circumstance, the metabolism poses a dilemma: What happens when diet fails, despite a patient's discipline? In such cases the metabolism becomes the focused site in which only surgical intervention can "fix" overweight patients who have exhausted all other options.

Dr. Ketkar was Mumbai's first weight-loss doctor, perhaps the city's best known as a result, but nonetheless his office was quite humble. Chairs faced mint-green walls plastered with 1970s-era posters of foods and their caloric values, such as one entitled "Calorie Reckoner." A small billboard had crumbly newspaper clips of Dr. Ketkar's successes with everyday Mumbaikars as well as Bollywood stars. Most of the articles noted how he doesn't accept referral money from other doctors and how low his charges are. What he did offer was an emphasis on personal responsibility: a standardized diet, roughly the same for all patients, whose success relied on fortitude. In Dr. Ketkar's office, individual responsibility kept diets (and by extension, weight loss) on track, a point his patients proudly echoed.

While I waited to interview Dr. Ketkar one morning, two middle-aged women entered the waiting room. As I began chatting with them, they realized that they recognized each other from previous visits and began sharing insider info. "My sister lost 34 kilos in six months," the first woman, in a blue polka-dot blouse, said to the other. "She was 119 kilos," the woman said, to the gasp of the second woman and of a third woman who sat down next to us. "She *must* be following his diet rigidly," the second woman said with approval. The first woman confessed that her attempts at diet had been less successful so far. "*Meri problem fruits hai* [my problem is fruit]—so much sugar!" She had gained much of her weight during pregnancy and hoped to "feel light" again with Dr. Ketkar's help.

"You don't really look that fat," the second woman said to her. "*I'm* fat." The first woman politely returned the compliment: "No! You're not fat!" This cycled on for several minutes.

A silent observer until this point, the third woman quietly asked the other two if they had personal trainers. No, they responded. Horribly expensive. They preferred to walk in the evenings, according to Dr. Ketkar's recommendation to walk one hour per day. "My friend lost fourteen kilos in three months just from walking," claimed the first woman. "Plus, trainers are very rigid and too hard to follow," said the second, not to mention the additional expense of gym memberships. They inquired about the third woman's weight loss so far. "I was eighty kilos, and now I'm seventy," she said, but she still felt sluggish. The first woman suggested that diet alone was inadequate; without exercise it would make one's skin dull. Dieting required mettle, but adding exercise entailed even farther reaches of effort.

The three women traded "weaknesses." "I have a real weakness for McDonald's burgers," the first said. "When I see one, I just can't help myself." The second tried to motivate her to resist indulgence, explaining that she herself used to love McDonald's but has convinced herself "to feel nauseous when she sees it." She recently lost her overweight fifty-two-year-old brother to a heart attack, then her mother to the same. "You can't know destiny, but at the same time, I don't want to live on insulin and suffer," she said. The first woman agreed and said that she had several family members whose problems crept up the minute they exceeded ninety kilos. "Crossing ninety is a sign of danger," she said. "All sorts of problems come up: heart, BP, cholesterol." The third woman shared that her weight problem was due to "vacuums" of little food intake during the day followed by huge meals in the evening. "We hog at night," she said of her family. "Our culture tells us to fast every week, because our body is a machine and we should keep servicing our body." But they didn't heed that call, fell prey to indulgence, and suffered as a result.

Anytime I waited to interview a physician—sometimes up to five hours so she could finish seeing her patients—I found myself in a space that at first blush might be considered liminal, as it was somewhere between the outside world and the inner sanctum of the clinic. It was the clinic, to be sure, but a different arrangement of persons and information than the doctor-patient arrangement that would eventually unfold. Dr. Ketkar's clinic used a time-tested mode of calling upon patients: the buzzer. A loud, urgent buzz would pierce the waiting room, and this was the signal for the receptionist to call the next patient into the doctor's examination room, even if the previous patient hadn't left. No time was left to waste. New patients sat down as the most recently seen patient packed up and left. I witnessed this from the vantage point of the waiting room and from inside the examination room, and I never became used to the buzz, always jumping a bit out of my seat as the doctor pressed the button by the desk.

A buzz bounced off the mint-green walls. Dr. Ketkar had called me into his consulting room at this point, and I said good-bye and good luck to the three women. He sat at an enormous wooden table, with two young nutritionists at one end filing papers and entering data into a computer. He began an interlaced personal and professional history the moment I sat down. "I added a new kind of medicine in India," he said, when he opened what he claimed was India's first modern medical weight-loss clinic in 1964. His own struggle with weight loss inspired his work. In 1960, as a young physician, he worked hard to reduce his weight by following a strict diet and decided he wanted to do the same for others. He trained as a pediatrician but studied the metabolism and clinical approaches to weight loss. He started "obesity camps," where he did education and outreach, and to date, he said, he had treated over three hundred thousand patients.

On the table lay a soft binder filled with pictures of his patients and little titles on the pages like "beautiful and healthy" and "feel the difference." He showed me some of the celebrity patients, including film stars Aamir Khan, Madhuri Dixit, and Rekha. Aamir Khan, he said, was especially diligent: "He ate small portions every thirty minutes," Dr. Ketkar said, which helped lead to his weight loss. This was the key to Dr. Ketkar's approach, the "diet" that the women in the waiting room discussed. It involves, quite simply, eating. No long breaks without food. High-protein biscuits as snacks if it's not time for a major meal. And one hour of walking, either all at once, or in fifteen-minute chunks. It was all outlined in his book, he explained, and pulled out a thin green hardcover volume called *Battle of the Bulge*.

I once asked how his patients might have changed over the years. Dr. Ketkar explained that the most evident change was their relationship to the practice of dieting. "They used to need coaxing and convincing," he said. "But now people come with the awareness about weight and diet," and they arrive at his office ready to diet. This readiness and its sense of potential help keep patients accountable and responsible. Being open to diets was a move of self-empowerment and was at the heart of the "new kind of medicine" Dr. Ketkar added to the Indian pharmacopeia. I asked if I could buy a copy of his book and paid him the three-hundred-rupee charge; before handing it over he autographed it on the title page with a reminder: "A proper diet is NO STARVATION." Then the buzzer.

A clinic waiting room like Dr. Ketkar's is a place in which the medical anthropologist commonly sits. In Mumbai, these rooms can be anything from an open-air corridor to an enclosed one connecting different rooms of a hospital's OPD (outpatient department), where staff physicians see their patients. Patients can wait in the room of exactly the same physician at her private clinic: the cost can be higher than the cost of seeing the doctor at the hospital, but the location might be more convenient. When I once tried to understand the calculus that patients did in terms of which hospital to attend, given that the city is blanketed with options, one physician pointed to the waiting room as an arbiter of decision making: "It's air-conditioned, and they can be comfortable and have some dignity." She articulated a different sense of waiting: dignified, calm, decisive.

Some of the waiting rooms I sat in were mostly silent, except for the cooing of babies or chattering of toddlers that patients brought with them. But often I observed the scenario that characterized Dr. Ketkar's waiting room: an exchange of information, a connection built between strangers, even an endorsement of medical procedures. In the waiting room for a bariatric surgery clinic I noticed that a billboard of news clips had become the centerpiece of social interaction. The billboard was against one wall, not particularly central to the spatial arrangement, yet as people paced around waiting for their turn to see the surgeon for a consult, they often stopped to read the clips. These were stories extolling the surgery, sometimes quoting the clinic's surgeons (in which case, the text would be highlighted). There were also diagrams of the digestive system, charts with population estimates of diabetics and obese people in India, and photos of patients who had successfully lost weight and/or reduced the severity of their diabetes. People would pace around the waiting room, stop by the billboard, and read through the articles. Often patients and those that accompanied them would talk about the surgical procedure, with the articles as a silent conversational partner. Some of the articles had detailed graphics of procedures, and the onlookers would put fingers to newsprint as they traced the outlines of the surgical cuts made in the stomach.

The printed step-by-step details, the news clippings of testimonials, and the endless magazine declarations of a chronic disease epidemic were also places where strangers met and exchanged ideas—a pretreatment sociality. For example, on one visit to the surgery clinic, a woman sat next to me with her friend and spoke excitedly about seeing the surgeon for her first consult. She wanted to have bariatric surgery to lose weight, as she had tried all sorts of diet and exercise programs, all to no avail. As she relayed her hopes and anxieties about the procedure to her friend, another woman sitting in the waiting room interrupted them and cut to the chase with terse nuggets of advice: "Follow the instructions they give you. Don't cheat! I used to be so fat, and after the surgery, my health has picked up." The first woman snapped to attention:

FW: Did it hurt?

SW: *Anything* surgical is painful. But don't wait. Don't. Just do it. It can't go wrong.

FW: I want to. I want to look good.

SW: Forget looking good! Your health is more important. Don't even think. Just do it! I lost fifty kilos; I used to have a huge stomach and throat. Just ask the doctor. And I did *major* research on [the surgery] before I decided to do it. You'll be happy.

FW: I will. I will.

In these rooms, therapy, care, and willpower emerged as relational fields forged between the walls and cemented between friends, news clippings, and even perfect strangers.

The Folly of *Fatafat* Weight Loss

In a windowless room at a medical conference in Mumbai about therapies for obesity, a woman named Neha narrated the surgery that reduced her stomach size, reconfigured her intestinal tract, and resulted in rapid weight loss. Her first slide showed a picture of a woman in a red *salwar kameez*, wearing a flat expression in front of a modest home in a Mumbai suburb. She laughed quietly at the picture of herself on the projection screen, which she didn't expect the audience of doctors to recognize because it depicted a "fat and unhappy" person before the surgery. "I was so overweight, at one point I realized that I had to do something extraordinary. . . . I had to work at some miracles myself," she explained. Neha underwent laparoscopic gastric bypass surgery because, as she put it, "I needed a miracle in my life to give me new life." Her friends and family were puzzled about this miracle, especially those who didn't know about the surgery. They thought she might have used some *fatafat* (quick, shortcut) method for weight loss. But Neha knew better: *fatafat* methods like celebrity diets or self-help books rarely imparted lasting results. She was tired of wasting money on *fatafat* schemes suffused with the assumption of instrumental willpower: if you try harder, then you'll do better. Neha didn't think her self needed this kind of cruel "help," because the source of her new life— her metabolism—could not be pinned down so easily. Unlike the patients described in chapter 4, Neha had already been through the ins and outs of dieting with little in the way of sustainable weight loss. Michel Foucault's observations (1988) about dietetics as a regimen built out of a "whole manner of forming oneself as a subject who had the proper, necessary, and sufficient concern for his body" (108) did not translate well in this context, when Neha had already pulled out all the stops to no avail.

What routes are possible when one has hit a biomedical brick wall? When the body doesn't seem to listen to the will of the will, what can be done? This chapter maps out how willpower becomes the grounds of metabolic living. Guided by beliefs that diets and medication are not always tenable long-term therapies, a growing number of experts have proposed a set of surgical procedures as a therapy and even a possible "cure" for metabolic disease.[1] Broadly speaking, surgeons cut, rearrange, and stitch up the gut in order to recalibrate the gut-brain axis itself. The procedure aims to make postsurgical patients less hungry, to have more balanced digestive hormonal regulation, to experience normalized insulin responses, and to lose weight rapidly. Quite literally, the body absorbs fewer macro- and micronutrients. As a result, different biochemical reactions occur. Signal pathways shift.

These reactions, in turn, result in normalized insulin levels such that a person with diabetes no longer has the physiological profile of a diabetic. Further, there is a large amount of weight loss that accompanies this biochemical tumult. Through this surgery, the body becomes its own instrument of therapy from the inside out. The surgeon intervenes on the body, with the idea that the metabolism then takes it from there. Postsurgery, a person could enjoy loosened ties to the diets and medication that led nowhere and might instead invest intimate attachments elsewhere. Metabolic surgery uses the metabolism as the anchor to ties "elsewhere." The surgery opens a material-discursive space in which intentionality— the will to get better and to become "normal"—has its moorings in the apparatus of the metabolism.

In metabolic surgery, persons are treatable: open to surgery's power to rearrange body, food, and medicine, and thus open to possibilities of absorption. Here is where the will becomes important, as willpower shuttles across a porous interchange between the body's interior and the world of objects outside it. At stake is rearrangement and reattachment rather than failure. If a pathological body's metabolism had grown too strong and was out of step with a person's will to change, the only way forward was to reconcile the two through a surgery on a set of attachments and arrangements with living. Metabolic attachments thus offer a frame of effort and effect different from one in which subjects are self-evident fleshy bubbles emptied of willpower or are persons who cannot escape overdetermined material dependencies. Throughout the chapter, I present stories of metabolic surgery, ranging from the surgeons who train in the procedure to the persons who pursue or refuse it.

Neha, whose story opened the chapter and to whom I return later, articulated a phrase in our conversations that captured what the surgery ultimately delivered: *badalte rishte*—a shift in life's arrangements.[2] Through rearrangements, the metabolism emerges as a site of willpower. The movements of organs and their attendant physiological aftereffects open up an echo chamber of sorts, where lived experiences of surgical intervention throw back elements of the history of metabolic science. In writing about Hans Jonas's philosophies of biology and biochemistry, Hannah Landecker explains that Jonas's writing on human metabolism reflects what for him were key features of the concept of metabolism in science. One is that for Jonas, "metabolism is a very particular kind of boundary. From it arises an individuation, an inwardness, and the possibility of selfhood." For Jonas, Landecker writes, "the facts of metabolism were no less than the basis of selfhood and the world" (Landecker 2013a: 217–18). This philosophical observation did not stay just with Jonas, as Landecker explains: it circulated in friendships with biologist Ludwig von Bertalanffy and then in von Bertalanffy's own research engagements with biochemist Rudolf Schoenheimer. What I want to point out here is "the possibility for selfhood" that metabolism has been understood to be historically. In my own encounters observing metabolic surgery, I began to question how even amid the supposed dissolving of all problems of sickness into metabolism, the question of selfhood never quite seemed to disappear.

## The Invisible Stomach

When gastric bypass surgery was first introduced in the United States in the 1950s, surgeons noticed that their obese patients—many of whom were also diabetic—had near-normal insulin responses soon after surgery. Diabetes nearly disappeared, sometimes as soon as days after surgery, in an unexpected outcome that accompanied weight loss. In the last fifteen years, as scientists have learned more about how intestinal hormones regulate hunger and metabolism, they have proposed theories that a particular hormone called GLP-1 (glucagon-like peptide 1) increases insulin secretion.

Because gastric bypass surgery directly routes food to the area of the intestine where GLP-1 is produced, researchers believe that the rerouted food causes intensified GLP-1 production. The increased GLP-1 levels help the diabetic body regulate insulin more effectively. Similarly, nearby areas of the intestine are thought to produce hunger-regulating hormones, such as ghrelin (see Couzin 2008: 438–40). When surgeons change the pace and amount of food that passes though the relevant intestinal passages, they can effectively change hormonal dynamics to dampen appetite and regulate elevated blood sugar levels that occur after eating. Surgical intervention in these areas, such as shortening a length of intestine, effects profound physiological change because of the intense, uniquely located metabolic mechanisms of these organs.

Thus surgeons and patients are ultimately hoping for a different overall bodily chemistry because of the intervention in this one specific part of the gut. This hope and rationale for intervention works with a specific understanding of the metabolism as the connective system of "the gut-brain axis," which refers to the links between the central nervous system (centered in the brain) and the enteric nervous system (rooted in the gastrointestinal organs). Intervention in the gut changes the pathways of signals in the gut and the brain and the passageways between them: eat less, you're sated. Narratives offered by post-op patients reinforce this idea. The surgery thus becomes a way of teaching scientists and surgeons and patients and observing anthropologists about the distributions of the metabolism. The embodied effects, inasmuch as they could be realized in language, teach about the rationale of the work that precedes them.

In contrast to a band around the stomach or a surgical reduction of the stomach pouch—both of which can be understood as mechanical— surgeries that effect changes in the intestines are metabolic because of the ways they effect changes in biochemical signals. This helps explain why surgeons I spoke with fashioned their work as a *metabolic* intervention rather than a *mechanical* one. Scalpels and retractors did mechanical work on the guts, but ultimately surgeons felt that the body itself turned a person toward horizons of weight loss. This was especially the case in operations that worked upon the intestines as sites of hormonal regulation. As this kind of procedure gains traction in India, a divergent set of surgical practices now group under the rubric of "metabolic." Differential absorption is the means and ends of the endeavor. It appears as a bodily system that has been reset. This change encompasses specific forms of agency tied to surgical intervention, but the reset entailed does not necessarily make the problem go away. As we will see, these metabolic changes can effect hydraulic tricks: they can transfer willpower from one set of medical practices to another—from the hands of the surgeon to the hands of the person taking pills and protein shakes to compensate for the surgery's aftereffects.

Given its wide-ranging physiological outcomes, surgeons have increasingly positioned metabolic surgery as therapy for ailments beyond diabetes and obesity, ranging from asthma to arthritis (Pories 2008). Some Indian physicians have suggested that long-term pharmaceutical treatments for diabetes and obesity are untenable because of their harsh side effects, further building the case for metabolic surgery as an acceptable intervention (see, e.g., *DNA Mumbai* 2009a, 2009b). One surgeon explained to me that the FDA in the United States was "very tough" in approving pharmaceutical therapies for weight loss, and "until you have more drugs, there is no other solution left" but surgical interventions for the very obese and the most dire of diabetic cases. Frankly, I was initially skeptical of the surgery's reach beyond Mumbai's elite and was surprised to learn that its patients spanned the city's fluid social, educational, and economic ranks. Whenever I asked friends and neighbors about the surgery, their fingers would tap the back-page ads of daily newspapers that implored the overweight reader to try "stapling" surgery or to think of weight-loss surgery as a good investment that could sidestep the costly complications of obesity. "Save rupees tomorrow by losing weight today!" the text below pictures of enormous bellies would announce.

The first time I observed a "public awareness session" to educate potential surgical patients, we began with a moment of silence. One week had passed since the terror attacks in Mumbai on November 26, 2008, and Dr. Prakash, the surgeon hosting a surgery information session, asked that we stand to remember the event, the victims, and the survivors. The dimmed lights and buzz of the slide projector buffered the audience of sixty in this downtown hospital auditorium from the cleanup and investigative efforts unfolding barely five hundred meters away. Dr. Prakash's presentation, entitled "Obesity and Diabetes: Lifetime Diseases? A Public Awareness Session on Obesity and Diabetes Surgery," introduced another national threat after the momentary memorial for the lives lost in the attacks. Over the next hour, he outlined the severity and possible reasons for obesity and diabetes in India and the various treatments available since their introduction in India in the early 1990s. His diagrams, statistics, and before/after photos of the obese turned slim divided the authorized from the rumored. Like all surgeons I met, Dr. Prakash made it clear at the public seminars that no surgery is free of risk and that surgery was neither an easy nor immediate replacement for medical therapies like insulin for patients with type 2 diabetes. Rather, he emphasized that "the risk is in the disease" and framed the long-term risks of metabolic disease as commensurable with its surgical treatment.

Dr. Prakash described the variety of procedures for metabolic surgery, using animated slides and diagrams to show different options for laparoscopic, "minimally invasive" techniques. First was the gastric band procedure, where the surgeon fixes an adjustable band round the upper part of the stomach, separating it into a smaller and larger pouch. This restricts the amount of food the patient can eat. It has relatively minor complications, he said, and is also good for diabetics: up to 50 percent of diabetics who opt for this procedure experience resolution of their diabetes postsurgery. The second laparoscopic option was sleeve gastrectomy, which he described as "very popular" in India because it can result in a 70 percent resolution rate for diabetics. In this procedure, the surgeon reduces the stomach to as little as 15 percent of its original size by removing a section along its curve and then stapling the cut edges together to create a smaller pouch. Lastly, there was the gastric bypass; like the sleeve gastrectomy, it reduces the size of the stomach pouch but additionally creates a shortcut from this smaller pouch to the lower reaches of the small intestine, effectively "bypassing" the upper lengths of the small intestine.

Inasmuch as surgery confers particular forms of agency, operations also call into question notions of standardized bodies, the uneven circulation of individuated body parts, ethics and faith, and the cultivated expertise of surgeons themselves (see Cohen 1999; Crowley-Matoka 2015; Hamdy 2012; Prentice 2013). These varied stakes suffused the room as Dr. Prakash opened the floor to questions and hands shot up across the audience. Most questions addressed the cost of the procedure, which he explained could range from 100,000 rupees ($2,100) for the traditional "open" (i.e., nonlaparoscopic) forms of surgery to 500,000 rupees ($10,500) for the laparoscopic-only procedures. He asserted that money should not be an obstacle to getting needed treatment and introduced a patient of his sitting on the dais, a middle-aged woman in a green sari. He described her as coming from "an average Maharashtrian family." She told her story briefly: she worked as a domestic servant, and was so overweight that she had problems doing the dishes or squatting to use the toilet. Her husband was a security guard, and they had little money. They asked their extended family for help; through donations they were able to afford the surgery because Dr. Prakash performed it as part of training for other surgeons, which allowed him to discount the price by half. Dr. Prakash emphasized that this woman never overate. Her weight just crept up over time. "Ninety percent of our patients have strong control," Dr. Prakash remarked of her case. "They never eat ice cream . . . they eat just two chapatis with their meals, and yet they still gain weight." Dr. Prakash asserted that the metabolism held its grip over patients, and only by loosening that grip via metabolic intervention could the body right itself again.

## Creating a Successful Therapy "Inside"

Some surgeons felt the risks associated with surgery were a small price to pay for what it offered their patients in terms of long-term therapy. One surgeon I shadowed, Dr. Karke, learned the metabolic surgical procedures because her own mother had died from complications of diabetes. Her case load averaged sixty patients a day (which I witnessed repeatedly during twelve-hour shifts), and her patients were not always of the middle class or elite but often were taxi drivers, domestic workers, and food hawkers. For Dr. Karke, the benefits of the surgery far exceeded those of weight loss or the reversal of diabetes. "There is a huge difference in quality of life," she said. "Absolutely huge. People cry because their fertility gets better, their medications go down, depression is out, fatigue is out. [Patients] tell me, 'Doctor, I could fit in my car today. Doctor, I could buy clothes today. I was ashamed before the surgery.'" When I asked Dr. Karke about the claims that the surgery was a "cure" for obesity and diabetes, she reminded me that "the science doesn't claim that the surgery *cures* diabetes. It claims that it *improves* it." This improvement could actually release patients from another stranglehold: that of endless pharmaceutical treatment. Dr. Karke explained that this was possible because the surgery ultimately works "from within." She likened the procedure to putting in a stent for a coronary patient. A stent made life livable but did not necessarily return a person to life before disease. "I can't make my gray hair black again, right?" she joked. And yet, she explained, "these treatments save lives." She constantly sees patients whose severity of diabetes and complications from excess weight far exceed the treatment possibilities of pharmaceuticals. "If you need a new valve in your heart, they replace the valve, and if you need a new rotator cuff, they replace the rotator cuff, but what if you need a new metabolism?" she asked. "That is the beauty of metabolic surgery. We change the control mechanisms from within. [We create] an in situ feedback mechanism which gets established after the operation, which medication from outside cannot do. It is a continued medical therapy from inside your body. You're creating a bodily therapy *inside*." For Dr. Karke, surgery was not a singular event but rather a continuous one, such that the body's intimacies between hormones, food stimulation, and "control" would ultimately rebalance themselves. The interiority of therapy and its constant work made it metabolic.

This theme of "control from within" and its influence over concepts of "success" structured many of the patient interactions I observed in Dr. Karke's practice. For example, a patient in her early thirties, Aditi, came into the office for her one-week postsurgical follow-up, accompanied by her parents. Aditi tossed a notebook onto the table: "My list of complaints." Penciled neatly in the lines of the book were "cramps," "body heat," "lethargy," and "back pain." Dr. Karke was concerned that Aditi wasn't taking in the required 3.5 liters of liquids each day. Aditi, who worked at a bank, came to the surgery by way of a sudden bout of pneumonia and an aftermath of weight gain. "The doctors told me that they were seeing me slip away," she explained to me. Her doctors prescribed steroids and appetite stimulants to treat the effects of pneumonia. Between the two drugs, she gained weight rapidly. Despite dieting and Ayurvedic treatments, she continued to gain weight. Her neighborhood doctor recommended that she consider metabolic surgery. "I wondered why I should get my stomach slit open," she said, so she waited a year and researched the procedure. She spoke with people who had undergone the surgery. "I wanted to come back to my own body," she said. It was a difficult return because of the sudden shift to eating so little and so differently: "But to see yourself as normal, it's all a small sacrifice." Dr. Karke asked Aditi how she was dealing with being in a family that loves to cook. Aditi responded that she avoids the temptation of food simply by leaving any room where food is being made and by avoiding lifting the lids of simmering food. As she left the consultation, she shook both of Dr. Karke's hands, saying "I love you for this."

Not all stories were ones of love and triumph. One of Dr. Karke's patients was a man in his late fifties, who still "had bad numbers" (cholesterol, lipids, fasting blood glucose, etc.) even six months after the surgery. He confessed to eating mostly rice and dal, which was not giving him enough nutrition. He also was drinking liquids along with his meal—another no-no. "This is wrong," Dr. Karke declared. "Your system can't take this." Mixing solids and liquids could cause a patient to vomit, and nutritional deficiency could have systemic ill effects. She brought her intern over and had the man repeat his dietary intake. Dr. Karke asked the intern what should be the course of action, to which the intern replied: change the diet. "No," Dr. Karke corrected him. She turned to the patient. "The long-term outcome depends on *you*." "You"—the metabolic person facing her across the desk—became the instrument of change. Renewal was certainly present in this conversation, and in those surrounding many other patients I observed, such as one woman whose weight loss and insulin levels were so stellar and who was so happy that Dr. Karke's entire clinical team came into the room to celebrate with her. "She's enjoying! She's happy! Not gloomy! A different person! Her family's happy!" the psychologist exclaimed. Dr. Karke was pleased: "*Life badal hai*," she said: The patient's life changed. But she still cautioned the patient that this life change requires "continuous work." The new, reattached metabolism's relationship to the will would work continuously, but there was a lingering responsibility. Dispersal and porosity could go only so far and at times like these flipped back into the frame of the medicalized individual, whose body was the instrument of therapy. Control was indeed happening from within, metabolically. Yet the porosity of the body could sometimes only be realized through individuated stories of tenuous success.

What about those who specifically opted to avoid the surgery? Saurab, in his midtwenties, was one such person who guided his metabolic trajectory away from surgery. We first met in a coffee shop close to his office. He sat down and first showed me pictures on his phone of his American friend, Dan. Saurab met Dan while working in a call center for a multinational bank; Dan was the trainer who taught the Indian workers "global English" ("You bite your *V*s, kiss your *W*s, and don't roll your *R*s," Saurab described as he demonstrated his global English phone voice.) Saurab described Dan as "morbidly obese" and explained that Dan decided to have metabolic surgery after he returned to the United States. Saurab knew all this because the two kept in close touch, especially around the topic of Dan's surgery: Dan frequently e-mailed photos and detailed descriptions of the surgery and healing process to Saurab. Saurab was not enthused about this option to remedy his own weight problem. Even though Dan lost a hundred pounds, Saurab refused to pursue surgery for himself. Many of his schoolteachers had suggested he do it—"*Lipo karelo*,"—"Get lipo," they'd say, using liposuction to stand in semantically for metabolic surgery. But Saurab didn't want surgery, because he was convinced that many of the surgeons were charlatans who offered only a temporary, high-priced fix. He wanted resolution to "life as a fat person," whereby he was too sweaty to sit next to on the train or to attract girls. But he was not willing to go under the knife for it.

Instead, Saurab wanted an option that relied primarily on diet and individual responsibility and, from his perspective, would ensure more permanent results because of his own moral and emotional investments. This is how he wound up at an obesity clinic where the mode of treatment was dieting. He had a cousin who had lost weight on the diet prescribed by the clinic's doctor, and Saurab was especially enthusiastic that the doctor didn't charge much for his consults (five hundred rupees a month, as opposed to the thousands charged by weight-loss clinics). This indicated to Saurab that the doctor was honest, not a charlatan pushing some corporate agenda. He arrived at the clinic at one hundred kilos, and with a cholesterol level of 252. One of his diagnostic laboratory tests computed his "body age" at fifty-four, meaning that physiologically he had the body of a man in his fifties—he was twenty-three at the time he took that test. A year later, at twenty-four, he had lost a considerable amount of weight and immediately prior to meeting me had gone to the lab to have his cholesterol tested again. He pointed to the spot where they sampled his blood. "I was damn scared by the whole thing," he said of the "body age" measurement. He adhered to the doctor's prescription for the diet: Eat food, all day, at least once an hour. He began with daily walks and now jogs daily as well, at a park near his home. On average, he lost three kilos a month since he began the diet.

This changed his self-perception completely. He grew up being teased, called *mota* (fat, in Hindi) or *jharia* (fat, in Gujarati) by schoolkids. He attributed his excess weight to too much "outside food": *vada pav* especially but also cheese sandwiches at afternoon teatime and alcohol at parties and bars. He was content as a call center worker because his customers didn't have to see him. But once he switched to a job in sales for a local newspaper, he felt constant disapproval from his clients and from his boss. They continued to encourage him to lose weight. Having done so, Saurab felt he's advanced professionally: "It matters if you're fat" in a job, he said, as far as discrimination goes. When I asked what he imagined himself doing in five years, as he approaches thirty, the answer he gave was not one of professional aspiration or of marriage but of weight: "I'll have reached my goal weight of being sixty-five kilos." Hours after our interview ended and I returned home, Saurab phoned me to let me know that the results from his lab tests that morning had come back. His lipid levels were much lower, as were his cholesterol and fasting blood glucose levels. He was so proud, he said. The lab diagnostics were concrete evidence of his accomplishments as a "successful" patient—no scalpel required. Saurab's story sets up how metabolic persons solidify through surgery, because his refusal to undergo the procedure kept his body in the domain of the mechanical. Had he elected the surgery, matters of fortitude and willpower could have been cast quite differently.

## Metabolic Persons, Metabolic Promises

In surgery the dynamic intimacies between the metabolism and will-power, although at times indistinguishable, formed the porous thresholds of power outlining a new, presumably healthier life.[3] Designating the metabolism as an operative site could shift the terrain of desire and disease by stabilizing the turbulence of progress and retrogress, success and failure, and therapy and folly. As Lawrence Cohen explains, an "'operation' is not just a procedure with certain risks, benefits, and cultural values" but also confers particular forms of agency in relation to medicalization (1999: 140). To work metabolically, "something extraordinary" had to be done, as Neha put it. That extraordinary work lay in the metabolism's willful attachments.

As noted earlier, the sciences of metabolism share a curious intersecting point with recent developments in science and technology studies, such as philosopher Annemarie Mol's study (2008) of diabetes, in which she asserts that "staying in metabolic balance does not depend on central control and a forceful will, but on dispersed coordination, inside and beyond the skin" (34). Mol's broader work explores questions of ontological dispersion and the necessary acts of coordination required to consolidate a singular medical object (in Mol's terms, "enactments"). In my observations of metabolic surgery, it seemed that surgeons and patients would certainly agree with Mol's claims about dispersed coordination. They also reminded me that a centralized, individuated, "forceful" will was precisely what was at stake in metabolic surgery. Distribution of power was what had gone awry because a person's metabolism gripped the body too strongly and was out of sync with the will. To rebalance the scales, metabolic surgery turned a person into the instrument of her own healing and proved that the metabolism was a crucial matrix of therapy, attachment, and transformative potential. The solution to excessive metabolic force was an intervention that in many senses tried to diminish its dispersion. Dispersion had its limits.

In India, those who undergo metabolic surgery almost always have already tried diet and lifestyle changes to lose weight. In their view and from the perspective of surgeons and of media grown obsessed with the procedure, excessively fat and sick bodies cannot be further disciplined by the efforts of diets or pharmaceuticals. This struck me at first as a compelling contrast to dominant public health and popular discourses, which asserted that pathological fatness was a failure of the will—how a person could not, despite her best efforts, lose weight by controlling food, diet, exercise, and even medication. But in the context of metabolic surgery, the dominant claim that obesity results from a failure of the will becomes perversely correct, because the procedure's advocates attested to the ways in which it was the metabolism that steered the body toward pathological fatness. A person could be metabolic inasmuch as she relied on diets for change, but should the kilos not come off, she was still considered a failure in matters of willpower. "Failure" as a touchstone of the medicalization of fat has its own problems, of course, inasmuch as failure resides not in fat people but in the very stigmatization of fat and in the systems of capitalism that emphasize consumption and then blame individuals for consuming excessively and improperly (Guthman 2011).

As the surgeries for metabolic illness (primarily obesity) have come into view for medical anthropology, scholars have taken up critical questions of success and failure. For example, Karen Throsby's research on obesity surgery in Britain describes the expansion of metabolic surgery there through policies premised on a hierarchy of effort and failure: the failure of extremely obese individuals to lose weight via more "conventional" approaches such as "lifestyle" (i.e., diet and exercise) and weight-loss drugs. In order to qualify for the surgery under the National Health Service, a patient must have failed in her efforts to lose weight by these means. In this way, Throsby (2008) explains, the NHS system demands a willingness to fail and an ownership of responsibility for weight-loss failure from its potential surgery subjects. This individualism is reflected in her interviews with patients who describe a "rebirth" that "signals the reconfiguration of the self as a disciplined subject, who is able to exercise control and restraint over consumption, and who is willing (and able) to take responsibility for the body" (108). Throsby interprets this "new me" discourse as an expression by weight-loss surgery patients of their attempts to get back to the "normal" work of disciplining the body. A new life is a renewed entry into life as before but with a different body, and medicalization through surgery is an enduring disciplinary relationship between biomedical power and the individual, instrumental subject.

What forms does the will take on in this context? The enduring ties between the intentionality and the metabolism's potential for change make the surgery different from simply a surgery that *creates* willpower. Rather, surgery creates a possibility for the will to become meaningful. Metabolic surgery normalizes the metabolism and makes it possible to speak again of the will after willpower has been deemed moot. As such, the "new me" promised through surgery depends not so much on a consolidated, medicalized subject as on a metabolic, porous one. The porous subject here is a metabolic person, in sickness and in health, and at stake are the things that persist as strength even after subjects have been deemed failures. Metabolic surgery mobilized the potential of a slimmer, more manageable body via an intervention on a dispersed force. But the actual results of the surgery materialized unevenly for surgery patients. Dispersal, in other words, was far from even, and the will came under scrutiny postsurgery as intensely as it had before. Many patients described their "transformed" postsurgical lives as indefinitely medicalized through compulsory medications and nutritional supplements. "Adherence" became the watchword. They had turned to metabolic surgery as a last-ditch alternative to dietary therapies but nonetheless became tied to regimens of vitamins and pills required to sustain the surgery's effects. Metabolic surgery ultimately reconnected patients to medicalized daily routines even as they hoped to be released from them.

## Short Cuts

The first live metabolic surgery I observed was at a training for surgeons interested in the procedure, which took place in a hotel ballroom. A banner-sized photo of a man with a bulging belly trying to fit a measuring tape anchored the stage. Two wall-sized projection screens flanking the dais came to life, porting the audience into the gut of a patient. First, an "outside" camera view showed white-gloved hands that palpated a stomach, marking places to insert the scope. Then we saw what the laparoscopic camera saw: the liver, the yellowish intestines, the surgeon's drill bit poking through a layer of white fat. The surgeon, a visiting American named Dr. Pitt, was in the operating room of a high-end corporate hospital in Mumbai, live-screening his procedure to the surgeons (and anthropologist) sitting several kilometers away in the hotel. The two spaces were connected

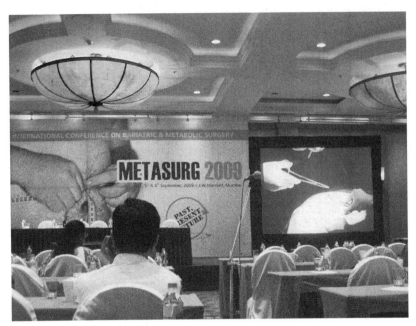

**FIG. 5.1** Metabolic Surgery Conference

by live video and audio so the surgeons at the training could ask questions and make comments as he performed the procedure in the OR. The surgery was the staging ground for teaching Indian surgeons the procedure, for corporations to market products associated with the surgery and its recovery process, and for the surgeons themselves to reflect on the potentials of changing the metabolism by operating on the gut.

Dr. Pitt asked an Indian surgical assistant to give the patient's history: "Twenty-nine-year-old girl, 167 kilos, BMI 51, strong history of family diabetes on both sides, no meds. This will demonstrate sleeve gastrectomy and how to prevent a second surgery." This procedure entailed removing a large portion of the patient's stomach and reducing its size so that only small amounts of food could be eaten and digested. Dr. Pitt showed the camera his tools and their hand placement: a liver retractor, spread out like three fingers, and an endoscope. The liver had some abnormal features, he said, as the camera view switched to inside the patient's body cavity. The retractor entered the picture, lifted the liver, and a pair of two-prong tongs pulled up the tissue underneath. He used an ultrasonic scalpel ("the harmonic"), which he maneuvered between two pinched nodes; its brand name was visible in the close-up view of the endoscope. After it clamped down, the harmonic dissected tissue with a muted humming sound. Small puffs of aerosolized matter sprayed out as the tool cauterized open edges of the cut into the stomach. In his instructions to the surgical team, Dr. Pitt was firm but friendly. When he finished the gastrectomy, he pulled the dissected stomach section out of the tubes, guiding it with retractors. An assistant fixed the outside camera onto a metal container on a side table, showing the stomach remnant, red and floppy. Dr. Pitt held up the stomach piece and explained how to handle events like a stapling misfire. "You don't want to have disasters in your first fifty or hundred patients. You need a lot of skills to do this technique," he said. An Indian surgeon at the meeting wanted to know if the harmonic made the procedure go faster. Dr. Pitt responded that it's not about speed, it's about safety, because the splenic artery can be easily damaged and "you'll get major hemorrhage." "It will not happen often," he said, "but the day it happens, you'll be sorry."

Dr. Pitt's assertion that "you need a lot of skills" spotlights the forms of expertise underlying metabolic surgery at the scale of organs and tissue. Once inside the body, the patient's self-control and lifestyle faded into a briefly recited history. Harmonics, sutures, staples, retractors, and their targets became the center of attention and the semiotic currency of metabolic disease in this context. These tools were complex objects: often during the surgery, Dr. Pitt would remark that certain brands of tools have been shown to be better for the procedure based on studies done in Germany or Israel. India made its mark only in moments when the foreign surgeon was dissatisfied with the tools available. In this space of transnational medical expertise, there was relative silence around the biological specificities of metabolic disease in India as opposed to anywhere else.

In contrast to the strong sense of the globally generic that backgrounded the morning's surgical demonstrations, the sessions following lunch framed surgery as the ideal means to redress the threats that trafficked between the fat body and national stability. One of the country's first metabolic surgeons noted that India is the "global hub" of obesity and diabetes, that surgery is the "next growth" in treatment possibilities, and that more and more clinicians are needed "to fight against this national epidemic that is killing our population at a premature age." His remarks were followed by the CEO of the hospital where the morning's live surgeries were conducted, who affirmed that "at some point in time, India will lead the world in diabetes and obesity" but there is hope because "India is being positioned on the world map as far as metabolic surgery is concerned." An insurance specialist told the surgeons that a high BMI can allow a private insurer in

India to deny coverage to a patient, but this is changing. Insurance regulations were being rewritten, he explained, so that after four years of continuous coverage an insurer cannot use a preexisting condition to deny a claim. Indian insurance companies were thinking "more long term" now: if more Indians are buying coverage beginning in their thirties and forties, metabolic surgery could be appealing to insurers because it would prevent future claims. Here, the metabolism would anchor a future-oriented temporality of security through insurance.

As assistants in the hospital across town put sutures in the girl's incisions exactly one hour after beginning the procedure, participants in the hotel meeting room wandered outside into the lobby area, where food, pharmaceutical, and medical technology companies had set up booths. Food companies shared samples of nutrient shakes and vitamin-enhanced snacks especially suited for post-op patients. Some medical device booths had surgical instruments set up in front of pieces of raw chicken so surgeons could get a simulated feel for the procedure. Another booth played prerecorded surgeries and animated demonstrations featuring the company's instruments on small TVs: the metabolism, commodified across the human body's bounds. The largest booth belonged to Ethicon Endo-Surgery, a division of Johnson and Johnson. The representative handed me a few pamphlets and explained that they were samples of the company's "Bariatric Edge" patient-outreach materials designed to educate potential patients about the procedure. One was a laminated double-sided card entitled "Bariatric Surgery: Losing 50% to 70% of excess weight is just the beginning."

On one side, the card shows a digital rendering of an obese woman whose translucent body reveals organs and bones. Arrows point to a variety of organs and show how bariatric surgery offers a host of cures: Migraines are reduced by 57 percent, depression by 47 percent, hypertension by 69 percent, "metabolic syndrome" by 80 percent (with an arrow pointing to the liver), and type 2 diabetes is 82 to 98 percent resolved. The other side of the card shows a man, with similar statistics linked by lines to his organs. Both have a red summary box at the bottom: "Quality of Life Improved in 95% of patients, and Mortality Reduced by 89% in five-year period." Straddling the boundary between marketing and education, the pamphlets show how obesity's comorbidities are easily locatable in the body, organ by organ, and how surgery can eradicate obesity's risks and allow you to "live your life to the fullest." As one of the pamphlets asserts, with surgery "Your new life can start today." As the pamphlet articulated risk down to individual body parts and disease sequelae, it illustrated the interiority of the metabolism and its indispensable role as the central platform for the expression of diabetes and obesity. The pamphlet summarized the disparate problems of specific organs: they are the elements of "life" and "mortality," and surgery is the intervention that will normalize them by rebalancing the metabolism.

## Side Effects

Dr. Prakash, who attended this training, expressed some concern about this aura of success around the surgery when I visited him for tea a few days later. We met first at his office in a hospital, and as we sat down to talk, he opened his mail. One especially large parcel took his attention for a few minutes, as his assistant struggled to cut open the knotted twine that sealed it. When the wrapping came off, Dr. Prakash pulled out a plastic-wrapped block of Johnson and Johnson "Bariatric Edge" pamphlets, the same ones I received from the company representative at the surgery training. He sighed, saying, "Now the multinationals, they don't only want your money, they want to control your thinking process. I've realized that we always used to wonder that they'll control this, control that, but that's the reality now. They're controlling media now, gradually. Publishing a booklet on obesity surgery, like this, is a way of telling someone 'You're sick. And you need treatment.' They tell people they're obese, and they're sick because they're obese, and they need surgery. And for that surgery, you come to us. And the media shows it." This conviction, he explained, guided him to conduct his "public awareness" seminars like the one I attended. He wanted himself, rather than a pharmaceutical company, to be a potential patient's source of information. In this space of opportunity, he worried that multinational pharmaceutical companies had become the arbiters of expertise, a phenomenon Joseph Dumit (2012) describes as a problem of biomedical conviction.

Trained as a general surgeon, Dr. Prakash initially wanted to specialize in liver transplants and studied transplant surgery in Europe in the 1980s. At the time, though, liver transplants were illegal in India. By the early 1990s, he decided he wanted to do laparoscopic surgery and learned about gastric bypass surgery. One doctor in India was doing the procedure, and so Dr. Prakash went to study with him. At the time, awareness about obesity was "extremely poor." Even up until 2001, he said that some people in the hospital would confuse "bariatric" with "pediatric." What he has been doing for the last five years with metabolic surgery is what he calls "concept selling." He shows people "scientific data" instead of "anecdotal data." He says that people will understand the scientific data and that science should be part of the public conversation around surgery. "Unfortunately," he said, "there is sometimes bad press about how bariatric surgery is life-threatening. And the way that people react to it is to avoid it, because they see that people can die from it." He saw himself less as selling the surgery than as giving information and explaining its risks, and he envisioned the doctor's consultation as the space where patients weigh the risks and benefits of surgery against the risks of staying obese. But although metabolic science has become a high-profile scientific and clinical field in the West, it has only recently been embraced in India.

I found it difficult to map a smooth historical transformation of sentiments about the surgery in my reading of Hindi, Marathi, and English news coverage of metabolic surgery in India. Instead, stories of caution and praise co-occurred for the first several years the surgery was publicized; then the pattern changed: positively themed stories appeared with greater frequency than the more negative, tabloid tales of surgeries gone awry. For example, in 2007, the English-language *Times of India* ran a series of articles about botched weight-loss reduction surgeries, such as the story of a "vivacious 18-year-old" who died in her sleep reportedly from surgical complications. In the article, surgery (and the surgeon) are the villains: "Purnima weighed 180 kg, considerably overweight even for her 6'4" frame. Stomach stapling is a surgery that the obese undergo to reduce the size of their stomachs which in turn limits their food intake. Soon after the surgery, Purnima told her family that agreeing to the bariatric surgery was the biggest mistake of her life. She was depressed after the surgery, her family says." Purnima's surgeon explained to the reporter that the surgery was "incidental" in relation to her death and that Purnima likely died of sleep apnea or pulmonary embolism. The news story concluded that Purnima "is not an isolated case" and noted a twenty-one-year-old who had died recently in Chennai following a similar procedure. Hindi news articles about bariatric surgery similarly cautioned against it, quoting doctors who asserted that it should be used only as a last resort (*Times of India* 2007; *Navbharat Times* 2010).

Along with cautionary tales came stories of satisfied patients who recounted how they turned to metabolic surgery after failed attempts to lose weight via dieting. These narratives formed an increasingly regular pattern of positive stories that counterbalanced tales of frightening, negative results. Journalists continued to weave death into the stories but named obesity itself rather than the surgery as the cause. Instead of stories of victimhood and deadly side effects, these public accounts of metabolic surgery showcased its *lack* of side effects. One story described obesity as the main problem for Jaipur's women, citing a study whose results indicated that 68 percent of urban women in Jaipur were obese, as were 36 percent of the women in the rural areas surrounding the city. The article first explained that bariatric surgery had been growing because of this rising obesity problem and then detailed different surgical procedures. It quoted a doctor who noted that 80 percent of his surgery patients were women. The surgery offered a lower risk of side effects (the story does not note a comparative procedure), with only one in two hundred patients having complications (*parishani ho sakti hain*). Emphasizing that the procedure was backed by research (*research mein yeh aaya samne*), the article concluded that if left untreated, obesity would result in problems ranging from snoring and joint pain to hypertension and diabetes; thus "doctors recommend the surgery" (*Patrika* 2010). From this perspective, obesity and diabetes were "silent killers" that took more lives than well-known killers like swine flu.

News stories also highlighted the plummeting cost of the procedure. The surgery performed on a fifty-four-year-old mother of two in New Delhi in 2008 "has given obese people a reason to smile," one article stated, because doctors performed it "at less than one-fourth the market rates" (*Indian Express* 2008). The reduced cost and increasing number of procedures "will go a long way in curing obesity-related issues," a doctor in Gujarat explained in another article (*Indian Express* 2009b). In February 2010, the Hindi newspaper *Navbharat Times* ran a story titled "Obesity surgery will be free." It described the situation of a man given the pseudonym Rajinder Sethi: "Thirty-eight-year-old Rajinder Sethi weighs 140 kg [308 lbs]. It gives him breathing trouble. In the last six months, he has [had] joint pain. His attempts at weight loss failed. His doctors told him that he needed to have surgery, which costs approximately a lakh of rupees [$2,200]. So Rajinder lost hope of losing weight, but now his dream of being slim will be fulfilled because the Delhi government-run LNGP Hospital has begun a metabolic [bariatric] surgery program, in which his treatment will be completely free" (*Navbharat Times* 2010). The article explained how epidemiological studies suggested that the number of low-income obese patients was rising quickly, and so doctors established a comprehensive obesity treatment program including surgery and counseling to patients with a BMI over

30. Since early 2010, several articles have emphasized that the surgery is within the reach of India's *aam admi* (common man). If not promised as free, the procedure was said to be in the reach of the *aam admi* because it costs less than fifty thousand rupees ($1,100), an amount deemed realistic because of imagined savings or willingness to go into debt (Bhaskar 2010).

Some reports elided the details of risk and focused instead on survival and transformation, such as the story of Chandra Sahu, an oil rig employee whose weight prevented him from boarding the helicopter out to the rig. Sahu's company paid for his gastric bypass surgery with donations from fellow employees; now he "is counting his blessings, which have come to him in the form of true friends and a caring employer" (*Mumbai Mirror* 2008). Love was often at the center of such stories. A laundry owner who underwent the procedure in 2007 told a reporter that he is "waiting for when he can take his wife out after leading an anti-social life for the last 15 years" (*Mid-Day*, n.d.). Such narratives fashion surgery as a platform for communitas and charity, a point where medicine, bodies, and labor intersect. They often position the surgery as a plausible public health intervention, describing it in terms as far-reaching as "Medicare for the Masses": "Manini Agarwal, 42, and Indrani Chaudhuri, 15 (names changed on request), were gaining kilos by the week. Both tried the usual remedial options, diet control and exercise, but couldn't shed a gram. On advice of doctors, they went for bariatric surgery and days later, their weight is back to normal." The article asserted that "more and more experts are banking on bariatric surgery as the surest way to treat obesity, which has risen to an alarming level in the country" and that "doctors say this quick rate of weight reduction is making bariatric surgery popular." A surgeon in Calcutta told the reporter, "Weight reduction through diet control or exercise fails in most cases. But in bariatric surgery, it is guaranteed" (*Calcutta Telegraph* 2007).This guarantee pointed out the gendered dimensions of the surgery. Its description was often linked to the quintessential Indian social hurdle of marriage, in which surgery could serve as a matchmaking aid. Worried that the scars of obesity surgery might "pose a hurdle in finding a suitable groom," a young woman in Ahmedabad opted for single-incision laparoscopic surgery, "which not only worked wonders by aiding to the weight loss process, but also ensured that her body had no scars." A Hindi article entitled "*Sab ek cut, aur vajan ho gaya kam*" (Just one cut, and your weight will lessen) praised single-incision laparoscopy and explained that "these days, there's a growing craze among unmarried girls who are focusing on this surgery that makes only one cut at the navel. Because of this, it leaves no mark." The single-incision method can be traced to 2009, when surgeons in Mumbai performed what was called "Asia's first" single-port laparoscopic bariatric sleeve gastrectomy surgery on a thirty-year-old woman from Trivandrum, who was in surgery for an hour and discharged the next day (*DNA Mumbai* 2009a).

Emphasizing low costs and high-probability results, media accounts positioned metabolic surgery as a plausible public health intervention that could work as a cure. The subheading of a 2007 article in the financial newspaper *Mint* read: "Recent research and debate seem to suggest that bariatric surgery could provide some answers and maybe a breakthrough cure for diabetes" (2007). One surgeon told a reporter, "Private insurance companies would start looking at covering bariatric surgery only if the government declared [obesity] as a serious concern and acknowledged that [surgery] is a lifesaving procedure" (*Loksatta* 2005). The increasing numbers of procedures helped cement the surgery's acceptability. An article in the English magazine *The Week* (2008) quoted a doctor whose early practice of the surgery in 2000 yielded only one patient every three months. "But today," he said, "I perform 10 to 12 bariatric operations every month, of which about 65 per cent are women between the age of 16 and 26." In a *Times of India* centerpiece that announced that 40 percent of India's middle classes are overweight, a Mumbai surgeon noted, "Two years ago barely one person a month would opt for bariatric surgery. Now we have five to six persons a week" (*Times of India* 2009b).

Over time, medical journal publications offered a complement to these media accounts and often offered a more skeptical view of the surgery's aftereffects. A 2013 paper in the *British Medical Journal* examined the many complex layers of bariatric surgery as a mode of treatment for diabetes in India. The author acknowledged postsurgical improvements in "quality of life" for patients. Further, the paper noted that while the mortality rates associated with a laparoscopic bariatric surgery are roughly equivalent to those of a laparoscopic cholecystectomy (gall bladder removal), the risks of malabsorption of nutrients, pulmonary embolus, and staple line leaks were a matter of concern. The paper also cited a Cochrane review of surgical intervention for obesity, which noted that in its review of twenty-two studies comparing surgery with nonsurgical interventions, "The direction of the effect indicated that people who had surgery achieved greater weight loss one to two years afterward compared with people who did not have surgery." But data quality was not consistent. The review noted, "From the information that was available to us about the studies, we were unable to assess how well designed they were. Adverse events and reoperation rates were not consistently reported in the publications of the studies. Most studies followed participants for only one or two years, therefore the long-term effects of surgery remain unclear."[4] The BMJ paper on surgery in India for diabetes, itself concluding on a note of pause, called for close thinking about questions of cost-effectiveness and the procedure's regulation in the Indian context (Varghese 2013).

The growing numbers of procedures also concerned some medical ethicists. Dr. Sanjay Nagral, a prominent physician and longtime editor of the Indian Journal of Medical Ethics, felt that "surgery should be the last option" for patients, that the procedure has been "oversimplified" to patients, and that the potential to gloss over its complications and enduring effects exists. This simplification has helped sway the narrative of metabolic surgery in public media toward a frequently gendered story more about life than death. The "new life" offered by the surgery is a life given to those who previously were distanced from the world, too heavy to work or to find a marriage match. In these narratives, surgery is the path toward resolution of illness not only for individuals but for the nation as well. As a local Mumbai politician who underwent the surgery put it, "I keep recommending it to people who need it." His surgeon agreed: "He was so happy with the result that he agreed to become a brand ambassador for bariatric surgery. Malik is happy to use his public image to spread the message of 'slim India, happy India'" (Times of India 2009a). Interpersonal testimony forged through descriptions of the body's transformation was key to channeling this potential happiness. As metabolic diseases were increasingly portrayed as threats, the ease and simplicity of their cure through surgery gained traction. A single incision and a few hours' stay have narrowed the metabolism to a locatable, easily altered object hardly different from the appendix in some accounts. Risk—and the relationship of individual will to risk—moved inward to a force that only a surgeon could rearrange.

The Only Way Out

The more I spoke to surgeons and asked about their patients, the more I came to understand how many of their patients were actually from outside India. For instance, the relationship between Saurab and Dan illustrates the ways that the surgery forged bonds across nations—how a biomedical commonplace connected persons from different worlds. As with many other surgical procedures, metabolic surgery's actual cost is much lower in

India than in the US or the UK. There is a range of reasons for this, including the low cost of medical supplies, lower labor costs, and the cost-based machinations of private and state-sponsored medical insurance, which are less applicable in India, where services are often cash-based. Metabolic surgery is one of many procedures falling broadly under the rubric "medical tourism," a phenomenon whereby persons travel to different countries for medical care because of comparatively lower costs. A prior research project on medical tourism initially clued me in to the rise in the number of metabolic surgeries performed in India, which in part can be credited to the influx of foreign patients.[5] When I began pursuing the topic of metabolic surgery as part of research on metabolic illness, I found that it was not difficult to meet patients "from abroad." In fact, these were often the ones that surgeons were most keen to introduce me to, so much so that at several points I mentioned that it was Indian patients that I was most interested in speaking with. This happened enough with one surgeon that I reasserted my gratitude for the linkups but wondered why he turned so quickly to the patients from the United States or the UK. Part of the answer was expected: they were "like me," he felt, making the encounter of the interview less awkward. But he also felt there was comfort in seeing someone familiar—that the presence of an American anthropologist would be a welcome breath of the West that the patients might otherwise be missing, no matter how modern or Western the space of the Indian hospital may seem.

As I met foreign patients, I was struck by the ways that India became the place to reconfigure their relations between willpower and weight. Peter was the first such patient I met. He met me at his hotel near Marine Drive, and he said he had begun going for short morning walks on the promenade to get out of bed. Coming from the UK for metabolic surgery in Mumbai, Peter had been in India for only a few weeks. This was not his first visit, however. He had volunteered with an NGO in India several years back and felt familiar enough with India to assertively reject the label "medical tourist" that he said some might apply to him as a foreigner coming for medical care in India. Peter described his obesity as a development in his adult life that would not ease no matter how much he tried. He certainly had the motivation. Having endured the loss of both parents as a child and his job and girlfriend as an adult following a debilitating car crash, he felt he could take on any burden. Throughout his life, Peter was told his intellectual capacity didn't amount to much, but he took the initiative to return to college as an adult and eventually earned several graduate degrees.

His willpower was put to the most stringent test when he was diagnosed with HIV. "Most people think that when you're HIV-positive, you're like a stick," he said, but not him. His antiretroviral medications caused him unremitting weight gain. He tried dieting, with no success. He starved himself, which did nothing for his weight and only made him sick. "I had a greater chance of dying from obesity than from HIV," he realized when he weighed nearly three hundred pounds and was diagnosed with diabetes.

Peter learned about metabolic surgery from Internet research; he wanted the sleeve gastrectomy procedure in particular. When he asked his physician in the UK about the surgery, the doctor adamantly refused because he said Peter needed a full, intact stomach to absorb his HIV medications. Peter was not deterred. He read a study of HIV-positive persons who underwent sleeve gastrectomy successfully, but no hospitals in the UK wanted to take the risk on him. "No one wanted to touch me," he said. The procedure was deemed "pioneering" and "risky." Moreover, his BMI was too low to qualify for any NHS coverage of the costs of surgery should he find a hospital willing to shoulder its risk. His only option was to binge-eat to gain weight and increase his BMI to meet the NHS minimum requirements. "Doctors in the West are driven by statistics and litigation," he said ruefully.

"Weight is willpower," his GP back home said, telling Peter that he needed to straighten out his emotions in order to lose weight. But Peter disagreed. His willpower ceased to matter as far as his weight was concerned, as no effort on his part was effecting change. Because he had visited India before, he knew about the growing number of metabolic procedures performed there; he also qualified for the surgery under the BMI guidelines used by most Indian surgeons. Through the Internet, he found Dr. Prakash and after several exchanges traveled to Mumbai for the surgery, which cost roughly a third of a comparable procedure in the UK. One week after the procedure, he lost twenty-eight pounds, and his insulin response to food normalized. Peter credits the surgery with breaking a destructive cycle of attachments to food in terms of eating and then trying to lose weight. "As you get fat, you withdraw from society," he said. Society promotes thinness, and to be a fat person living in a thin society is painful, "a double whammy" for him being both HIV-positive and fat. He felt stigmatized and consigned to his house being HIV-positive, and being overweight, the forced retreat drove him to eat even more. He believes the surgery will move him out of the house and into an ordinary rhythm of living in the outside world.

Peter had come alone to India for his surgery, but other foreign patients brought in family members for support. This was the case with Amy and Dina, a mother-daughter couple that I met in the lobby of their hotel in South Mumbai. When I spoke with the mother, Amy, I first asked how she came to India for the surgery she had undergone just days before. "She'd had it, too, and I was having problems with my diabetes," Amy replied, pointing at Dina. I was confused, but Dina interjected, explaining that she herself had had the surgery (gastric bypass) in India several years back. Dina convinced Amy to do it, too. "It'll be nice to be smaller," Amy said, "but the diabetes was the real reason." She was already off all of her medications for diabetes (she had been diabetic for five years). She wanted to be able to drive around Dina's kids, her grandchildren. "I don't want them to be ashamed of me," Amy said. "You know they love you, and they let you know they love you, but you know that they aren't real happy to say 'this is my grandma.'"

Insurance was another factor that brought her to India: "I guess I splurged on myself," she said. At sixty-two, Amy was fully insured, but metabolic surgery was not covered by her plan. It was "ridiculous," she said, that no matter how severe her diabetes, she could not get the surgery covered. Amy worked at a bank and had discussed her situation with some of her clients who were doctors; they believed that if U.S. insurance plans covered the procedure, doctors "would be overwhelmed with the people that would do it all at once." She was not yet sixty-five either, and so Medicare was out of the question. She calculated that the surgery would cost thirty-five to forty-five thousand dollars in the United States, and that did not even cover lab tests and the required presurgical education sessions ("and I don't really need to hear those things again"). The total cost of her procedure in India was nine thousand dollars, and her only other expense was the plane ticket. Amy felt the quality of care was extremely high. "I mean, you always hear people saying 'oh, people die from that surgery,'" she said, and she personally knew two people back in the United States whose spouses died from complications of metabolic surgery. But her surgeon in India had a much better success rate and had performed far more operations. Her procedure wasn't without minor complication, though. "It hurt like hell," she admitted, which surprised her because Dina never had any pain. Amy pointed to Dina again: "That kid was a frank breech," she said of Dina's birth. "I almost died. But this was worse." But she felt that even in the most painful moments during her surgery in Mumbai, a hospital staff member was there to care for her. And she's not diabetic anymore, she emphasized again. "You try convincing Blue Cross/Blue Shield of that," she joked.

While Amy had gained weight later in life related to her adult-onset diabetes, Dina had been heavy all her life. In high school, boys would promise that "we might really have something together" if she lost twenty pounds. "Then I ended up gaining more weight, gained it all back, and every time you gain weight it brings friends and then you end up heavier than before," Dina explained. She was an employee of the city government, and in her early forties she looked into the option of metabolic surgery in her home town. Insurance didn't cover it. She even tried using her connections in the town, to no avail. She continued to gain weight following a hysterectomy, then more when she quit smoking. "I was trapped—I was hidden down there, and you couldn't see the real me," she said. She was passed over for promotions at her job, which she attributed to discrimination based on her appearance. But then a friend of hers who also wanted to do the surgery discovered the option of medical tourism. Dina and her friend made a pact to go to India together. Her friend, though, worked for a military contractor and was suddenly sent to Iraq, leaving Dina alone. Deciding to go ahead with the plan, she went to India alone. Upon meeting her surgeon in India, she told him, "I'm the same person but I'm trapped inside this large body and can't get out." She said. "I wanted the surgery so badly, it was my only way out."

As much as I had heard about and witnessed scalpels and laparoscopes moving through the body, it was striking to witness how metabolic surgery created global channels, too. The metabolism was the site of rearrangements for the will; the brain-gut axis of therapy had a geopolitical axis as well.

Medicinal *Atyachaar*

A few weeks following the conference where we met, Neha called me. She was going to be "in town," meaning Central/South Mumbai, and wanted to meet there, as opposed to trying to coordinate a meeting near her home, which was hours away in traffic. Because of its proximity to the city's central railway station, we met at McDonald's. The lively crowd around us, mostly teenagers and office workers, ate off plastic trays covered by paper liners that announced "McDonald's balances its food for you!" underneath a picture of a Filet-O-Fish with labeled arrows pointing to the bun ("carbohydrates"), the lettuce ("fibres"), the fish ("proteins"), and the tartar sauce ("fat").

In recalling the developments over the course of her life that led up to her surgery, Neha, now thirty, expressed conflicted sentiments. Becoming heavy was a more recent change; until the end of high school, she was skinny. Then she started putting on weight and "moved into a sedentary lifestyle." She described herself as extremely studious and as spending lots of time with her books; it was during study times that her mother pampered her with food: "Before I could realize it, I was obese. I was putting on six or seven kilos a year." She noted that from an early age, she was fixated on eating. "Normal people eat to live," she said. "But superobese people live to eat. I still love to eat food, but it's a matter of internal control." Looks had never been a priority for her. But a doctor's visit confirmed that she had a thyroid problem, and so she "passed the buck" of her weight onto the thyroid problem. Eventually she joined a gym, buying the most expensive membership she could afford, but it didn't work. She entered a destructive cycle: she was happy once she lost weight, but she associated happiness with food, and then she would indulge. "Food is the best reward, I learned," she said, "but it left emotional cobwebs," meaning that food made such strong impressions on her sense of self that she couldn't see where one ended and the other began.

With no success at the gym or with dieting and feeling time slipping through her fingers, she tried other approaches to losing weight. She went to a health farm in Pune, famous for "scientific" Ayurvedic approaches to weight loss and body purification. She wanted "to deal with obesity as a disease" rather than as an aesthetic issue. But it didn't work. She became depressed and felt distant from her family and their support, so she ran away from the health farm and came back to Mumbai. She tried diets endorsed by celebrities. She tried corporate weight-loss programs. "Luckily, I was married already," she said. She didn't have to worry about finding a husband, unlike her overweight cousin, for whom the family still can't find a match. Trying to lose weight became a dead end for Neha: "I decided to live with this body for the rest of my life. I gave up. I became fatalistic. I closed out relationships, distanced myself from anyone who would give me suggestions about how to lose weight."

Then a trusted friend and a cousin both mentioned that they knew patients who had undergone gastric bypass surgery. Neha decided that "it was God's design" that these two reminders came at the same time from two people she trusted deeply. She also learned about the surgery from online obesity-surgery bulletin boards, where you can post a profile and communicate with potential and past patients. She thought seriously about it: "I thought, maybe you can buy life." She wanted it done in December, before New Year's, because she didn't want an obese body in the forthcoming year, and after visiting several surgeons settled on Dr. Prakash. The timing was very meaningful to her: "It's a cliché, and my husband jokes about it, but it *is* a birth, a miracle. I don't know how else to describe it. I can just feel a new body." Since the surgery, she has lost nearly sixty kilograms and is working toward losing more by her birthday. Her digestion and breathing have improved. "I met this friend called adipose, but now I'm making space for new friends. Before, it was me and my fat and my other friend, food." But now more porous, she had made room for other people and was planning a weekend trip with girlfriends for no particular reason except to get out of the city. Before the surgery, she only would have come home to her husband after work.

However, the medicines she must take following the surgery are extensive. She called her daily routine "medicinal *atyachaar*," meaning tyranny or torture by medicine. It's *atyachaar*, she explained, because she has to take nutritional supplement pills throughout the day and always has to think, "Did I pack my medicines?" Moreover, the torture comes in the constant reminder that she's medicating herself: "I try to say to myself, it's not medicine, it's nutritional supplements." "Supplements" enhance a new metabolism rather than remediate a sick one. In this frame, cure relies on enrichment of the new rather than reparation of the old. Enrichment describes well how Neha has refined her everyday life in a future-forward sense in surgery's aftermath. Monitoring the medications, going to the gym, and keeping track of food now takes up all of her time. She keeps a diary, which has several check boxes that she evaluates every evening: swim, gym, diet, medicines, protein shake. Prior to the surgery, she had "a complaining body, an achy body. It was an ill body. But I've become active now. My body has become lighter." The trade-off, however, is the "medicinal *atyachaar*," as she emphasized again: "My whole day works around my medicines. . . . I've had to come to terms with the fact that I'll be taking these supplements for life." But the tyranny of pills was the trade-off for seeing her new body in the mirror as a result of the surgery. She had few complaints about the procedure, although she found it difficult to wear certain kinds of clothes to show off her body because of sagging skin left in some places after the weight loss. She thought her body would tone up, but she was coming to terms with the possibility it wouldn't. She wanted cosmetic surgery to take care of it but explained, "I come from a middle-class family, I can't afford that." She had already spent a large sum of money on the metabolic surgery procedure itself.

An unexpected outcome of the surgery was that it reconnected Neha to her spirituality. She described herself as a religious and spiritual person but one who had a tough time maintaining faith because of the psychological challenges of being obese. But she had faith in her doctor, faith in her husband's support, and faith in her body to cooperate with the surgery. One of our several meetings occurred in the middle of Navratri, a nine-day period of fasting and reflection for Hindus. As a child, she would have only liquids during Navratri, choosing to forgo solid food as part of her fast. As she grew older, she would either avoid fasting entirely or would fast because she saw it as an opportunity to crash-diet. But the surgery connected her elsewhere. She took out a small plastic container from her purse and showed me the handful of dried fruits and nuts she had been eating during the day as her version of fasting. But she was also looking forward to Dusshera, the tenth day that concludes Navratri's nine days of fasting. She could "indulge" then. Her friend was fasting, too, so she had a "fasting buddy," and they would break the fast on Dusshera together. This would be Neha's first indulgence in her new body.

Neha's example shows the capacity for intimacies to be crafted between a willful self, a sick body, and an operation to fix both via the metabolism. Her words to describe her body moved from a register of distance wrought by heaviness to one of closeness that emerged with a sense of being light. It was heaviness that erected walls between her body, her family, and her friends—and had it not been for her husband, she would have been walled off from finding love and security in marriage as well. Her surgery has helped her to unbrick those walls. One reading of Neha's narrative might be as a story of rebirth in which she emphasizes miraculous genesis and the pursuit of life goals otherwise forestalled by obesity. Surgery in this frame incorporates subjects who are not remedied as much as they are renewed through a metabolic intervention. The narrative of renewed will, crafted through a language of "fixing" and "rebirth," points to a failure by overweight people to achieve health in their first bodily incarnation.

Such a reading, however, risks missing how much Neha emphasized the *atyachaar*, the torture, of the surgery's aftermath amid this rebirth. Our interviews in Mumbai unfolded as *atyachaar* gained more traction in the city's parlance, perhaps because of the soundtrack from the film *Dev*

D, which includes a song called "Emotional Atyachaar." The hero in this 2009 adaptation of the 1917 Bengali novel *Devdas* experiences "emotional torture" amid unrequited love and alcohol addiction. In 2009, "Emotional Atyachaar" leapt from song title to urban argot to reflect a conflicted inner state with tinges of addiction, even becoming the title of a TV show that unearths romantic infidelity and helps its cast members (and presumably its viewers) avoid future "emotional atyachaar" should they suspect a cheating partner. *Atyachaar* describes tyranny's chronic presence and tenuous attempts to dispel it rather than a singular act of vertical power from a vague overseer. The will was speakable again but came with several attachments. Neha looked to metabolic surgery to be let off the hook; she was, but she was hung on another lifelong hook in the process: the *atyachaar* that now outlined her attempt to disentangle a world in which willpower was still inextricably tied to weight.

## A Shift in Arrangements

"Life doesn't merely move and change, it exchanges," writes Michel Serres. For Serres, exchange occurs "by means of the metabolism, and the diverse transactions with the environment" (2011: 51). Metabolic persons attest to the visceral porosity of the body in this exchange. They announce forces of courage, love, fear, and desire cascading through the body's energetic channels, even as a medical diagnosis has consolidated that body as a singular success or failure. Yet as Serres reminds us, "All power must, in every circumstance, stop short of the body's integrity" (2011: 52). There is something about dispersal and decentralization that eventually runs into a hitch. Bodily integrity does not just dissolve into the metabolism without a lingering reminder of the changes it takes for the self to move into different alignments with the gut.

Metabolic surgery offered a different kind of porous thriving amid efforts to dispel weight. Surgery tempered the metabolism so that metabolic persons could once again be in the thrall of external attachments. At the same time, some of those new attachments involved prescribed drugs and timed meals in order to sustain the surgery's benefits and echoed the kinds of regimented life before the surgery that prompted a flight path in the first place. These shifting connections joining the will, the metabolism, and medicine illustrate the problematic promises and realities of healing the suspected ills of consumption and of alternative vectors of metabolic life besides mere success or failure. In his writings about illness and cure,

Georges Canguilhem (1991) notes that the reactions of the sick person to sickness "are not the residue of previous normal behavior . . . they are reactions which never turn up in the normal subject in the same form and in the same conditions" (184). Cure for illness is what Canguilhem calls "a shift in arrangements": not a reversal of processes that unfold in the course of sickness and thus not the inverse of injury but rather a rearrangement of the unique order of life cultivated by the sick subject for whom disease reverberates in everyday and often banal moments. The enactment of cure occurs through new, more general disturbances, a set of conditions of normalcy that for Canguilhem "lies hidden" in the compromised subject.

Neha's invocation of *badalte rishte*, a change in relationships following her surgery, articulates some of the rearrangements at stake for metabolic persons seeking this path to cure. So do the visceral rearrangements that happen between the surgeon's hands, their laparoscopic appendages, stomach pouches, and hormone levels. Metabolic rearrangements complicate an assumption of medicalization as life's singular, unobstructed outcome. Rearrangements point out the uneven dispersal of the will as a person recuperates and regroups. The surgical patients I observed and spoke with in Mumbai took extensive measures to avoid medicalization through dieting, even as they embraced an intensive, intimate form of medicalization through surgery and then wound up feeling trapped in postoperative bodily regimens. Goal-oriented pursuits only of life and health were exactly what the surgery was supposed to overcome. They wanted to disconnect their relations to dieting and reconnect with friends, family, and faith, and they saw surgery as the best means to do so. The contours of a will impossible to realize in relation to health came under the knife. Once sutured to the metabolism, the will was speakable again. This explained why surgery could treat and possibly "cure" metabolic disease in ways that diet or exercise schemes could not. "Cure" meant being healed in terms other than a rigid language of willful, healthful ambition. Putting cure into practice involved dampening an aggravated metabolism so that the willful subject might again have a say in the extent of her porosity to the world. The question "Do I have enough will to cure the problem?" must, like the metabolic person, be porous enough to accommodate another question: "Is this a rearrangement I can live with?" For even in its less despotic forms, the metabolism still demands the attention of both will and world, in conditions both torturous and vitalizing, offering both improvement and *atyachaar*.

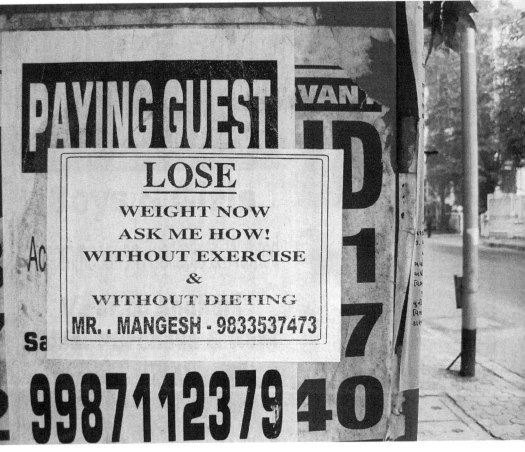

**FIG. C.1** Weight loss ad, Bandra

Bulldozers breach Manuli's streets. Mumbai's civic authorities deemed several of its beachfront hutments unlawful due to lack of permit payments, and bulldozers crashed them down, with a noise that woke people up in the early hours and triggered their *tenshun*. The plague crosses amid the rubble were spared and continued to cast shadows over homes with curtains for doors. Televisions lit the entryways from the inside. One evening's light source came from a televised special called "Is obesity now one of urban India's silent killers?" In front of the camera sat prominent metabolic disease specialists and a man several months out of his successful metabolic surgery. The host of the show began the program with a provocation: "We are asking 'How fat is too fat'? Is obesity one of urban India's silent killers? SMS us Yes/No at 56388 in India, 6388 if you are in the UAE, or 63880 if you are in the UK. You can also log on to EntertainmentTonight .com during tonight's debate live as we speak." In the format of a debate, the demands to make metabolic living comprehensible could work only as a text message and only in terms of a single relation of pathological overflow: Yes or no? Is there or is there not a problem? Like the weight-loss crosses that opened this book's introduction, fat's presence or absence set the conditions for life.

Let us consider not the host of the program nor the doctors seated in a face-off nor even the patient brought in to testify. Let us instead consider the camera itself. In the question above—is there or is there not a problem?—there is a misrecognition of what might be understood as the *aperture effects* of chronic disease discourses. In a camera lens, as the aperture opens wider, the depth of field of the picture decreases. The subject appears more crisp, and the background more blurry. But the camera can only zoom in so far, and so the person and the body are stand-ins for the metabolism. Here, the problem of framing is representational and material both, one of epistemology and ontology. One element of the picture—the subject—becomes highly detailed in this wide-aperture shot. All that coexists with the subject in the frame dissolves into haziness.[1] This kind of hyperfocus and background blurring characterizes much of the chronic disease discourse in India and elsewhere. Representationally, what comes into focus is the rise of the new urban middle class and its habit of overconsumption, believed to logically lead to illness. Public health discourses integrate these logics to assert a rationale for prevention and treatment programs (see Crane 2013). With an emphasis on transition, the subject in focus is one of change: from undernourishment to overnourishment, from under- to overconsumption. In these popular epidemiologies that tie fatness to sickness, the subject of accumulation explains the causes of chronic disease. Any number of risk factors float in the background, but the consuming subject stands at the fore. Materially, the dynamics of biology and affect condense into a body, fattened or thinned, that works as a substitute of sorts: the metabolism's stuntman. Metabolism, skin, and the experiential worlds of desire and aversion connected to substances remain disparate.

Attunement to absorption has different aperture effects. It twists the lens. It blurs the subject a bit, while giving the background some crispness. Absorption stretches across the domains of the body and environment and across the material and the biopolitical, precisely because these domains already stretch across and overlap each other in representation and in experience. In times when the stakes of long life hinge on bodies and environments suffused with substances, my research suggests that we ask how and why life comes to reside in fat or in specific patterns of food. To ask this question requires conceiving of persons who *have* metabolisms and understanding the lived features of metabolism presupposed in the "have." Such features include ways that metabolism is distributed in and outside a singular body; ways that it operates across bodies and environments, because those domains are unequally but mutually porous; and ways that it stretches beyond humans, for the substances humans ingest or absorb have past and potential metabolic and political activity themselves. Absorption twists the lens to see these features lived out in real time in persons who turn objects into themselves. It clarifies why the solid subject and blurry background hold so much power to explain ideas about the contexts, causes, and consequences of metabolic illness in India and elsewhere. One might say that it is not so much that persons and metabolisms are mismatched. Rather, we could make a stronger statement that it is an abiding analytic that is out of alignment with all the things metabolisms are and do across shifting arrangements of bodies, substances, and environments.

My principal concern in this book has been to develop an ethos of absorption at the interfaces between food and living. Each chapter has narrated absorptive patterns concerned with metabolism: its constitution, its moments of concreteness or abstraction, its locational coordinates, its shareability, what satisfies or aggravates it, and its ends. Inquiry into ideas and experiences of absorption allows food to be important to the story of metabolic illness but disallows food's exclusive reign as an end unto itself. Attention to food's movements in and out of bodies and surroundings demonstrates how persons and food interrelate in ways besides instrumental eating. The implication of this analytic is a more nuanced way to witness how passages between organisms and environments do cultural, social, and political work. It is an entry point into technoethical questions, such as "What counts as food and when does it mean life?" as well as questions about method and narrative, such as "How might we account for the complexity of vital substances, while staying close to the thoroughly human elements of appetite, nutrition, and illness?"

I have argued that metabolic illnesses are symptoms of, first, porosity between bodies and environments and, second, degrees of openness of understanding metabolisms. In metabolic living's material, subjective, and conceptual terms, one can see and hear and smell and touch and taste appeals to biochemistry, metaphors of machines, and eddies of strengthened and weakened willpower. In the case of the *vada pav*, we saw that urban politics plays a key role in defining the parameters of what food is and does. Scales in Mumbai's train stations, taken alongside scales of a national body mass index for Indians, can question claims that fatness always equals sickness, that substance transmutes fully into the attrition of life, and that metabolic disorders kill only in terms of a body consuming too much. The plastic enrobing packaged foods and the brick in the chili powder the plastic is supposed to deter destabilize easy answers about what it means to be sick from food.

As metabolic illness increasingly occupies global health interest and investment, what is needed is a perspective on metabolisms and their disorders different from one grounded in concerns about overconsumption. Metanarratives such as "globesity" and its mapping onto India cannot precisely account for the variable and relational entanglements of illness's connected objects, experiences, and environments. Conceptually, overconsumption closes doors when it comes to metabolic matters, because it remains moored in questions of proportion and excess. Through the lens of consumption, material-experiential worlds can appear only as equal-opposite vectors, such as indulgence and illness or risk and reward. Obesity and diabetes should not be approached as "diseases of modernity" without either "diseases" or "modernity" better specified, because this classification too often stands in for expressions of willful overconsumption. Small cutouts of the amounts of rice a person eats, cascades of pills and injections of insulin, and the stitches of a postsurgical gut challenge us to understand how the metabolism cannot be taken for granted as a unit that is equally shared, equally disturbable or restorable, or equally the "thing" that people talk about when they talk about ordered and disordered eating. Flattening the metabolism in this way risks an analytical and narrative overreliance on a general theory of consumption. To be clear, I am not calling for removing consumerism or consumption from the picture; in fact, my argument has often tracked across grounds of individuated desires for material goods and for a life sustained by aspirations characterized by fashion, beauty, possession, upward class mobility, and symbolic capital. Rather, I have emphasized absorption in order to describe persons living in environments of illness. These persons are fully enmeshed in the byproducts of modern life (see Fortun 2012). Through absorption, we might consider how to relay that description without presuming that metabolisms match persons and places, and to elaborate how food and fat traverse unexpected pathways before and after they turn into disease (see Farquhar 2002). The constant rescripting of what counts as metabolic illness creates a broad spectrum of possible meanings for clinicians and persons experiencing obesity and diabetes to work with. From its links to *tenshun* and stress of the city to the ways metabolism comes to be a proxy for willpower in metabolic surgery, this dynamic has profound implications for people who experience a moving target of expert knowledge that informs bodily intervention.

Anthropology engaged with metabolism adds to the conceptual and material history of this moving target. Intensifying concerns about obesity have prompted a reckoning with the metabolism in recent years, but the metabolism has anchored dynamic conversations between the biological and social sciences since the nineteenth century. "Metabolism is not a concept floating above time, influenced by metaphor and imprinted by context . . . metabolism is *in* history," Hannah Landecker writes, and "the alimentary and the therapeutic are being pressed into new relations of meaning and value in ways that reconfigure both food and medicine" (Landecker 2013b: 497–99). Detailing the history of the concept of metabolism, Landecker observes that "while many ask the question of what causes metabolic disorder . . . we should reverse the formulation and ask instead what metabolic disorder is causing; specifically, what are its knowledge effects?" (2013b: 498). In attempting to follow this suggestion, I have explored where, when, and how the capacity to change impacts knowledge and forms of life. I have approached metabolism ethnographically as a pattern at work. How its relations condense into *a metabolism* or *the metabolism* or *an Indian metabolism* are matters of absorption. "Metabolic" in "metabolic living" reminds us that as substances bleed between the body and the world, they effect changes upon how both domains interrelate. I recognize that hanging this book's analytic work on metabolism adds further questions to a concept whose instability is my ethnography's prerequisite. This indeed may be deemed a limitation of the research. Nonetheless, this approach is intentional. Any appreciable concluding thoughts on metabolism cannot pull on its emergency brake, for whether in flesh or in theory, metabolism is in constant motion as people abide and reorganize their passages between substances and vitality.

During a trip to Delhi toward the end of my fieldwork, I treated my friend Rekha to dinner as a thank-you for letting me stay with her. She asked if we could go to her favorite restaurant in an outdoor middle-class market brimming with activity on a warm Friday evening. Hawkers sold jeans from open-air stalls; carts sold kebabs, biryanis, Chinese stir-fries, and Delhi's famous *chaat* (snacks), all grouped together to fashion a food court. The setting was a modest counterpoint to the three megamalls we passed in the car on the way to the restaurant, sprawling structures that glowed with spotlit signs for high-end boutiques. One ad reminded passersby to embrace the spirit of "shoptimism" during the lean economic times of the 2008 global financial crisis.

As Rekha and I walked out of the restaurant after dinner, a girl in a dusty dress approached. "Hello, madam," she said sweetly to Rekha, hand extended to signal a request for money. "*Nahin* [no]" Rekha said, and kept walking. The girl followed, moving her hand repeatedly from her mouth to pat Rekha on the arm. "*Bilkul nahin*—absolutely not!" Rekha said firmly. Frustrated, the girl put her hands on her hips, stood firm, and shouted, "I'm just asking for food—who said I was asking for your life?" (*Khana hi mang raha hai, kaun sa jaan mang raha hai?*) A pause, then Rekha quietly handed over her leftovers from dinner, wrapped in tinfoil boxes and plastic bags. In the car on the way home, she said she felt bad about being stern initially. She relented because she was stunned by the girl's candor. Shaking her head in amazement, Rekha repeated the girl's words, in English but for the word *jaan*, meaning "life": "Who said I was asking for your *jaan*?" In that encounter, *jaan* was a counterpoint to a box of leftover rice, a condition of living that included but exceeded food.

The question of what kind of *jaan* living with and without food entails was a question that stayed with me after the encounter with Rekha. I returned from Delhi to Mumbai and then to Manuli. Under the watch of the crosses, men and women wade into the sea for work and for ritual, to get fish, to wash clothes, and to immerse idols. Persons net the sea for sustenance. Yet the sea nets life, too. It absorbs bodies over time. I was told many stories about fishers who had drunk too much *desi daru* (country liquor) with their *chakna* (snacking often coupled with drinking alcohol) to steel themselves against the tides for the day's work. "I don't know what happened that day," Aunty Cecilia's grandson, Thomas, told me of his cousin Wilfred, who had drowned one morning while fishing. Wilfred was known to be a skillful drinker: he could navigate the sea, collect shells, and net fish after a long night of drinking or a morning "breakfast" gulped down. But one morning he went into the sea and didn't return. "Maybe the sea swallowed him," Thomas thought. Over many months, the family had tried to intervene in Wilfred's habit of drinking *daru*. Everyone knew it was adulterated; people who drank cheaper versions of it might go blind or even die from ethanol poisoning. Thomas tried to get Wilfred to switch to whiskey, to little avail. "This is my wife," Thomas recalled Wilfred saying of his *daru*, the night before he drowned. It was a substance he cared for, and one that cared for him. In the neighborhood, there were equivalences between food and pharmaceuticals (see chapter 3). But in this instance a different sort of food came to the fore: a liquid sustenance that was omnipresent but whose mortal effects materialized as persons whose bloated bodies washed on the shore.

Thomas described other ways in which the sea stretched the boundaries of the skin. Like many men in the neighborhood, he had worked on oil rigs in the Gulf. A man would stay for several months, send money home, and return to Mumbai from time to time to be with family. Thomas had rotating shifts in Saudi Arabia, Dubai, and Qatar. He complained of a permanent cough he developed and attributed it to the chemical spray in the mechanic's area that showered him day in and day out. When I first interviewed Thomas, we talked about his rhythms of eating, of fish and rice when he was in Mumbai and whatever the cook on the rig prepared when he was on one of his work trips. The international makeup of the crews on the rigs meant the menus were quite diverse; he got to know and love foods from the Philippines, from Thailand, and elsewhere. Men worked together and ate together—and the meals were often centered around beef (Thomas loved steak). The overlaps between masculinity, meat, and labor (on the rig but also affectively, between workers) anchored our conversations about any given "typical" day on the rig. But as I got to know Thomas better, our discussions about rhythm and time shifted. More and more, he discussed the time he spent in or out of the protective suit he had to wear against the chemicals he was exposed to. Thomas showed different pictures—not just those of men eating together but of men working together, sluicing chemical solutions from one hose to another, tightening and loosening the valves controlling the flows, looking somewhat awkward in thick yellow protective suits. There were photos of him and his friends taking soda breaks, suits half undone. Mealtimes, like sleep, were some of the only times spent out of the suit. The heat was searing on any given day, and the offshore rig offered little shade. To be encapsulated in a heavy canvas suit was awful, Thomas explained, but necessary; who knew what the cascade of chemicals would do to you over time? Substance and time had complex and uncertain relations to metabolisms in what we might understand as windows of exposure, windows filled with steak and spray.

Across the book's chapters, I have maintained that there is a temporal consequence to the idea that people are their metabolisms, individually and in aggregate. Cultural figures like the thin-fat Indian condense the past and the present risk of disease. The processed housewife is the gatekeeper of the family's health in times of changing food markets. These figures are made to produce evidence about the passing of time in relation to illness, even though, as we can see with Thomas's example, bodies in Mumbai do not stay put. Nonetheless, these cultural figures "clock" Mumbai's vitality and mortality. They show how the selective porosity between bodies and environments is a story about time as much as it is a story about illness. They suggest future directions for the ways medical anthropology can better engage matters of chronicity in terms of substances that signal life-giving and life-draining actions. This is important for a better understanding of global health in the era of HIV, cancer, and other disease formations with long-term experiential and material features (see Redfield 2013). So too is it resonant with the questions posed in medical anthropology about exposure, toxicity, and the attrition of life in the context of environmental crises (see Fortun 1998 and Petryna 2003).

To further an anthropology of life's metabolic dimensions, perhaps we might think about *world clocks*. With this term, I mean to conjure the idea of bodily time zones with temporal alignments and disjunctions that we do not understand fully but deploy nonetheless.[2] The world clock allows multiple temporal horizons to converge while retaining the specificity of the local. Sometimes we forget about world clocks, thinking the time "here" and "now" is the same everywhere. In other moments, moments of comparison, we might remember the most commonly reckoned method of global temporal difference, Greenwich mean time: "Mumbai is 10.5 hours ahead of eastern standard time right now," I might think. With this metric, time here and time there can be different but coexistent.[3] The asynchrony of bodies and lives in one place is a cue to think with the complex chronicities of metabolic illness. Different forms of time often condense into a seemingly singular thing like metabolism in order to be portable and meaningful. Several examples from this book show how the time of the body and the time of the city converge, consolidate, and circulate. Recall the amount of time left for productivity, as the doctors and epidemiologists in Chapter 1 expressed concerns that diabetes was increasingly afflicting India's young and productive group. We also see time at work in the phenomenon of readiness, a temporal condition inflecting how packaged foods move in and out of homes. World clocks govern the lines outside Trinity Hospital and inside its hallways, the different time frames that Dr. Samant and Dr. Chitre each worked with in relation to the pancreas or to the circulatory system. Later, we saw that *atyachaar* works as a kind of chronicity in which body, food, medical intervention, and willpower are in tense relation. In the introduction, I posed the idea that it is more accurate and productive to think of persons who have metabolisms rather than persons who are their metabolisms. This allows us to understand how people may share physical space but do not necessarily inhabit the same metabolic world. Thinking of absorptive bodies and environments as constituting world clocks can offer insight into the conditions under which time works as an important bodily resource and form of expression of both health and illness. It also offers a way to consider the merits and flaws of the demands people face to fold their knowledge and experience into globally comparative forms of evidence.

Moving through these local articulations of long- and short-term injuries, it becomes clear that the "chronic" in "chronic disease" is the time for science to digest itself, and our bodies are differentially featured on the menu. Expertise about metabolism changes across knowledge production in epigenetics, clinical medicine, urban governance, diabetology, endocrinology, nutrition science, and surgery. World clocks show us our inability to know precisely *when* metabolism is (in addition to not knowing precisely *what* it is and *who* must authenticate it). They concentrate our thinking on what must be concealed or arranged together in order to gain enough confidence to say, "Over time, eating this will eventually kill you" or "Over time, eating this will eventually save you." The body accumulates and diminishes through absorption as toxic substances seep into its cells and into the seas that feed it. World clocks open up questions about absorption's temporal trajectories across substances, bodily injuries, and technoscience.[4]

Metabolic living is a way of living through, asking about, and critiquing the composition and permeabilities of these trajectories.[5] It is also a way of thinking differently about persons in health circumstances, because of the conventional assumption in many medical discourses of a singular world for an identical mass of bodies. For instance, in these refrains, persons are caught in "the built environment" or succumb to "lifestyle" practices that render them fat and sick. I have attempted to parse alternatives to such singularities by describing the makeup of diverse metabolic worlds and by pointing out how environments are "a field of experiences and enterprises," as suggested by Georges Canguilhem.[6] I envision a both-and engagement with organisms and environments.[7] With this conceptual guide I hope that conversations about metabolic illness concerned with *the environment* can emphasize the relational emplacement of persons and objects (for critiques of the term "environment" in relation to obesity in the United States, see Guthman 2011, Kirkland 2011). Recall the television commercial for noodles in this book's introduction. If bodies share space but not entire worlds because metabolisms are not uniform, anthropologists might describe the makeup and relational paths of these differentiated worlds. Some lead to better health, and some literally dead end. To return to Hannah Landecker's assertion, the metabolism is *already* in objects, persons, and environments. The challenge that follows is to examine how people grapple with and live out the emplacement and displacement of a world within a world.[8]

My study of metabolic living reveals an overlap of the politics of life, knowledge, desire, and substance. Metabolic disorder is an ethnographic object that tells us much about the kinds of desires produced in popular and anthropological efforts to elucidate the relations between foods, fats, bodies, and environments. It would be an understatement to say that fatness in times of obesity has provoked intense popular and scholarly inquiry, albeit mostly in Euro-American settings.[9] Although this book has drawn on scholarly engagements with obesity and diabetes to ask what fat looks like when viewed "from the South," I do not take these conditions as already legible, globally mobile, and happily settled down in an unexpected place such as India. I have worked anthropologically to build alternatives to a common trope in global health discourse and research whereby the vernacular reads as self-evident, such that the "in India" part speaks for itself. It never does. My concern with "metabolic disease in Mumbai" ultimately has been directed at the preposition itself—"in"— as I have narrated stories of metabolic living. This kind of prepositional analysis foregrounds absorption and permeability in a specific ethnographic case study. It also highlights Mumbai's material dynamism, such that "metabolic" is again not a metaphorical reading of the city but rather a quite literal one. The city is built upon shifting sands, some reclaimed, some eroding away.[10] Finally, this study raises questions about what anthropology itself seeks to absorb: what, where, when, and who engrosses and fattens it. For metabolic living—metabolic *jaan*—entails grappling with the magnetism of intimate attachments. When that magnetism is disturbed, a question arises: How do we live with rearrangements of persons, substances, and places over time?

*Introduction*

1. I have changed the neighborhood's name, along with the names of its residents and other persons and institutions involved in this book. The distinction between "Mumbai" and "Bombay" is a complex one, with political and historical entailments that stretch back even before the official name change in 1995; see Hansen 2002. Many of the residents in the neighborhood use "Bombay" and "Mumbai" interchangeably, sometimes as a function of the language being spoken. I attempt to reflect these patterns wherever possible. The work of Kalpish Ratna (Kalpana Swaminathan and Ishrat Syed) first brought the Bombay plague's manifestation in Bandra to my attention; see Ratna 2008, 2010, 2015. For additional engagements with the plague in India, see Arnold 1987, 1993; Klein 1988; and Kidambi 2004.

2. Philosopher Catherine Malabou calls transitions "theoretical fissures." "Problematically, they are not recognized as such and thus "run the risk of being overwhelmed by brute, naïve ideology," she writes (2008: 63).

3. This model, presented as somewhat infallible during my own graduate public health education, explains dietary trends in human history as a five-pattern process that moves through regimes of plant-based foraging, famine, famine's reduction and the rise of processed food intake, and the eventual final, ideal pattern of "healthy" food intake and subsequent reduction in chronic diseases. The nutrition transition model nests within ideas about "the epidemiological transition," a shift from predominant burdens of infectious disease to those of chronic disease. See Popkin 2001; Popkin et al. 2001; Popkin and Gordon-Larsen 2004. For critiques of these models, see Nichter and Van Sickle 2002;

Gutierrez and Kendall 2000; Barrett et al. 1998; Inhorn 1995; and Trostle and Sommerfeld 1996. In her ethnography of cancer in Botswana, Julie Livingston (2012: 34) addresses the telos of the epidemiological transition at length.

4. Political scientist Leela Fernandes persuasively argues for thinking of the new middle class in India "as part of a state-led project (and problem) of development rather than as an expanding consumer group that has naturally been produced by economic growth" (2009: 220). Fernandes lauds scholarship in anthropology and media studies that has focused on the public sphere and public culture to better understand expressions of class identity and consumer desire (Mazzarella 2003, 2006; Rajagopal 2001; Appadurai 1996; Mankekar 1999; Breckenridge 1996). However, she notes (222) that studies of public culture "tend to associate new consumption practices with the expansion of privatized spaces" and have an "implicit tendency to locate consumption as a site of individual, privatized strategies that are shaped by these processes of privatization". Fernandes suggests that the problem with a "public culture" approach is twofold. First, it undertheorizes the influences and discourses of state-led development over middle-class consumption. Second, it reproduces an erroneous assumption that the middle classes belong to the market, while the rural and urban poor belong to the state and its development schemes. This is a quite helpful critique, although in light of my own intervention it has a key limitation. It allows the state to work in unexpected places, but still the analytic of consumption itself remains unquestioned—it merely shifts places. On the middle classes in India and their historical and contemporary dynamics, also see Goswami 2004; Srivastava 2007; Jeffrey 2010; Lukose 2009.

5. See, e.g., Joshi et al. 2012; Patel et al. 2011; Misra et al. 2011; Kinra 2004.

6. Jean Comaroff (2007) usefully calls this phenomenon a "medicament"—a clash between public health officials, pharmaceutical companies, insurance companies, and health activists over the comparative merit and urgency of the issue.

7. According to national surveys, eating habits indeed do vary across social classes. See, e.g., http://www.thehindu.com/news/national/eating-habits-vary-across-classes-nsso/article6178320.ece.

8. Landecker's historical and contemporary work on metabolism guides my thinking; it inspires questions about environmental absorption more pertinent to my topic of study than does the act of digestion. For a detailed analysis of digestion in South Asia, see Roy 2010.

9. Here I draw on Latour's notion of composition "from discontinuous pieces." In his "Compositionist Manifesto," Latour observes that we find ourselves in a situation where "consequences overwhelm their causes, and this overflow has to be respected everywhere, in every domain, in every discipline, for every type of entity" (2010: 484). Later: "For a compositionist, nothing is beyond dispute. And yet, closure has to be achieved. But it is achieved only by the slow process of composition and compromise, not by the revelation of the world of beyond."

10. Haraway (2008: 46) points out this thread of Marx's theory as central to her thinking: "Of all philosophers, Marx understood relational sensuousness [of relationships underlying use and exchange value], and he thought deeply about the metabolism between human beings and the rest of the world enacted in living labor." Landecker (2013a) explains the specificity of science that influenced Marx's thinking here: it was German scientists theorizing how the metabolism works, in contrast to French scientists.

11. A discussion in 1958 about the relationship between culture and economic development included anthropologists M. N. Srinivas and Milton Singer, who opined that "there are practical values held by the Hindu peasant strong enough to give welcome support to economic reform." Everyday cultural practices were key to this question. Anthropologist Milton Singer (1972: 188) observed that the central problem for "traditional" Indian society was how to sustain their "cultural metabolism" and "continue converting the 'raw' and 'uncooked' events of history into 'cooked' and assimilable 'cultural traditions.'"

12. See Nichter 2001 and Langford 2002. Nichter examines in Ayurvedic care contexts how matters of indigestion surface as stress. For engagements with Nichter on this front, see Ecks 2014: 83.

13. Analyses that trace back to Pierce are compelling, but I have chosen a different route for my own material. For work in this tradition, see Meneley 2008; Keane 1997; and Weiss 1996. For an analysis in this vein in South Asia, see Hull 2012. I follow Karen Barad's definition of an apparatus as fundamentally part of both the object being observed and the agencies of observation (2007: 119). By extension, I find Barad's use of the term "phenomenon" as an observation-dependent object a strong analytic for conceptualizing the metabolism. My use of "pattern" stems from the work of Gregory Bateson, who considers a pattern to be "an aggregate of events or objects which will permit in some degree such guesses when the entire aggregate is not available for inspection" (2000: 413). Bateson wrote of cybernetics and hydraulics, of stimuli and reflexes. He described the metabolic nature of systems of stimulus and response in his cybernetic models of human perception and behavior. "If I kick a dog," Bateson wrote, "his immediately sequential behavior is energized by his metabolism, not by my kick. Similarly, when one neuron fires another, or an impulse from a microphone activates a circuit, the sequent event has its own energy sources" (2000: 409). Note here the echo of Bateson's engagement with metabolism in Latour's cybernetics-inspired concept of the black box, where a circuitous, almost mechanized process gains life. This illustrates the salience of metabolism to contemporary concepts of "hybrids" (such as Haraway's cyborg or Latour's black box), precisely because of Bateson's influence on science studies (Tresch 1998).

14. One of the reasons I emphasize "living" and not just "life" is summed up well by Susan Leigh Star (1991): "I think it is both more analytically interesting and more politically just to begin with the question, cui bono? Than

to begin with a celebration of the fact of human/nonhuman mingling" (43). Cui bono—for whose benefit?—is a question within reach when analysis is focused on the constriction and widening of people's ways of living.

15. Of course, conceptions of epidemics change over time and with political contextual variation, evidenced most familiarly in the case of AIDS (Rosenberg 2002; Briggs 2003; Epstein 1998; Biehl 2007; Farmer 1992; Fassin 2008). On the outbreak narrative, see Wald 2008. Even the Bombay plague outbreak of 1896 sparked an interpretive tangle; see Ratna 2008, 2010.

16. Perspectives on causality reflect perspectives on "real-world" possibilities for change. As Karen Barad notes: "Causality is not interactional, but rather intra-actional. Making policy based on additive approaches to multiple causes, misses key factors in avoiding epidemics such as providing inexpensive forms of safe food for the poorest populations and the elimination of industrial forms of the mass killing of animals" (Dolphijn and van der Tuin 2012).

17. For a compelling example in the case of brain imaging, see Dumit 2004.

18. I am deeply grateful to Joseph Dumit for pointing out this contrast to me; it unlocked all sorts of doors to new ways of thinking.

19. As Ed Cohen (2009: 70) explains, via Locke, being and having a body are property relations.

20. So too has scholarship on traditional forms of healing in South Asia addressed arrangements of the body's constituent parts and wholes; see Craig 2012. On the ontological contingencies of "traditional" medicine elsewhere, see Langwick 2011; Zhan 2009.

21. To be clear, my framing of fat and of fatness in this book sustains a critique of the fear of fat developed by critical scholarship about obesity. Metabolic living is meant both to speak to fat-phobia and to open up moral models tightly fixed to body size. However, I also want to be careful here to avoid casually importing specific political formations (such as queer and feminist movements in the US that link up with fat rights) into India (where to the best of my knowledge, fatness is not articulated as a "right").

22. See Sen 1983; Patnaik 2007; Deaton and Drèze 2009; Arnold 1988, 1993. On famine as a modern formation, see McLean 2004. On famine as a mode of Indian historiography, see Mukherjee 2015.

23. One way this move to put science studies and area studies into conversation has materialized has been as "postcolonial science studies." See, e.g., Anderson 2002, Anderson 2008, Hecht 2012.

24. This raises several questions about the usefulness of the concept of "urban health"—which I do not employ in this book, because the urban and the healthy are both constantly subject to change and also have amalgamated relations.

25. Robert Tattersall (2009) notes that current definitions surrounding states of diabetes differ from previous invocations of "prediabetic," which in the mid-twentieth century could refer to children whose parents both had diabetes (160).

26. For ethnographic work on fishers, also see Subramanian 2009; for Mumbai-specific case studies, see Subramanian 2010.

27. Elsie Baptista's ethnography of Bombay's East Indians remains the only holistic ethnographic study of the community that I was able to find; it is still held in the library of the Bombay East Indian Association, blocks from where I lived. It is striking in its details and includes several sections specifically devoted to food practices and cuisine. The literature on Christianity and Catholicism in India is extensive; see, e.g., Raj and Dempsey 2002. A history of the East Indians written and published online by community members both incorporates and diverges from Baptista's research; see http://www.east-indians.com/historygeography.htm.

28. See Metzl and Kirkland 2010, particularly essays by Vincanne Adams and Lauren Berlant.

29. On the ontological and material turns in STS, see Lynch 2013 and Paxson and Helmreich 2014.

30. The metabolism is not quite like language, a system that can be used self-referentially.

31. Annemarie Mol's study of medical ontologies considers the metabolism in this light, such that "diabetes" is distributed across its actors (diabetics and their caregivers) and objects (insulin pens, socks). According to Mol, "Staying in metabolic balance does not depend on central control and a forceful will, but on dispersed coordination, inside and beyond the skin" (Mol 2008: 34). I agree with Mol's point about dispersion but am less sure about coordination as a suitable political formation. In Mumbai, as I hope to show throughout the book, things may coordinate but often there are extremely divergent interests in play. To say that food companies coordinate with the opportunity presented by chronic disease by offering functional foods is correct, but the term "coordinate" risks flattening and even eclipsing power relations quite central to the story.

32. On this count, metabolic living offers a different standpoint than "coproduction," whose deployment I find can risk leaning too heavily on the lot of the sufferer to speak to the instability of science, a burden I am not interested in demanding of my interlocutors, who already have enough fires to put out in the everyday.

33. It is important to account in small ways for my hunger, my eating, and my body in relation to food from these inquiries. How do you ask about what the body and food do to each other in another person even as *you* sit across from that person chewing, digesting, feeling? I have found Gregory Bateson's thoughts helpful here, as Bateson sought to understand how to write about the mind while acknowledging that he did so as a thinking being. See Bateson 1991: 283–85.

34. As Julie Livingston (2012) notes, this of course impinges upon questions of the extent of disease: "We cannot know the extent to which a long-standing burden of disease is now being unearthed through the expansion of services

and public awareness, and the extent to which actual rates are rising. Most likely, it is a combination of the two" (11).

35. A political economy of matters of concern (as articulated by Latour) is what Lynch (2013) seems to be calling for: "We would want to treat 'matters of concern' not as a master category. . . . We would look for instance in which 'matters of concern' are locally relevant and locally contested" (456).

36. There is an additional challenge: I do not suggest that people in Mumbai demonstrate an ineluctably uniform "local" manifestation of a "global" health transformation such that the case closes around national borders. Mumbai is a deeply and historically globalized setting: "From its inception, Bombay has been closely linked to the world market," write Sujata Patel and Alice Thorner (1995: xiv). As location pertains to global health, see Brada 2011.

*Chapter 1. The Thin-Fat Indian*

1. See, e.g., Jirtle and Skinner 2007; Bateson et al. 2004. For a social critique of epigenetics and epigenomics, see Papadopoulos 2011 and Landecker and Panofsky 2013. Also see Alter 2014; Fortun 2008; Fullwiley 2011; Lock 2013.

2. Neel 1962. Neel is not always painted in the most positive of lights. Nancy Scheper-Hughes (2006) notes that his theories are "just so stories" that cement indigenous peoples into representations of inherent pathology (xx).

3. For political histories of famine in India, see Arnold 1988.

4. On the stabilization of an organism's boundaries, see Fleck 1979.

5. For critical engagements with plasticity, see Malabou 2008; Papadopoulos 2011; Rees 2010. To varying ends and through various tactics, these authors examine the political entailments of the "flexibility" of the brain and in terms of the metabolism as an organic system. This is a caveat well articulated in Wilson 2004 and Wilson 2015. On development systems theory in biology, see West-Eberhard 2003. On the plasticity of the cell, see Landecker 2007: 92.

6. See Kuzawa and Quinn 2013. Kuzawa elaborates from a biological anthropological perspective how the inverse relation between birth weight and adult cardiometabolic disease can be understood as a problem of memory.

7. Scale "is the spatial dimensionality necessary for a particular kind of view, up close or from a distance, microscopic or planetary," writes Anna Tsing (2005: 58).

8. For reflections on the explosion of number and its capaciousness across the social, see Guyer et al. 2010 and Patel 2007. For medical anthropologists, bodily enumerations do complex cultural and ontological work; see Biehl 2007; Mol 2002.

9. As Julie Chu writes about her observations of numbers in Chinese temples, "Numbers did not have to add up to some elegant figure here. Instead, they needed to overflow as public spectacle, unfolding one after another in a recursive and resonating pattern" (2010: 137).

10. The 2012 film *Shanghai* also spins an ironic twist on this term of national

grandiosity in the song "Bharat Mata Ki Jai": "*Sone ki chiḍiya, dengue malaria*" (The golden bird [of India], [now infected with] dengue and malaria).

11. While some vernacular-language papers assign their reporters to health care stories, more often I found that health news was syndicated and translated from its original English. This was made possible because many of the wider-circulation vernacular papers were part of a conglomerate, along with English papers, magazines, and television channels. Within a media corporation, stories could circulate internally, requiring only translation specific to the language of the region in question.

12. Radhakrishnan 2009: 457. Radhakrishnan also points out that "the comparative act, in enabling a new form of recognition along one axis, perpetrates dire misrecognition along another." Comparisons of thinness and fatness, then, are only one axis running through the plastic body. Radhakrishnan uses the example of the city to further his point: "I would argue, for example, that the 'global city' is the product of a comparatist coup: a coup that commits the global city to the rationale of transnational flows rather than to the rhythms and needs of the intranation," he writes. In a different sense, the thin-fat Indian can also be taken as a figure of what Peter Sloterdijk calls a "territorial fallacy" (2013: 151). Globesity and the thin-fat Indian are in an off-center relation. Globesity evokes terrestrial globalization, but the thin-fat Indian is a landed figure. That land has strong vernacular resonance in the Indian setting, as it is the ground between city and village, which filters into studies like Dr. Yajnik's carried out in rural Maharashtrian villages and then producing hypotheses that guide clinical application in cities. Imprints of thinking comparison in terms of location appear in anthropology in Boas 1887.

13. *Tenshun* appears in several ethnographies of healing and distress in South Asia. See, e.g., Chua 2014: 52; Cohen 1998: 194–99; Ecks 2014: 87; and Halliburton 2009: 195. These scholars point out how tension, or worry, circulate through layers of felt experience, diagnostic psychology/psychiatry, and circulatory disorders ranging from imbalanced sugar levels to depression to hypertension, or "BP" (blood pressure).

14. In Bombaiyya Hindi, the city's vernacular mash-up, English words inserted themselves into conversations otherwise strung together from Hindi, Marathi, Gujarati, and Tamil; in Manuli, it could be peppered with Konkani, too, because of the many Goans living in the neighborhood.

15. Cohen (2000) also notes the ubiquity of "tenshun" and particularly "BP" as an illness category in his fieldwork in North India, although he observed specific gendered differences in its meaning. In my own observations in Mumbai, BP seemed to affect men and women similarly.

16. See Lawrence Cohen's discussion of the body of the peasant in medical anthropology in Inhorn and Wentzell 2012.

17. Ian Hacking (2006) argues that the BMI is a cheap alternative to knowing the distribution of population-level obesity: "Yes, self-identification is imperfect information. But it is cheap. It is comparable to the BMI, the Body Mass

Index, which the current obesity panic has made a household phrase. Adiposity, the ratio of body fat to body mass, is the important health indicator, but it is fairly expensive to measure by any current technique—and thus comparable to a personal DNA readout. But the BMI is very cheap: stand on a scale, stand under a device that measures height, press two buttons on a calculator (or use one of the innumerable online BMI calculators), and there you have your BMI. . . . A national study of adiposity would have been more informative and would have cost about a million times more" (88).

18. Dr. Mehta, as an Ayurvedic physician, traffics in categorical body types that might very well be understood as metabolic types, but he made no mention of this in our interaction.

19. Historian Sander Gilman (2010), in writing about the "Hindoo boy" obesity case study, notes that Dr. Don's invocation of the "Fat Boy" is likely a reference to the character of Fat Joe, also known as the Fat Boy, in Charles Dickens's *Pickwick Papers* (1836): "The echo of Dickens in this colonial report is clear" (11).

20. A group of scholars have converged around the Barker hypothesis as a site of critique; some find it liberatory because of its possibilities to think through emergence; others have found that it demands too much of mothers and their bodies (this critique was later revisited). The challenge with these works is that, however unintentionally, they take the world of possible analysis as the West. *Tenshun* is not on the radar. For Dr. Kartik, it is; and while I absolutely agree with these scholars that a feminist critique is necessary, I also want to point out how clinicians work with absorption (and not maternity) as a first-order axiom of critiquing something like "fetal programming."

21. Here Dr. Kartik's thoughts on accommodation overlap semantically with such terms in developmental biology and biological anthropology as "phenotype accommodation" and "phenotypic inertia." See Kuzawa 2013.

22. See Mol 2002: "If the outcomes of diagnostic techniques are taken to stand for different objects, however, these may be aligned again to form a single one. The form of coordination that comes into play here is that of adding things together" (68).

23. Georges Canguilhem (2008) writes the following about the body as a product: "The body is a product insofar as its activity of insertion in a specific milieu, its (selected or imposed) way of life, sport, or work, contributes in fashioning its phenotype, that is, in modifying its morphological beginning and structure in individualizing its capacities. It is here that a certain discourse finds occasion and justification: the discourse of hygiene, a traditional medical discipline, recently recovered and travestied by the sociopolitical-medical ambition of regulating the lives of individuals" (473). See Landecker 2007 for a detailed explanation of these conditions.

24. Berlant's broader conclusion is that "long-term problems of embodiment within capitalism, in the zoning of the everyday and the work of getting through it, are less successfully addressed in the typical temporalities of

crisis" (2007). See Kirkland 2011 for a critique of Berlant's deployment of "environment" here. Also see Povinelli 2011 for thinking about the "lethality of liberalism" that is not about catastrophe but rather about the "slow rhythms of lethal violence" that wears persons down (153).

## Chapter 2. The Taste No Chef Can Give

1. Appadurai's conditions for gastropolitics are as follows: "Gastro-politics . . . can arise for a variety of reasons, but there are three types of situations that are likely to engender conflict: when one or more of the relevant principles is inherently ambiguous; when two of the principles are in apparent contradiction in a particular context; and when, though the principles are clearly grasped, incumbents of key roles are in conflict over actual gastronomic compliance with the expectations associated with these roles" (1981: 495–98).
2. For an examination of this question from the perspective of sex work, see Shah 2014.
3. Mumbai has many street foods that might be known as "the favorite." This is certainly the case for *bhel puri*, a puffed rice and chutney snack. Some claim *vada pav* as a Maharashtrian food, and *bhel puri* has a lineage connected to groups ranging from Gujaratis to others as far away as West Bengal. To call the *vada pav* Mumbai's favorite food is in some senses to claim Maharashtra as the "natural" root of Mumbai's street food, although the influences from other regions are readily apparent.
4. Navaro-Yashin (2012) is working through a critique about actor-network theory (ANT) here, and I largely concur with her that ANT's "things-first" mantra has resulted in ethnographic quandaries such that "if the human has not altogether disappeared in ANT frameworks, accounts of it have become extremely impoverished" (163–64). This is a sentiment I also find in Arjun Appadurai's reflections on ANT: "In its preoccupation with the agency of the device, [ANT] has evacuated from its accounts of sociality all the things that make human sociality so fascinating in the first place" (2013: 258).
5. In the case of Mumbai, which had long had a Maharashtrian middle class (centered on Shivaji Park and in the neighborhoods of Lalbaug and Parel for the more working classes), such distinctions are critical.
6. While the fried potato patty alone (a *batata vada*) can be found across the city, the potato patty sandwiched in bread (the *vada pav*) is often found in the working-class neighborhoods surrounding the mills of the city's center and in the neighborhoods where former mill workers have resettled. But it has also spread to other areas of the city and can be found around college campuses, outside office buildings, and on busy thoroughfares.
7. See Cohen (2010) on the politics of recognition and relation at stake in becoming publicized in India. See Hansen (2001: 16) and Sen (2007) about negotiating sympathy and field methodology with the Shiv Sena.
8. See PTI (2009) for the text of Thackeray's speech in Marathi and English.

9. For coverage of the event, see Koppikar 2009 and Allen 2008.

10. There is also an invocation here of the rural Sindhi countered against the urban Mumbaikar. As Weiss (2011) explains, food has a powerful ability to show how "the distinctiveness of place shifts with respect to the social relations of interlocution" (444).

11. See Ries (2009) on the ideologies of nationalism that cohere through food and, in this shared case, potatoes. Many scholars of Shiv Sena politics and of Hindutva have pointed out this linkage between Hindu nationalism and consumerism since India's economic liberalization (Appadurai 2000; Rajagopal 2001). Appadurai (2000: 645) notes that Bal Thackeray was pleased to welcome Michael Jackson to his home and clinched a deal with Enron, which had been interested in energy initiatives in Maharashtra. In this way, the "transformation of Bombay into Mumbai is part of a contradictory utopia in which an ethnically cleansed city is still the gateway to the world." For other studies of the Shiv Sena, see, e.g., Bedi 2007; Eckert 2004; Katzenstein 1979; Masselos 2007; and Prakash 2010.

12. On people as infrastructure, see Simone 2004.

13. For a detailed discussion of the gendered, embodied politics of vegetarianism, see Alter 2000a; Donner 2008; Ghassem-Fachandi 2009; and Roy 2010.

14. See Paxson (2013) on the concept of "microbiopolitics" in this light.

15. This seemed an odd way to describe the food, as calling someone "healthy" in Hindi is often a euphemism meaning that the person is chubby.

*Chapter 3. Readying the Home*

1. Monteiro, in this venue and elsewhere, called it "ultra-processing." See Monteiro and Cannon 2012.

2. On the cultural figure of the market woman and matters of propriety in other geographic contexts, see de la Cadena 2000; Weismantel 2001.

3. The term "functional foods" was the newest label for what previously were called "nutraceuticals": food products (including drinks) that have some added nutritional benefit. For an overview of functional foods, including their history and questions about their blurred medicine/food qualities, see Chen 2008.

4. An extensive set of studies examines tensions between inside and outside, home and world, and public and private as constitutive of modern Indian social, cultural, and political life. See, e.g., Chakrabarty 1991; Das 2007; Kaviraj 1997; Procida 2003. Veena Das (2007: 179) offers a helpful critique of Chatterjee's division between *bahir* and *ghar* by pointing out that the "signature of the state" is "re-created and not only outside such forms of sociality" of inside and outside that Chatterjee's dichotomy proposes. For gendered and queer readings of domesticity, see Price (2002) on the production of structures of feeling around the home that help make invisible the violence enacted in the name of naturalizing a sense of safety where (primarily men's)

needs can be anticipated and met. The work of Arlie Hochschild (1983) is fundamental to outlining the problems of domestic labor and an affective economy in the American context, much of which also reverberates within Indian appeals to Western, middle-class domesticity marked by two working parents but persistent obligations of the female partner to care for the husband, children, and the extended family.

5. This work is reminiscent of Margaret Mead's writing on "nutritional gatekeepers," the women who carefully police ingestion in American households (1943).

6. Vanaspati, or vanaspati ghee, also works culturally as the manufactured fat of the West, as opposed to a vernacular indulgence, as in this nostalgic reflection: "You know what's the perfect symbol of India's *bindaas* [fearless, daredevil] gung ho spirit, its cussed refusal to mimic the West, and its unpredictability? It's ghee. India has always loved ghee, or pure butterfat. Ayurveda says ghee is great for increasing self-awareness and intelligence, besides getting a complexion and voice to die for. Ghee is soothing and delicious. It evokes memories of dripping rotis, drenched rice, and bowls of dal with a half-inch layer floating on top. Those innocent days before we learnt to eat alien palm oil and soya bean oil" (Srinivas 2009). In this rendering, ghee belongs to the innocent vernacular, while vanaspati—often made from palm oil—is "alien."

7. I concentrate here on *naqli* food, but for an extensive analysis of "fake" drugs, see Peterson 2014. The word *milawat* ("mixed") is used in everyday Mumbai speech in both Hindi and Marathi along with the English-derived word *adulterashun* to describe the unwanted compromise of proper food with other substances. When describing a particular item of food that is adulterated, one is more likely to use *milawat*'s adjectival form, thus *milawati dudh*, "adulterated milk." This usage is also common with drugs deemed counterfeit or adulterated: *milawati dava*, "adulterated medicine." The overlaps here between "adulterated" and "fake" show the importance of a substance's possible corruptibility and efficacy to its ontological realness. *Naqli* works to foreground authenticity and belonging, as ethnographers of brands and their counterfeits in India have detailed (Cohen 2007; Mazzarella 2003; Nakassis 2012).

8. The force of biomedicine here is where functional foods become part of a much longer history of adulteration in India. It is also in this light that I examine both adulterated and functional foods as what Sidney Mintz calls "drug-foods" (1985).

9. I did not have the opportunity to speak with milk sellers themselves, but Joseph Alter's ethnography *Knowing Dil Das* offers insights into milk adulteration from their point of view. Alter's ethnography is based on the life of a milkman named Dil Das, whom Alter knew since his own childhood, spent in the North Indian hill town of Mussorie. Alter (2000b) devotes an entire chapter of the book, "Dairying," to Dil Das's stories about life as a *dudhwala* (milkman). Milk adulteration and the milk economy more broadly represent what he calls "the gastropolitics of postcolonial India": "In coming to represent health and wealth among those who consume it, milk, for those who produce and sell it,

has become a fluid channel through which resources are being drained away," he writes (111). Scandals were profitable for the nexus but that profit was in liquid relation to the health of families. Alter notes that "it is virtually commonplace among urban consumers to categorically accuse rural producers of diluting the milk they sell with water" (101). He points out that milkmen themselves complain about how "watery" milk can be, a property blamed as much on the wet grass that buffaloes consume as on criminal middlemen. Alter writes that "all milkmen do dilute the milk they sell with some water," and that the variability of butterfat content from animal to animal provides a cover for the practice of adding a ratio of roughly 25% water that is the tacit threshold for diluting "without getting caught" (101). Alter's analysis of milk adulteration, told from the perspective of Dil Das and other milkmen, brings to light the instability of local, regional, and national milk economies. He explains that milk adulteration is one way in which farmers and local milkmen brace themselves against the contingencies of price fluctuations, and of the loss of labor-contributing family members to life events such as marriage and illness. Alter also notes the embodied consequences of milk adulteration: "The commodification of dairying has meant, ironically, that very little milk is being consumed by the children of those who produce it, while their labor directly contributes to the girthy status of middle-class tourists and the physical fitness of missionary youth. . . . Given the multiplex significance of milk as a vital fluid in the gastropolitics of postcolonial India it seems that what might simply be characterized as an economic injustice is also, and more significantly, embodied as a hierarchy of health, within the core and periphery of Mussorie's milk shed" (111). For a global cultural history of milk, see DuPuis 2002; for a discussion of dairy adulteration in China, see Tracy 2010.

10. This was something rather exceptional in terms of propriety, because in most of my relations to neighbors, if they had a cook/housekeeper it was a woman. The kitchen was a space where Manu—a man in his fifties who had been Jyoti's servant for thirty years—and I could be alone together, a shared experiential space that I would never be allowed in the usual configuration in Manuli of a female cook (much less a younger woman).

11. This emphasis on individual responsibility poses a solution to what novelist Rana Dasgupta (2005) lists as the ultimate threats to Indian middle-class life: "germs, crime, poverty, [and] unwise consumer decisions" (77).

12. While it is an issue of contemporary concern, it also has historical precedent. In his study of the school lunch as a modern social institution, historian James Vernon (2005) explains how food-adulteration scandals in mid-nineteenth-century Britain "energized investigations into the properties of food and the biochemical processes of the human body while simultaneously cementing the connection of these forms to agencies of the state" (271).

13. There is some flexibility for individual countries in terms of labeling; in India, companies print a green circle on products that are halal.

14. The full section reads thus: "The Central Government, the State Governments, the Food Authority and other agencies, as the case may be, while implementing the provisions of this Act shall be guided by the following principles, namely: (1) (a) endeavour to achieve an appropriate level of protection of human life and health and the protection of consumer's interests, including fair practices in all kinds of food trade with reference to food safety standards and practices; (b) carry out risk management which shall include taking into account the results of risk assessment and other factors which in the opinion of the Food Authority are relevant to the matter under consideration and where the conditions are relevant, in order to achieve the general objectives of regulations; (c) where in any specific circumstances, on the basis of assessment of available information, the possibility of harmful effects on health is identified but scientific uncertainty persists, provisional risk management measures necessary to ensure appropriate level of health protection may be adopted, pending further scientific information for a more comprehensive risk assessment; (d) the measures adopted on the basis of clause (c) shall be proportionate and no more restrictive of trade than is required to achieve appropriate level of health protection, regard being had to technical and economic feasibility and other factors regarded as reasonable and proper in the matter under consideration; (e) The measures adopted shall be reviewed within a reasonable period of time, depending on the nature of the risk to life or health being identified and the type of scientific information needed to clarify the scientific uncertainty and to conduct a more comprehensive risk assessment; (f) in cases where there are reasonable grounds to suspect that a food may present a risk for human health, then, depending on the nature, seriousness and extent of that risk, the Food Authority and the Commissioner of Food Safety shall take appropriate steps to inform the general public of the nature of the risk to health, identifying to the fullest extent possible the food or type of food, the risk that it may present, and the measures which are taken or about to be taken to prevent, reduce or eliminate that risk; and (g) where any food which fails to comply with food safety requirements is part of a batch, lot or consignment of food of the same class or description, it shall be presumed until the contrary is proved, that all of the food in that batch, lot or consignment fails to comply with those requirements."
15. These products do have an energized market in India, however. In particular, Amway has launched a line of nutraceuticals and protein powders that has seen initial market success among higher-income groups in the urban centers; see Mukherjee 2009.
16. On the "blockbuster" drug, see Dumit 2012.
17. Ahead of time, I asserted my own position as interested in market research work but also critical of it. This seemed of little importance to the research firm, as long as I never specified company names or products. Many of the staff were trained in qualitative research in sociology at local universities; indeed, many were graduate students themselves.

18. He also thought its aesthetics were "too NRI," meaning "non-resident Indian," using a film reference about feel-good romances of the 1990s that worked out possibilities for Indian life abroad: "Too much *Kol Ho Na Ho* or any other Karan Johar film," as he put it.

19. As Andrew Lakoff (2007) explains in his analysis of biosecurity and "preparedness" in the US, "preparedness is oriented to crisis situations and to localized sites of disorder or disruption . . . the key site of vulnerability is not the health of a population but rather the critical infrastructure that guarantees the continuity of political and economic order" (271). Lakoff's perspective is helpful here, because if we think of inside/outside divides as "critical infrastructure," we can shift the stakes of survival from those exclusive to the health of the public to more intimate, homeward vulnerabilities.

*Chapter 4. Lines of Therapy*

1. Dr. Bhatt saw a range of patients, especially diabetics. Many of his clients included type 1 (juvenile) diabetics. Because I limited my study to type 2 diabetes, I did not take notes or speak with any minors with type 1 diabetes who entered the room. Thus "diabetes" here refers solely to type 2.

2. For ethnographic studies of medical nutrition therapy (MNT) and its vernacular resonances, see Ferzacca 2000, 2004; Manderson 1981; Yates-Doerr 2012, 2015.

3. What occurs in conversations using *andar* and *bahar* is actually a complex overlap between *andar se* (from the inside), *bahar se* (from the outside), and the additional term described in chapter 3, *ghar se* (from the house). Here is where spatial domains of inside and outside find resonance with somatic domains of inside and outside—not a perfect overlap but a resonance, and one almost always with *se* (from, emergent from) to emphasize source and vector.

4. In addition to detailing a given "traditional" medical system, these works attest to the multiplicity of medical traditions in South Asia, including that of biomedicine.

5. See Zhan (2009) on this contingent globality at the interface of traditional and contemporary forms of medical practice.

6. On the politics of biomedical definitions of addiction, see Bourgois and Schonberg 2009 and Garcia 2010.

7. Angela Garcia (2010: 18) makes a distinction that is useful here: "Thus while relapse is understandable and even expected (at least from the medical point of view), the relapsed addict is ultimately assigned blame for the relapse and is therefore seen as lacking the will to recover."

8. See Ecks (2014) on the tangled relations between ingestion, digestion, and mind in contemporary India. Ecks discusses the phenomenon of "eating drugs" in his ethnography of mental health care in Kolkata; the resonance between food and drugs is key to his study and pertinent to my analysis here,

although the lines of association I explore diffuse beyond clinical contexts (both biomedical and Ayurvedic, which are what Ecks primarily engages).

9. See Tattersall (2009: 114) for a discussion of Novo Nordisk and its relation to India.

10. Taken further, this line of gendering women's bodies as more absorbent and thus accepting of more foreign substances than men's would dovetail with post-Dumontian moments of thinking substance in South Asian studies. Such forms of thinking are compelling to me when put into conversation with feminist studies of material difference, because this convergence creates a challenge of representational politics.

11. At the time of writing, the prices for varying brands of drugs often prescribed for type 2 diabetes are as follows:

> Metformin: 10 tabs ranging from 15 to 30 rupees
> Older formulations of sulfonylureas, such as glibenclamide: 10 rupees for a strip of 10 tabs
> Newer formulations of sulfonylureas, such as glimipride: 100–200 rupees
> Combination of metformin and glimipride: 30–50 rupees
> Prandial hypoglycemics (nateglinide, repaglinide): 30–50 rupees for a strip of 10 tabs
> Pioglitazone: 60–80 rupees for a strip of 10 tabs
> Acarbose: 45–60 rupees for a strip of 10 tabs
> Voglibose: 20–30 rupees for a strip of 10 tabs
> Human insulin: 40 units: ca. 160 rupees
> Insulin pens: 500–3,000 rupees
> Victoza pen: 3,000–4,000 rupees

I thank Dr. Kalpana Swaminathan for gathering this information.

12. Julie Livingston describes in vivid detail the kinds of decisions patients face around amputation of cancerous tissue. "Amputation," she writes, "is a moment when the tremendously social nature of the human body as experienced outside the clinic comes up against the individuated body that biomedicine takes as its object. It is a moment when decisions hinge on sacrificing a part of the body in the hope of cure, time, or relief" (2012: 89).

13. See Belasco 1993; Dixon 2009; Scrinis 2013. The language of citizenship has its own problems, inasmuch as it invokes an assumed (Euro-American) relation between the state and nutrition, colored by body size.

14. In volume 2 of *The History of Sexuality*, Foucault (1988) offers a lengthy discussion of regimens of food and pleasure and works with a concept that he terms "dietetics." "The purpose of diet," he writes, "was not to extend life as far as possible in time nor as high as possible in performance, but rather to make it useful and happy within the limits that had been set for it" (105). Foucault points out that "dietetics was a technique of existence in the sense that it was not content to transmit the advice of a doctor to an individual, who would then be expected to apply it passively" (107). Dietetics offered "a rational framework

for the whole of [the free man's] existence," whereby a regimen through diet and sex works as "a concrete and active practice of the relation to self" (107).

15. As Ian Whitmarsh notes, "A focus on 'compliance and non-compliance' flattens difference by restricting behaviors to a field of one criterion, muting other forms of contrast and connection" (2009: 470).

## Chapter 5. Gut Attachments

1. I refer to this set of procedures as "the surgery" for simplicity, although as I explain later, there are multiple procedures that fall into the category of bariatric/metabolic surgery. For a history and description of the procedures, see Pories 2008: S89–S96. For a discussion about how surgery becomes framed as a viable option alongside diets and surgery, see Boero 2010.

2. I translate the Hindi *rishta* as "arrangement," in the context of Neha's utterance as relations under reconfiguration. *Rishta* may also be translated as "relationship," either in general or implying an intimate or familial connection.

3. The permeable will thus offers one provisional answer to the question about location implied in Lauren Berlant's (1998) query, "What happens to the energy of attachment when it has no designated place?" (285).

4. For the *Cochrane* review, see Colquitt et al. 2014. For additional meta-analyses of surgical procedures for obesity, see Gloy et al. 2013.

5. See Solomon 2011. In that project, I was interested in the development of corporate hospitals. But years later, when I pursued metabolic surgery, I saw again what I had seen before: special arrangements in place for visitors, cultural intermediaries, and a framing of globally generic biomedicine with the touch of Indian care.

## Conclusion. Metabolic Mumbai

1. Mol (2002: 124) also discusses camera movements. Saunders (2008) elaborates visuality in medicine at length, reminding us of the ways that Benjamin and Goffman offer compelling sources to contemplate distances between the body and projected images of it. For Ralph (2014), "framing" has immense political potential at the scale of injured communities. Inspired by these thoughtful works, my own sense of "framing" derives from Saunders in order to assert that across the bridge between the camera's "eyes" to our own, both the representational and the visceral are at stake. I also take a cue from Cavell (2005: 72), who in a frame-by-frame study of Fred Astaire's dance, wonders "Just how and where has this man managed this metamorphosis or quasi-metempsychosis (not finding a new body but finding his body anew?)" To find the metabolism anew as comprehensive frames shift, I suggest, is to find it differently in imagination and in biology.

2. Deployment with partial understanding is a gesture toward Bruno Latour's "black box" (1987: 130–31). For thoughts on "clock time," see Stengers 1997.

On the knowledge politics of Indian standard time in relation to the violence of science, see Viswanathan 1987.

3. It is important to note here how Greenwich mean time has its own history. It is noteworthy that Bandra's plague crosses, commemorating the plague in the 1890s, sat in one place but in several different time zones over the years. During the late nineteenth century, as Jim Masselos (2000) explains, a complex debate took shape over the differences between "Bombay time" and "Indian mean time" in the context of a global synchronization around Greenwich mean time. The city of Bombay shifted time zones, while most other parts of India hewed to a particular standard. It was not until later that the city synchronized with the rest of the country. For thoughts on "deep time" as it relates to biology, see Franklin 2014. I offer the world clocks analytic mindful of the kinds of power differences that time can produce in terms of race and coloniality; see Fabian 2014.

4. I offer "accumulation through absorption" here as a way into thinking about the bodily dimensions of neoliberalism. For a conversation on this front, see Harvey and Haraway 1995. On toxicity, see Hecht 2009 and Silverman 2012.

5. These trajectories might be thought of as "entanglements," in the spirit of Nading's (2014) discussion of the term and the ethnographic possibilities of following trails.

6. Canguilhem discusses his concept of the environment in several essays. I use his definition sketched in Canguilhem 1991: 284 and in the essay "The Living and Its Milieu" (Canguilhem 2008).

7. I agree with Yael Navaro-Yashin (2012: 18) that "a human-centered perspective must not be eradicated but complemented with an object-centered one" because "the environment exerts a force on human beings in its own right." In her work on spaces of memory and conflict, Navaro-Yashin asks a series of compelling questions: "Why assume a separation between interiority and exteriority? Why conceive of human beings as distinct from the environments, spaces, and objects with which they coexist, correlate, or cohabit? Likewise, why presume that interiority (conceptualized as a separate entity) will always reign supreme, that it will, through its projection onto the 'outer' world, determine everything? This would be a limited approach." I concur with her conclusion about the limitations of separating the inside and the outside, but I move this idea in a different direction because I intend to question the very conditions that enclose the inside from the outside. Navaro-Yashin further claims that "if the human has not altogether disappeared in ANT frameworks, accounts of it have become extremely impoverished" (164). Arjun Appadurai (2013) seems to concur with this sentiment. In revisiting his *Social Life of Things*, he expresses his "unease" about actor-network theory (ANT), inasmuch as this theoretical framework "takes a huge sociological tax on earlier ideas of sociality in order to extend the idea of sociality to the empire of things. The tax is this: like all pendulums, ANT has now fixed itself at the other end of the pendulum, and, in its preoccupation with the agency of the device, has evacuated from

its accounts of sociality all the things that make human sociality so fascinating in the first place. . . . In other words, the cost of extending the idea

of sociality in this manner to the empire of things has been to require a truly narrow picture of sociality, shorn of those things that make human sociality worth studying" (258). He continues: "The primary problems with images of object agency, network, and the device is not just that they tend to lose the soul of objects, in spite of their intention to reanimate the object, but that they have no real grip on the deepest problem of objects, which is their capacity to create contexts" (258). Metabolism, however abstractly or concretely realized, both demands and produces context, if by context one means a frame of reference.

8. I thank Peter Redfield for this turn of phrase, which twisted the aperture of this book in many wonderful ways.

9. Guthman 2011 engages this scholarship in detail.

10. Mathur 2009 offers an architectural perspective on building a city in and on an estuary.

Abu-Bakare, A., G.V. Gill, R. Taylor, and K. G. M. M. Alberti. 1986. Tropical or malnutrition-related diabetes: A real syndrome? *Lancet* 327.8490: 1135–38.

Adams, Vincanne. 2013. *Markets of Sorrow, Labors of Faith: New Orleans in the Wake of Katrina.* Durham, NC: Duke University Press.

Allen, Jonathan. 2008. Shiv Sena fights back with *vada pav*. *Reuters*, May 23.

Alter, Joseph S. 1999. Heaps of health, metaphysical fitness: Ayurveda and the ontology of good health in medical anthropology. *Current Anthropology* 40 (S1): S43–S56.

Alter, Joseph S. 2000a. *Gandhi's Body: Sex, Diet, and the Politics of Nationalism.* Philadelphia: University of Pennsylvania Press.

Alter, Joseph S. 2000b. *Knowing Dil Das.* Philadelphia: University of Pennsylvania Press.

Alter, Joseph. 2004. *Yoga in Modern India: The Body between Science and Philosophy.* Princeton, NJ: Princeton University Press.

Alter, Joseph S. 2014. Nature cure and Ayurveda: Nationalism, viscerality and bio-ecology in India. *Body & Society* 21 (1): 3–28.

Anand, Nikhil. 2011. Pressure: The politechnics of water supply in Mumbai. *Cultural Anthropology* 26 (4): 542–64.

Anand, Nikhil, and Anne Rademacher. 2011. Housing in the urban age: Inequality and aspiration in Mumbai. *Antipode* 43 (5): 1748–72.

Anderson, Warwick. 2002. Introduction: Postcolonial technoscience." *Social Studies of Science* 32 (5/6): 643–58.

Anderson, Warwick. 2008. *The Collectors of Lost Souls: Turning Kuru Scientists into Whitemen.* Baltimore: Johns Hopkins University Press.

Anjaria, Jonathan. 2006. Street hawkers and public space in Mumbai. *Economic and Political Weekly* 41 (21): 2140–46.

Anjaria, Jonathan. 2009. Guardians of the bourgeois city: Citizenship, public space, and middle-class activism in Mumbai. *City & Community*, 8 (4): 391–406.

Appadurai, Arjun. 1981. Gastro-politics in Hindu South Asia. *American Ethnologist* 8 (3): 494–511.

Appadurai, Arjun. 1988. How to make a national cuisine: Cookbooks in contemporary India. *Comparative Studies in Society and History* 30 (1): 3–24.

Appadurai, Arjun. 1996. *Modernity at Large: Cultural Dimensions of Globalization*. Minneapolis: University of Minnesota Press.

Appadurai, Arjun. 2000. Spectral housing and urban cleansing: Notes on millennial Mumbai. *Public Culture* 12 (3): 627–51.

Appadurai, Arjun. 2013. *The Future as Cultural Fact: Essays on the Global Condition*. London: Verso.

Arnold, David. 1988. Touching the body: Perspectives on the Indian plague, 1896–1900. In *Selected Subaltern Studies*. Ed. Ranajit Guha and Gayatri Chakravorty Spivak, 391–426. Oxford: Oxford University Press.

Arnold, David. 1988. *Famine: Social Crisis and Historical Change*. London: Blackwell.

Arnold, David. 1987. Touching the body: Perspectives on the Indian plague, 1896–1900. In Ranajit Guha (Ed.), *Subaltern Studies V*. New Delhi: Oxford University Press.

Arnold, David. 1993. *Colonizing the Body: State Medicine and Epidemic Disease in Nineteenth-Century India*. Berkeley: University of California Press.

Arnold, David. 2009. Diabetes in the tropics: Race, place and class in India, 1880–1965. *Social History of Medicine* 22 (2): 245–61.

Associated Press. 1964. In India: Food adulteration is big racket. *Free Lance-Star*, August 5.

Baptista, Elsie W. 1967. *The East Indians: Catholic Community of Bombay, Salsette and Bassein*. Bombay: Bombay East Indian Association.

Barad, Karen Michelle. 2007. *Meeting the Universe Halfway: Quantum Physics and the Entanglement of Matter and Meaning*. Durham, NC: Duke University Press.

Barker, D. J. P. 2007. The origins of the developmental origins theory. *Journal of Internal Medicine* 261 (5): 412–17.

Barrett, Ronald, Christopher Kuzawa, Thomas McDade, and George Armelagos. 1998. Emerging and re-emerging infectious diseases: The third epidemiologic transition. *Annual Review of Anthropology* 27: 247–71.

Bateson, Gregory. 1991. *A Sacred Unity*. New York: HarperCollins.

Bateson, Gregory. 2000. *Steps to an Ecology of Mind*. Chicago: University of Chicago Press.

Bateson, Patrick, David Barker, Timothy Clutton-Brock, Debal Deb, Bruno D'Udine, Robert A. Foley, Peter Gluckman, Keith Godfrey, Tom Kirkwood, and Marta Mirazón Lahr. 2004. Developmental plasticity and human health. *Nature* 430 (6998): 419–21.

Bedi, Tarini. 2007. The dashing ladies of the shiv sena. *Economic and Political Weekly* 42 (17): 1534–41.

Belasco, Warren. 1993. *Appetite for Change*. Ithaca, NY: Cornell University Press.

Berlant, Lauren. 1998. Intimacy: A special issue. *Critical Inquiry* 24 (2): 281–88.

Berlant, Lauren. 2007. Slow death (sovereignty, obesity, lateral agency). *Critical Inquiry* 33 (4): 754–80.

Berlant, Lauren. 2010. Risky bigness: On obesity, eating, and the ambiguity of 'health.' In Jonathan Metzl and Anna Kirkland (Eds.), *Against Health: How Health Became the New Morality*. New York: New York University Press.

Bhaskar, Dainik. 2010. Sab ek cut, aur vajan ho gaya kam [Just one cut and your weight will drop]. *Dainik Bhaskar*, March 10.

Biehl, João. 2007. *Will to Live: AIDS Therapies and the Politics of Survival*. Princeton, NJ: Princeton University Press.

Biehl, João, and Adriana Petryna. 2013. *When People Come First: Critical Studies in Global Health*. Princeton, NJ: Princeton University Press.

Boas, Franz. 1887. The study of geography. *Science* 9 (210): 137–41.

Boero, Natalie. 2010. Bypassing blame: Bariatric surgery and the case of biomedical failure. In *Biomedicalization: Technoscience, Health, and Illness in the US*. Ed. Adele Clarke, Laura Mamo, Jennifer Ruth Fosket, Jennifer Fishman, and Janet Shim, 307–30. Durham, NC: Duke University Press.

Bourgois, Philippe, and Jeff Schonberg. 2009. *Righteous Dopefiend*. Berkeley: University of California Press.

Brada, Betsey. 2011. "Not here": Making the spaces and subjects of "global health" in Botswana. *Culture, Medicine and Psychiatry* 35 (2): 285–312.

Breckenridge, Carol. 1995. *Consuming Modernity: Public Culture in Contemporary India*. New York: Oxford University Press.

Briggs, Charles. 2003. *Stories in the Time of Cholera: Racial Profiling during a Medical Nightmare*. Berkeley: University of California Press.

*Calcutta Telegraph*. 2007. Medicare for masses: Bariatric boon to cut kilos. July 4.

Candea, Matei, and Giovanni da Col. 2012. The return to hospitality. *Journal of the Royal Anthropological Institute* 18 (supp. S1): S1–S19.

Canguilhem, Georges. 1991. *The Normal and the Pathological*. Trans. Carolyn R. Fawcett. New York: Zone Books.

Canguilhem, Georges. 2008. *Knowledge of Life*. New York: Fordham University Press.

Carsten, Janet. 2001. Substantivism, anti-substantivism, and anti-antisubstantivism. In *Relative Values: Reconfiguring Kinship Studies*. Ed. Sarah Franklin and Susan McKinnon, 29–53. Durham, NC: Duke University Press.

Cavell, Stanley. 2005. *Philosophy the Day after Tomorrow*. Cambridge, MA: Harvard University Press.

Chakrabarty, Dipesh. 1991. Open space / public place: Garbage, modernity and India. *South Asia: Journal of South Asian Studies* 14 (1): 15–31.

Chanda, Mamata. 2009. FSSAI likely to establish food safety courts soon. *Food and Beverage News*, October 16.

Chatterjee, Partha. 1993. *The Nation and its Fragments: Colonial and Postcolonial Histories*. Princeton, NJ: Princeton University Press.

Chen, Nancy N. 2008. *Food, Medicine, and the Quest for Good Health*. New York: Columbia University Press.

Chu, Julie. 2010. The attraction of numbers: Accounting for ritual expenditures in Fuzhou, China. *Anthropological Theory* 10: 132–42.

Chua, Jocelyn. 2014. *In Pursuit of the Good Life: Aspiration and Suicide in Globalizing South India*. Berkeley: University of California Press.

Cohen, Ed. 2009. *A Body Worth Defending: Immunity, Biopolitics, and the Apotheosis of the Modern Body*. Durham, NC: Duke University Press.

Cohen, Lawrence. 1999. Where it hurts: Indian material for an ethics of organ transplantation. *Daedalus* 128 (4): 135–65.

Cohen, Lawrence. 1998. *No Aging in India: Alzheimer's, the Bad Family, and Other Modern Things*. Berkeley: University of California Press.

Cohen, Lawrence. 2007. Song for Pushkin. *Daedalus* 136 (2): 103–15.

Cohen, Lawrence. 2010. Ethical publicity: On transplant victims, wounded communities, and the moral demands of dreaming. In *Ethical Life in South Asia*. Ed. Anand Pandian and Daud Ali, 253–74. Bloomington: Indiana University Press.

Colquitt, Jill, K. Pickett, E. Loveman, and G. Frampton. 2014. Surgery for weight loss in adults. *Cochrane Database of Systematic Reviews* 8: Article CD003641.

Comaroff, Jean. 2007. Beyond bare life: AIDS, (bio)politics, and the neoliberal order. *Public Culture* 19 (1): 197–219.

Conlon, Frank F. 1995. Dining out in Bombay. In *Consuming Modernity: Public Culture in a South Asian World*. Ed. Carol A. Breckenridge, 90–127. Minneapolis, MN: University of Minnesota Press.

Coole, Diana and Samantha Frost. 2010. *New Materialisms: Ontology, Agency, and Politics*. Durham, NC: Duke University Press.

Couzin, Jennifer. 2008. Bypassing medicine to treat diabetes. *Science* 320: 438–40.

Craig, Sienna R. 2012. *Healing Elements: Efficacy and the Social Ecologies of Tibetan Medicine*. Berkeley: University of California Press.

Crane, Johanna Tayloe. 2013. *Scrambling for Africa: AIDS, Expertise, and the Rise of American Global Health*. Ithaca, NY: Cornell University Press.

Crowley-Matoka, Megan. 2015. *Domesticating Organ Transplant: Familial Sacrifice and National Aspiration in Mexico*. Durham, NC: Duke University Press.

Daniel, E. Valentine. 1984. *Fluid Signs: Being a Person the Tamil Way*. Berkeley: University of California Press.

Das, Veena. 2007. *Life and Words: Violence and the Descent into the Ordinary*. Berkeley: University of California Press.

Das, Veena. 2014. *Affliction: Health, Disease, Poverty*. New York: Fordham University Press.

Das, Veena, and R. K. Das. 2007. How the body speaks: Illness and the lifeworld among the urban poor. In *Subjectivity: Ethnographic Investigations*. Ed. João

Biehl, Byron J. Good, and Arthur Kleinman, 66–97. Berkeley: University of California Press.

Dasgupta, Rana. 2005. *Tokyo Cancelled*. New York: Black Cat.

Deaton, Angus, and Jean Drèze. 2009. Food and nutrition in India: Facts and interpretations. *Economic & Political Weekly* 44 (7): 42–65.

de la Cadena, Marisol. 2000. *Indigenous Mestizos: The Politics of Race and Culture in Cusco, Peru, 1919–1991*. Durham, NC: Duke University Press.

Desai, Shweta. 2009a. Culinary fights: Cong, Sena to battle it out at BMC next week. *Indian Express*, February 20.

Desai, Shweta. 2009b. No space for Shiv *vada pav* stalls beyond civic zones. *Indian Express*, July 31.

Desai, Shweta. 2009c. Shiv *vada pav* to miss launch date once more. *Indian Express*, April 27.

Descola, Philippe. 2013. *Beyond Nature and Culture*. Chicago: University of Chicago Press.

Dickey, Sara. 2000. Permeable homes: Domestic service, household space, and the vulnerability of class boundaries in urban India. *American Ethnologist* 27 (2): 462–89.

Dirks, Nicholas. 2001. *Castes of Mind: Colonialism and the Making of Modern India*. Princeton, NJ: Princeton University Press.

Dixon, Jane. 2009. From the imperial to the empty calorie: How nutrition relations underpin food regime transitions. *Agriculture and Human Values* 26 (4): 321–33.

*DNA Mumbai*. 2009a. Scar-less surgery for treating obesity. September 26.

*DNA Mumbai*. 2009b. Surgery can check morbid obesity. October 5.

Doctor, Vikram. n.d. Streetfood. Unpublished manuscript.

Doctor, Vikram. 2008. An attitude to serve: Why Marathi food lost out. *Economic Times*, May 17.

Dolphijn, Rick and Iris van der Tuin. 2012. *New Materialism: Interviews & Cartographies*. Ann Arbor, MI: Open Humanities Press.

Don, W. G. 1859. Remarkable case of obesity in a Hindoo boy aged twelve years. *Lancet* 73 (1858): 363.

Donner, Henrike. 2008. New vegetarianism: Food, gender and neo-liberal regimes in Bengali middle-class families. *South Asia: Journal of South Asian Studies* 31 (1): 143–69.

Dumit, Joseph. 2004. *Picturing Personhood: Brain Scans and Biomedical Identity*. Princeton, NJ: Princeton University Press.

Dumit, Joseph. 2012. *Drugs for Life: How Pharmaceutical Companies Define Our Health*. Durham, NC: Duke University Press.

Dupré, John, and Maureen A. O'Malley. 2013. Varieties of living things: Life at the intersection of lineage and metabolism. In *Vitalism and the Scientific Image in Post-Enlightenment Life Science, 1800–2010*. Ed. Sebastian Normandin and Charles T. Wolfe, 311–44. New York: Springer.

DuPuis, E. Melanie. 2002. *Nature's Perfect Food: How Milk Became America's Drink*. New York: New York University Press.

Eckert, Julia. 2004. Urban governance and emergent forms of legal pluralism in Mumbai. *The Journal Legal Pluralism and Unofficial Law* 36 (50): 29–60.

Ecks, Stefan. 2014. *Eating Drugs: Psychopharmaceutical Pluralism in India*. New York: New York University Press.

Edmonds, Alexander. 2010. *Pretty Modern: Beauty, Sex, and Plastic Surgery in Brazil*. Durham, NC: Duke University Press.

Epstein, Steven. 1998. *Impure Science: AIDS, Activism, and the Politics of Knowledge*. Berkeley: University of California Press.

Fabian, Johannes. 2014. *Time and the Other: How Anthropology Makes Its Object*. New York: Columbia University Press.

Farmer, Paul. 1992. *AIDS and Accusation: Haiti and the Geography of Blame*. Berkeley: University of California Press.

Farquhar, Judith. 2002. *Appetites: Food and Sex in Postsocialist China*. Durham, NC: Duke University Press.

Farquhar, Judith. 2009. The park pass: Peopling and civilizing a new old Beijing. *Public Culture* 21 (3): 551–76.

Fassin, Didier. 2008. *When Bodies Remember: Experiences and Politics of AIDS in South Africa*. Berkeley: University of California Press.

Fernandes, Leela. 2009. The political economy of lifestyle: Consumption, India's new middle class and state-led development. In *The New Middle Classes: Globalizing Lifestyles, Consumerism and Environmental Concern*. Ed. Hellmuth Lange and Lars Meier, 219–36. New York: Springer.

Ferzacca, Steve. 2000. "Actually, I don't feel that bad": Managing diabetes and the clinical encounter. *Medical Anthropology Quarterly* 14 (1): 28–50.

Ferzacca, Steve. 2004. Lived food and judgments of taste at a time of disease. *Medical Anthropology* 23 (1): 41–67.

Finkelstein, Maura. 2015. Landscapes of invisibility: Anachronistic subjects and allochronous spaces in mill land Mumbai. *City & Society* 27 (3): 250–71.

Fischer-Kowalski, Marina. 1998. Society's metabolism. The intellectual history of materials flow analysis, part I, 1860–1970. *Journal of Industrial Ecology* 2 (1): 61–78.

Fleck, Ludwig. 1979. *Genesis and Development of a Scientific Fact*. Chicago: University of Chicago Press.

Fortun, Kim. 1998. *Advocacy after Bhopal: Environmentalism, Disaster, New Global Orders*. Chicago: University of Chicago Press.

Fortun, Kim. 2012. Ethnography in Late Industrialism. *Cultural Anthropology* 27 (3): 446–64.

Fortun, Michael. 2008. *Promising Genomics: Iceland and DeCODE Genetics in a World of Speculation*. Berkeley: University of California Press.

Foucault, Michel. 1988. *The Use of Pleasure*. Vol. 2 of *The History of Sexuality*. New York: Vintage Books.

Franklin, Sarah. 2014. Rethinking reproductive politics in time, and time in UK reproductive politics: 1978–2008. *Journal of the Royal Anthropological Institute* 20 (supp. S1): 109–25.

Fruzzetti, Lina, and Akos Ostor. 1982. Bad blood in Bengal: Category and affect in the study of kinship, caste, and marriage. In *Concepts of Person: Kinship, Caste, and Marriage in India*. Ed. Lina Fruzzetti and Akos Ostor. Cambridge, MA: Harvard University Press.

Fullwiley, Duana. 2007. Race and genetics: Attempts to define the relationship. *BioSocieties* 2 (2): 221–37.

Fullwiley, Duana. 2011. *The Enculturated Gene: Sickle Cell Health Politics and Biological Difference in West Africa*. Princeton, NJ: Princeton University Press.

Gandy, Matthew. 2004. Rethinking urban metabolism: Water, space and the modern city. *City* 8 (3): 363–79.

Garcia, Angela. 2010. *The Pastoral Clinic: Addiction and Dispossession along the Rio Grande*. Berkeley: University of California Press.

Ghassem-Fachandi, P. 2009. The hyperbolic vegetarian: Notes on a fragile subject in Gujarat. In *Being There: The Fieldwork Encounter and the Making of Truth*. Ed. John Borneman and Abdellah Hammoudi, 77–112. Berkeley: University of California Press.

Gianani, Kareena. 2009. The Indian woman is not okay. *DNA Mumbai*.

Gilman, Sander L. 2008. *Fat: A Cultural History of Obesity*. London: Polity.

Gilman, Sander L. 2010. *Obesity: The Biography*. Oxford: Oxford University Press.

Gloy, V. L., M. Briel, D. L. Bhatt, S. R. Kashyap, P. R. Schauer, G. Mingrone, H. C. Bucher, A. J. Nordmann. 2013. Bariatric surgery versus non-surgical treatment for obesity: A systematic review and meta-analysis of randomised controlled trials. *British Medical Journal* 347: f5934.

Goswami, Manu. 2004. *Producing India: From Colonial Economy to National Space*. Chicago: University of Chicago Press.

Grosz, Elizabeth. 2004. *The Nick of Time: Politics, Evolution and the Untimely*. Durham, NC: Duke University Press.

Guthman, Julie. 2011. *Weighing In: Obesity, Food Justice, and the Limits of Capitalism*. Berkeley: University of California Press.

Guthman, Julie, and Melanie DuPuis. 2006. Embodying neoliberalism: Economy, culture, and the politics of fat. *Environment and Planning D: Society and Space* 24 (3): 427–48.

Gutiérrez, Emily C. and Carl Kendall. 2000. The globalization of health and disease: The health transition and global change. In Gary L. Albrecht, Ray Fitzpatrick, and Susan Scrimshaw (Eds.), *The Handbook of Social Studies in Health & Medicine*. London: Sage.

Guyer, Jane, N. Khan, J. Obarrio, C. Bledsoe, J. Chu, S. Bachir Diagne, K. Hart, et al. 2010. Introduction: Number as inventive frontier. *Anthropological Theory* 10 (1–2): 36–61.

Hacking, Ian. 2006. Genetics, biosocial groups & the future of identity. *Daedalus* 135 (4): 81–95.

Halliburton, Murphy. 2009. *Mudpacks and Prozac: Experiencing Ayurvedic, Biomedical, and Religious Healing*. Walnut Creek, CA: Left Coast Press.

Hamdy, Sherine. 2012. *Our Bodies Belong to God: Organ Transplants, Islam, and the Struggle for Human Dignity in Egypt.* Berkeley: University of California Press.

Hansen, Thomas Blom. 1999. *The Saffron Wave: Democracy and Hindu Nationalism in Modern India.* Princeton, NJ: Princeton University Press.

Hansen, Thomas Blom. 2002. *Wages of Violence: Naming and Identity in Postcolonial Bombay.* Princeton, NJ: Princeton University Press.

Hansen, Thomas Blom, and Oskar Verkaaik. 2009. Urban charisma: On everyday mythologies in the city. *Critique of Anthropology* 29 (1): 5–26.

Haraway, Donna J. 2008. *When Species Meet.* Minneapolis: University of Minnesota Press.

Harris, Marvin. 1978. India's sacred cow. *Human Nature* 1 (2): 28–36.

Harvey, David, and Donna Haraway. 1995. Nature, politics, and possibilities: A debate and discussion with David Harvey and Donna Haraway. *Environment and Planning D: Society and Space* 13: 507–27.

Hecht, Gabrielle. 2009. *The Radiance of France: Nuclear Power and National Identity After World War II.* Cambridge, MA: MIT Press.

Hecht, Gabrielle. 2012. *Being Nuclear: Africans and the Global Uranium Trade.* Cambridge, MA: MIT Press.

Hochschild, Arlie Russell. 1983. *The Managed Heart: Commercialization of Human Feeling.* Berkeley: University of California Press.

Holtzman, Jon. 2009. *Uncertain Tastes: Memory, Ambivalence, and the Politics of Eating in Samburu, Northern Kenya.* Berkeley: University of California Press.

Hull, Matthew S. 2012. *Government of Paper: The Materiality of Bureaucracy in Urban Pakistan.* Berkeley: University of California Press.

IANS. 2009a. 68% working women suffer lifestyle diseases: ASSOCHAM. *Times of India*, March 7.

IANS. 2009b. India's obese population goes up by 70 million. *Mid-Day*, July 15.

*Indian Express.* 2008. Now, weight-loss surgery comes cheap at RML. November 24.

*Indian Express.* 2009a. Bariatric surgery an effective cure: Experts. May 25.

*Indian Express.* 2009b. City docs perform Asia's first sleeve gastrectomy. September 30.

Ingold, Tim. 2011. *Being Alive: Essays on Movement, Knowledge and Description.* London: Routledge.

Inhorn, Marcia. 1995. Medical anthropology and epidemiology: Divergences or convergences? *Social Science & Medicine* 40 (3): 285–90.

Inhorn, Marcia, and Emily Wentzell. 2012. *Medical Anthropology at the Intersections: Histories, Activisms, and Futures.* Durham, NC: Duke University Press.

International Institute for Population Sciences (IIPS) and Macro International. 2007. *National Family Health Survey (NFHS-3), 2005–2006: India: Volume II.* Mumbai: IIPS.

Iversen, Vegard, and P. S. Raghavendra. 2006. What the signboard hides: Food, caste, and employability at small South Indian eating places. *Contributions to Indian Sociology* 40 (3): 311–41.

Jain, Sarah S. Lochlann. 2013. *Malignant: How Cancer Becomes Us.* Berkeley: University of California Press.

Jeffrey, Craig. 2010. *Timepass: Youth, Class, and the Politics of Waiting in India.* Stanford, CA: Stanford University Press.

Jirtle, Randy L., and Michael K. Skinner. 2007. Environmental epigenomics and disease susceptibility. *Nature Reviews Genetics* 8 (4): 253–62.

Johnson, Andrew M.F. and Jerrold Olefsky. 2013. The origins and drivers of insulin resistance. *Cell* 152: 673–84.

Joshi, Shashank and Rakesh Parikh. 2007. India—diabetes capital of the world: Now heading towards hypertension. *Journal of the Association of Physicians of India* 55: 323–24

Joshi, Shashank R., V. Mohan, S. S. Joshi, Jeffrey I. Mechanick, and Albert Marchetti. 2012. Transcultural diabetes nutrition therapy algorithm: The Asian Indian application. *Current Diabetes Reports* 12 (2): 204–12.

Katzenstein, Mary. 1979. *Ethnicity and Equality: The Shiv Sena Party and Preferential Policies in Bombay.* Ithaca, NY: Cornell University Press.

Kaviraj, Sudipta. 1997. Filth and the public sphere: Concepts and practices about space in Calcutta. *Public Culture* 10 (1): 83–113.

Keane, Webb. 1997. *Signs of Recognition: Powers and Hazards of Representation in an Indonesian Society.* Berkeley: University of California Press.

Khare, R. S. 1976. *The Hindu Hearth and Home.* New Delhi: Vikas.

Khare, R. S. 1992. *The Eternal Food: Gastronomic Ideas and Experiences of Hindus and Buddhists.* Albany: State University of New York Press.

Kidambi, Prashant. 2004. "An infection of locality": Plague, pythogenesis and the poor in Bombay, c. 1896–1905. *Urban History* 31: 249–67.

Kinra, Sanjay. 2004. Commentary: Beyond urban-rural comparisons: Towards a life course approach to understanding health effects of urbanization. *International Journal of Epidemiology* 33 (4): 777–78.

Kirkland, Anna. 2011. The environmental account of obesity: A case for feminist skepticism. *Signs* 36 (2): 463–85.

Klein, Ira. 1988. Plague, policy and popular unrest in British India. *Modern Asian Studies* 22 (4): 723–55.

Koppikar, Smruti. 2009. The Shivaji flavour. *Outlook India*, July 27.

Kulick, Don, and Anne Meneley. 2005. *Fat: The Anthropology of an Obsession.* New York: Tarcher/Penguin.

Kuzawa, C. W., and E. A. Quinn. 2009. Developmental origins of adult function and health: Evolutionary hypotheses. *Annual Review of Anthropology* 38: 131–47.

Kuzawa, C. W., and E. A. Quinn. 2013. You are what your mother ate? *American Journal of Clinical Nutrition* 97: 1157–58.

Lakoff, Andrew. 2007. Preparing for the next emergency. *Public Culture* 19 (2): 247–71.

Landecker, Hannah. 2007. *Culturing Life: How Cells Became Technologies.* Cambridge, MA: Harvard University Press.

Landecker, Hannah. 2011. Food as exposure: Nutritional epigenetics and the new metabolism. *BioSocieties* 6 (2): 167–94.

Landecker, Hannah. 2013a. The metabolism of philosophy, in three parts. In *Dialectic and Paradox: Configurations of the Third in Modernity*. Ed. Ian Cooper and Bernhard F. Malkmus, 193–224. Bern: Peter Lang.

Landecker, Hannah. 2013b. Postindustrial metabolism: Fat knowledge. *Public Culture* 25 (3): 495–522.

Landecker, Hannah, and Aaron Panofsky. 2013. From social structure to gene regulation, and back: A critical introduction to environmental epigenetics for sociology. *Annual Review of Sociology* 39: 333–57.

Langford, Jean. 2002. *Fluent Bodies: Ayurvedic Remedies for Postcolonial Imbalance*. Durham, NC: Duke University Press.

Langwick, Stacey Ann. 2011. *Bodies, Politics, and African Healing: The Matter of Maladies in Tanzania*. Bloomington: Indiana University Press.

Latour, Bruno. 1987. *Science in Action*. Cambridge, MA: Harvard University Press.

Latour, Bruno. 2005. *Making Things Public: Atmospheres of Democracy*. Cambridge, MA: MIT Press.

Latour, Bruno. 2010. An attempt at a "compositionist manifesto." *New Literary History* 41 (3): 471–90.

Lavin, Chad. 2009. The year of eating politically. *Theory & Event* 12 (2). DOI: 10.1353/tae.0.0074

Leslie, Charles. 1976. *Asian Medical Systems: A Comparative Study*. Berkeley: University of California Press.

Livingston, Julie. 2012. *Improvising Medicine: An African Oncology Ward in an Emerging Cancer Epidemic*. Durham, NC: Duke University Press.

Lock, Margaret. 2013. *The Alzheimer's Conundrum: Entanglements of Dementia and Aging*. Princeton, NJ: Princeton University Press.

Lock, Margaret, and P. Kaufert. 2001. Menopause, local biologies, and cultures of aging. *American Journal of Human Biology* 13 (4): 494–504.

*Loksatta*. 2005. Anesgrik lattpanna [Unnatural fatness]. August 29.

Lukose, Ritty A. 2009. *Liberalization's Children: Gender, Youth, and Consumer Citizenship in Globalizing India*. Durham, NC: Duke University Press.

Lynch, Michael. 2013. Ontography: Investigating the production of things, deflating ontology. *Social Studies of Science* 43 (3): 444–62.

Malabou, Catherine. 2008. *What Should We Do with Our Brain?* New York: Fordham University Press.

Malinowski, Bronislaw. 1944. *A Scientific Theory of Culture and Other Essays*. Oxford: Oxford University Press.

Manderson, Lenore. 1981. Traditional food classifications and humoral medical theory in peninsular Malaysia. *Ecology of Food and Nutrition* 11 (2): 81–93.

Manderson, Lenore, and Renata Kokanovic. 2009. "Worried all the time": Distress and the circumstances of everyday life among immigrant Australians with type 2 diabetes. *Chronic Illness* 5 (1): 21–32.

Manderson, Lenore, and Carolyn Smith-Morris. 2010. *Chronic Conditions, Fluid States: Chronicity and the Anthropology of Illness*. New Brunswick, NJ: Rutgers University Press.

Mankekar, Purnima. 1999. *Screening Culture, Viewing Politics: An Ethnography of Television, Womanhood, and Nation Postcolonial India*. Durham, NC: Duke University Press.

Mann, A., Annemarie Mol, Priya Satalkar, Amalinda Savirani, Nasima Selim, Malini Sur, and Emily Yates-Doerr. 2011. Mixing methods, tasting fingers: Notes on an ethnographic experiment. *HAU: Journal of Ethnographic Theory* 1 (1): 221–43.

Martin, Emily. 1994. *Flexible Bodies: Tracking Immunity in American Culture from the Days of Polio to the Age of AIDS*. Boston: Beacon.

Marriott, McKim. 1968. Caste ranking and food transactions: A matrix analysis. In *Structure and Change in Indian Society*. Ed. Milton Singer and Bernard S. Cohn. New York: Wenner-Gren Foundation for Anthropological Research.

Marriott, McKim. 1989. Constructing an Indian ethnosociology. *Contributions to Indian Sociology* 23 (1): 1–39.

Masselos, Jim. 2000. Bombay time. In *Intersections: Socio-cultural Trends in Maharashtra*. Ed. Meera Kosambi, 161–86. New Delhi: Orient Longman.

Masselos, Jim. 2007. *The City in Action: Bombay Struggles for Power*. New Delhi: Oxford University Press.

Mathur, Anuradha. 2009. *Soak: Mumbai in an Estuary*. New Delhi: Rupa.

Mazzarella, William. 2003. *Shoveling Smoke: Advertising and Globalization in Contemporary India*. Durham, NC: Duke University Press.

Mazzarella, William. 2006. Internet X-ray: E-Governance, transparency, and the politics of immediation in India. *Public Culture* 18 (3): 473–505.

McLean, Stuart. 2004. *The Event and Its Terrors: Ireland, Famine, Modernity*. Stanford, CA: Stanford University Press.

Mead, Margaret. 1943. The factor of food habits. *Annals of the American Academy of Political and Social Science* 225: 136–41.

Meneley, Anne. 2008. Oleo-signs and quali-signs: The qualities of olive oil. *Ethnos* 73 (3): 303–26.

Metzl, Jonathan, and Anna Rutherford Kirkland. 2010. *Against Health: How Health Became the New Morality*. New York: New York University Press.

Ministry of Law and Justice, Government of India. 2006. Food Safety and Standards Act. New Delhi.

*Mint*. 2007. Bariatric surgery: It's a big deal. October 9.

Mintz, Sidney. 1985. *Sweetness and Power: The Place of Sugar in Modern History*. New York: Penguin.

Mintz, Sidney, and C. M. Du Bois. 2002. The anthropology of food and eating. *Annual Review of Anthropology* 31: 99–119.

Misra, Anoop. 2003. Revisions of cutoffs of body mass index to define overweight and obesity are needed for the Asian-ethnic groups. *International Journal of Obesity* 27 (11): 1294–96.

Misra, Anoop, Rekha Sharma, Seema Gulati, et al. 2011. Consensus dietary guidelines for healthy living and prevention of obesity, the metabolic syndrome, diabetes, and related disorders in Asian Indians. *Diabetes Technology & Therapeutics* 13 (6): 683–94.

Mol, Annemarie. 2002. *The Body Multiple: Ontology in Medical Practice*. Durham, NC: Duke University Press.

Mol, Annemarie. 2008. *The Logic of Care: Health and the Problem of Patient Choice*. New York: Routledge.

Mol, Annemarie, and Jessica Mesman. 1996. Neonatal food and the politics of theory: Some questions of method. *Social Studies of Science* 26 (2): 419–44.

Monteiro, Carlos A., and Geoffrey Cannon. 2012. The impact of transnational "big food" companies on the South: A view from Brazil. *PLoS Medicine* 9 (7): e1001252.

Montoya, Michael J. 2011. *Making the Mexican Diabetic: Race, Science, and the Genetics of Inequality*. Berkeley: University of California Press.

Mukherjee, Janam. 2015. *Hungry Bengal: War, Famine, and the End of Empire*. Oxford: Oxford University Press.

Mukherjee, Pradipta. 2009. Amway, Dabur to sweat it out over vitamins, dietary supplements. *Business Standard*, May 8.

Mukhopadhyay, Bhaskar. 2004. Between elite hysteria and subaltern carnivalesque: The politics of street-food in the city of Calcutta. *South Asia Research* 24 (1): 37–50.

*Mumbai Mirror*. 2008. Colleagues, employer round up help for obese rig worker. October 27.

Nading, Alex M. 2014. *Mosquito Trails: Ecology, Health, and the Politics of Entanglement*. Berkeley: University of California Press.

Naemiratch, Bhensri, and Lenore Manderson. 2006. Control and adherence: Living with diabetes in Bangkok, Thailand. *Social Science & Medicine* 63 (5): 1147–57.

Nakassis, Constantine V. 2012. Counterfeiting what?: Aesthetics of brandedness and BRAND in Tamil Nadu, India. *Anthropological Quarterly* 85 (3): 701–21.

Nandakumar, Prathima. 2007. Bangalore gorges on junk food. *Times of India*, November 13.

Nandy, Ashis. 2004. The changing popular culture of Indian food: Preliminary notes. *South Asia Research* 24 (1): 9–19.

Nandy, Ashis. 2007. *Time Treks: The Uncertain Future of Old and New Despotisms*. New Delhi: Permanent Black.

Natu, Nitasha. 2009. Milk adulteration racket busted, 11 arrested. *Times of India*, November 20.

Navaro-Yashin, Yael. 2012. *The Make-Believe Space: Affective Geography in a Postwar Polity*. Durham, NC: Duke University Press.

*Navbharat Times*. 2009. Sehat ka dushman hai vanaspati ghee [Vanaspati ghee is the enemy of health], February 20.

*Navbharat Times*. 2010. Motapa ki surjeri muft mein hogi [Obesity surgery will be free], February 26.

Neel, James V. 1962. Diabetes mellitus: A "thrifty" genotype rendered detrimental by "progress"? *American Journal of Human Genetics* 14: 353–62.

Nichter, Mark. 1981. Negotiation of the illness experience: Ayurvedic therapy and the psychosocial dimension of illness. *Culture, Medicine, and Psychiatry* 5 (1): 5–24.

Nichter, Mark. 2001. The political ecology of health in India: Indigestion as sign and symptom of defective modernization. In *Healing Powers and Modernity: Traditional Medicine, Shamanism, and Science in Contemporary Asia*. Ed. Linda H. Connor and Geoffrey Samuel, 85–108. Westport, CT: Greenwood Press.

Nichter, Mark and David Van Sickle. 2002. The challenges of India's health and healthcare transitions. In *India Briefing: Quickening the Pace of Change*. London: ME Sharpe, 184–85.

Niewöhner, Jörg. 2011 Epigenetics: Embedded bodies and the molecularisation of biography and milieu. *BioSocieties* 6: 279–98.

Ohmann, Richard. 1988. History and literary history: The case of mass culture. *Poetics Today* 9 (2): 357–75.

Osella, Caroline. 2008. Introduction. *South Asia* 31 (1): 1–9.

Pandya, Karina. 2010. Make lunch matter. *Hindustan Times*, June 28.

Papadopoulos, Dimitris. 2011. The imaginary of plasticity: Neural embodiment, epigenetics and ecomorphs. *Sociological Review* 59 (3): 432–56.

Patel, Aakar. 2009. Why Indians are stressed and unhealthy. *The News*, January 25.

Patel, Geeta. 2004. Homely housewives run amok: Lesbians in marital fixes. *Public Culture* 16 (1): 131–57.

Patel, Geeta. 2007. Imagining risk, care, and security: Insurance and fantasy. *Anthropological Theory* 7: 99–117.

Patel, Sujata, and Alice Thorner. 1995. *Bombay: Metaphor for Modern India*. Delhi: Oxford University Press.

Patel, Vikram, Somnath Chatterji, Dan Chisholm, Shah Ebrahim, Gururaj Gopalakrishna, Colin Mathers, Viswanathan Mohan, Dorairaj Prabhakaran, Ravilla D. Ravindran, and K. Srinath Reddy. 2011. Chronic diseases and injuries in India. *Lancet* 377 (9763): 413–28.

Patell, B. F. 1896. *History of the Plague in Bombay*. Bombay: Caxton Works.

Patnaik, Utsa. 2007. *The Republic of Hunger and Other Essays*. New Delhi: Three Essays Collective.

*Patrika*. 2010. Citi women ki parishani obesiti [Obesity problems for city women]. February 22.

Paxson, Heather. 2013. *The Life of Cheese: Crafting Food and Value in America*. Berkeley: University of California Press.

Paxson, Heather and Stefan Helmreich. 2014. The perils and promises of microbial abundance: Novel natures and model ecosystems, from artisan cheese to alien seas. *Social Studies of Science* 44 (2): 165–93.

Peterson, Kristin. 2014. *Speculative Markets: Drug Circuits and Derivative Life in Nigeria*. Durham, NC: Duke University Press.

Petryna, Adriana. 2003. *Life Exposed: Biological Citizens After Chernobyl*. Princeton, NJ: Princeton University Press.

Popenoe, Rebecca. 2003. *Feeding Desire: Fatness, Beauty and Sexuality among a Saharan People*. New York: Routledge.

Popkin, Barry M. 2001. The nutrition transition and obesity in the developing world. *Journal of Nutrition* 131 (3): 871–73S.

Popkin, Barry, and P. Gordon-Larsen. 2004. The nutrition transition: Worldwide obesity dynamics and their determinants. *International Journal of Obesity* 28: S2–S9.

Popkin, Barry, S. Horton, S. Kim, A. Mahal, and J. Shuigao. 2001. Trends in diet, nutritional status, and diet-related noncommunicable diseases in China and India: The economic costs of the nutrition transition. *Nutrition Reviews* 59 (12): 379–90.

Pories, W. J. 2008. Bariatric surgery: Risks and rewards. *Journal of Clinical Endocrinology & Metabolism* 93 (11, supp. 1): S89–S96.

Povinelli, Elizabeth A. 2011. *Economies of Abandonment: Social Belonging and Endurance in Late Liberalism*. Durham, NC: Duke University Press.

Powdermaker, Hortense. 1960. An anthropological approach to the problem of obesity. *Bulletin of the New York Academy of Medicine* 36 (5): 286–95.

Prakash, Gyan. 1999. *Another Reason: Science and the Imagination of Modern India*. Princeton, NJ: Princeton University Press.

Prakash, Gyan. 2010. *Mumbai Fables*. Princeton, NJ: Princeton University Press.

Prentice, Rachel. 2013. *Bodies in Formation: An Ethnography of Anatomy and Surgery Education*. Durham, NC: Duke University Press.

Price, Joshua M. 2002. The apotheosis of home and the maintenance of spaces of violence. *Hypatia* 17 (4): 39–70.

Procida, Mary A. 2003. Feeding the imperial appetite: Imperial knowledge and Anglo-Indian discourse. *Journal of Women's History* 15 (2): 123–49.

Protevi, John. 2013. *Life, War, Earth: Deleuze and the Sciences*. Minneapolis: University of Minnesota Press.

PTI. 2009. Shiv Sena launches the poor man's burger Shiv *vada pav*. DNA *Mumbai*, June 18.

Radhakrishnan, R. 2009. Why compare? *New Literary History* 40 (3): 453–71.

Raj, Selva J., and Corrine G. Dempsey. 2002. *Popular Christianity in India: Rising between the Lines*. Albany: SUNY Press.

Rajagopal, Arvind. 2001. *Politics after Television: Hindu Nationalism and the Reshaping of the Public in India*. Cambridge: Cambridge University Press.

Ralph, Lawrence. 2014. *Renegade Dreams: Living through Injury in Gangland Chicago*. Chicago: University of Chicago Press.

Rapp, Rayna. 1999. *Testing Women, Testing the Fetus: The Social Impact of Amniocentesis in America*. New York: Routledge.

Ratna, Kalpish. 2008. *Uncertain Life and Sure Death: Medicine and Mahamaari in Maritime Mumbai*. Mumbai: Maritime History Society.

Ratna, Kalpish. 2010. *The Quarantine Papers*. New Delhi: HarperCollins India.

Ratna, Kalpish. 2015. *Room 000*. New Delhi: Penguin.

Reaven, Gerald. 1988. Role of insulin resistance in human disease. *Diabetes* 37: 1595–608.

Redfield, Peter. 2013. *Life in Crisis: The Ethical Journey of Doctors without Borders.* Berkeley: University of California Press.

Rees, Tobias. 2010. Being neurologically human today: Life and science and adult cerebral plasticity (an ethical analysis). *American Ethnologist* 37 (1): 150–66.

Ries, Nancy. 2009. Potato ontology: Surviving postsocialism in Russia. *Cultural Anthropology* 24 (2): 181–212.

Rosenberg, Charles E. 2002. The tyranny of diagnosis: Specific entities and individual experience. *Milbank Quarterly* 80 (2): 237–60.

Roy, Parama. 2010. *Alimentary Tracts: Appetites, Aversions, and the Postcolonial.* Durham, NC: Duke University Press.

Salaman, Radcliffe N. 1985. *The History and Social Influence of the Potato.* Cambridge: Cambridge University Press.

Sanders, Barry F. 2008. *CT Suite: The Work of Diagnosis in the Age of Noninvasive Cutting.* Durham, NC: Duke University Press.

Scheper-Hughes, Nancy. 2006. Foreword: Diabetes and genocide—beyond the thrifty gene. In *Indigenous Peoples and Diabetes: Community Empowerment and Wellness.* Ed. Mariana Ferreira and Gretchen Lang. Durham, NC: Carolina Academic Press.

Schlosser, Eric. 2005. *Fast Food Nation: The Dark Side of the All-American Meal.* New York: Houghton Mifflin Harcourt.

Schwartz, Hillel. 1986. *Never Satisfied: A Cultural History of Diets, Fantasies, and Fat.* New York: Free Press.

Scrinis, Gyorgy. 2013. *Nutritionism: The Science and Politics of Dietary Advice.* New York: Columbia University Press.

Sedgwick, Eve Kosofsky. 1993. *Tendencies.* Durham, NC: Duke University Press.

Sen, Amartya. 1983. *Poverty and Famines: An Essay on Entitlement and Deprivation.* Oxford: Oxford University Press.

Sen, Antara Dev. 2010. A healthy dose of poison. *Deccan Chronicle,* September 18.

Sen, Atrayee. 2007. *Shiv Sena Women: Violence and Communalism in a Bombay Slum.* Bloomington: Indiana University Press.

Serres, Michel. 2011. *Variations on the Body.* Minneapolis: Univocal.

Shah, Svati P. 2014. *Street Corner Secrets: Sex, Work, and Migration in the City of Mumbai.* Durham, NC: Duke University Press.

Sharma, Sanchita. 2009. Nutrition labels a must from March. *Hindustan Times,* February 5.

Siddhaye, Ninad. 2010. Milk adulteration racket busted in Maharashtra. DNA, March 21.

Silverman, Chloe. 2012. *Understanding Autism: Parents, Doctors, and the History of a Disorder.* Princeton, NJ: Princeton University Press.

Simone, AbdouMaliq. 2004. People as infrastructure: Intersecting fragments in Johannesburg. *Public Culture* 16 (3): 407–29.

Singer, Milton. 1972. *When a Great Tradition Modernizes: An Anthropological Approach to Indian Civilization*. New York: Praeger.

Sinha, Kounteya. 2007. Why stress can lead to obesity. *Times of India*, July 3.

Sinha, Kounteya. 2009. Indian cooking oils unfit. *Times of India*, February 4.

Sloterdijk, Peter. 2011. *Bubbles*. Cambridge: Semiotext(e).

Sloterdijk, Peter. 2013. *In the Interior World of Capital*. Cambridge: Polity.

Smith-Morris, Carolyn. 2006. *Diabetes among the Pima: Stories of Survival*. Tucson: University of Arizona Press.

Solomon, Harris. 2011. Affective journeys: The emotional structuring of medical tourism in India. *Anthropology and Medicine* 18 (1): 105–18.

Srinivas, Nidhi. 2009. Ghee says "Jai Ho." *Economic Times*, April 5.

Srivastava, Sanjay. 2007. *Passionate Modernity: Sexuality, Class, and Consumption in India*. New Delhi: Routledge.

Staples, James. 2003. Disguise, revelation and copyright: Disassembling the South Indian leper. *Journal of the Royal Anthropological Institute* 9 (2): 295–315.

Staples, James. 2004. Delineating disease: Self-management of leprosy identities in South India. *Medical Anthropology* 23 (1): 69–88.

Star, Susan Leigh. 1991. Power, technology, and the phenomenology of conventions: On being allergic to onions. In *A Sociology of Monsters: Essays on Power, Technology, and Domination*. Ed. John Law. New York: Routledge.

Stengers, Isabelle. 1997. *Power and Invention: Situating Science*. Minneapolis: University of Minnesota Press.

Stoller, Paul. 1989. *The Taste of Ethnographic Things: The Senses in Anthropology*. Philadelphia: University of Pennsylvania Press.

Subramanian, Ajantha. 2009. *Shorelines: Space and Rights in South India*. Stanford, CA: Stanford University Press.

Subramanian, Sanjay. 2010. *Following Fish: Travels around the Indian Coast*. New Delhi: Penguin.

Sujata C. 2010. Be a kitchen detective. *The Hindu*, July 13.

Sunder Rajan, Kaushik. 2006. *Biocapital: The Constitution of Postgenomic Life*. Durham, NC: Duke University Press.

Suryanarayan, Deepa. 2009. Mumbai children top junk food eating charts. *DNA*, September 11.

Sutton, David E. 2010. Food and the senses. *Annual Review of Anthropology* 39: 209–23.

Swyngedouw, Erik. 2006. Circulations and metabolisms: (Hybrid) natures and (cyborg) cities. *Science as Culture* 15 (2): 105–21.

Tattersall, Robert. 2009. *Diabetes: The Biography*. Oxford: Oxford University Press.

Thompson, Charis. 2005. *Making Parents: The Ontological Choreography of Reproductive Technologies*. Cambridge, MA: MIT Press.

Throsby, Karen. 2008. Happy re-birthday: Weight loss surgery and the "new me." *Body & Society* 14 (1): 117–33.

*Times of India*. 2007. Load-shedding ops rise five-fold in city. March 29.

*Times of India*. 2009a. Bariatric surgery gives politician new vigour. October 25.

*Times of India.* 2009b. Weight loss surgery possible in city. February 20.

TNN. 2010a. 51% BEST staffers obese, says study. *Times of India,* February 16.

TNN. 2010b. Stress leaves city on the brink. *Times of India,* March 19.

Tracy, Megan. 2010. The mutability of melamine: A transductive account of a scandal. *Anthropology Today* 26 (6): 4–8.

Tresch, John. 1998. Heredity is an open system: Gregory Bateson as descendant and ancestor. *Anthropology Today* 14 (6): 3–6.

Trostle, James and Johannes Sommerfeld. 1996. Medical Anthropology and Epidemiology. *Annual Review of Anthropology* 25: 253–74.

Tsing, Anna Lowenhaupt. 2005. *Friction: An Ethnography of Global Connection.* Princeton, NJ: Princeton University Press.

UNI. 2009. RPI will have Bhim *vada pav* if Sena has Shiv *vada pav*: Athavale. *OneIndia.com,* May 17. http://www.oneindia.com/2008/05/17/rpi-will-have -bhim-vada-pav-if-sena-has-shiv-vada-pav-athavale-1211151857.html. Accessed Sept 14, 2015.

Valentine, Gill. 1999. Eating in: Home, consumption and identity. *Sociological Review* 47 (3): 491–524.

Varghese, Ron Thomas. 2013. The advent of bariatric surgery for diabetes in India. *British Medical Journal* 347: f3391.

Varma, Rashmi. 2004. Provincializing the global city: From Bombay to Mumbai. *Social Text* 22 (4): 65–89.

Vedwan, Neeraj. 2007. Pesticides in Coca-Cola and Pepsi: Consumerism, brand image, and public interest in a globalizing India. *Cultural Anthropology* 22 (4): 659–84.

Vernon, James. 2005. The ethics of hunger and the assembly of society: The techno-politics of the school meal in modern Britain. *American Historical Review* 110 (3): 693–725.

Vernon, James. 2007. *Hunger: A Modern History.* Cambridge, MA: Harvard University Press.

Viswanathan, Shiv. 1987. From the annals of the laboratory state. *Alternatives* 12: 37–59.

Wald, Priscilla. 2008. *Contagious: Cultures, Carriers, and the Outbreak Narrative.* Durham, NC: Duke University Press.

*Week, The.* 2008. Underbelly of beauty. November 23.

Weintraub, Judith. 1974. Adulterated foods causing serious problems in India. *New York Times,* January 28.

Weismantel, Mary. 2001. *Cholas and Pishtacos: Stories of Race and Sex in the Andes.* Chicago: University of Chicago Press.

Weiss, Brad. 1996. *The Making and Unmaking of the Haya Lived World: Consumption, Commoditization, and Everyday Practice.* Durham, NC: Duke University Press.

Weiss, Brad. 2011. Making pigs local: Discerning the sensory character of place. *Cultural Anthropology* 26 (3): 438–61.

Weiss, Brad. 2012. Configuring the authentic value of real food: Farm-to-fork, snout-to-tail, and local food movements. *American Ethnologist* 39 (3): 614–26.

West-Eberhard, M. J. 2003. *Developmental Plasticity and Evolution*. Oxford: Oxford University Press.

White, Leslie. 1943. Energy and the evolution of culture. *American Anthropologist* 45 (3): 335–56.

Whitmarsh, Ian. 2009. Medical schismogenics: Compliance and "culture" in Caribbean biomedicine. *Anthropological Quarterly* 82 (2): 447–75.

Wiegman, Robyn. 2012. *Object Lessons*. Durham, NC: Duke University Press.

Wilson, Elizabeth A. 2004. Gut feminism. *Differences: A Journal of Feminist Cultural Studies* 15 (3): 66–94.

Wilson, Elizabeth A. 2015. *Gut Feminism*. Durham, NC: Duke University Press.

Yadav, Kiran. 2008. A fresh index. *Financial Express*, November 30.

Yajnik, C. S., and J. S. Yudkin. 2004. The Y-Y paradox. *Lancet* 363: 163.

Yates-Doerr, Emily. 2012. The weight of the self: Care and compassion in Guatemalan dietary choices. *Medical Anthropology Quarterly* 26 (1): 136–58.

Yates-Doerr, Emily. 2015. *The Weight of Obesity: Hunger and Global Health in Postwar Guatemala*. Berkeley: University of California Press.

Zhan, Mei. 2009. *Other-Worldly: Making Chinese Medicine through Transnational Frames*. Durham, NC: Duke University Press.

Note: Italicized numbers indicate a figure; n indicates an endnote

absorption: as basis for understanding metabolic disease, 5; agents of, 6; bad copy as product of sociocultural malabsorption, 46, 61; bodily of stress, 49, 62–64; externally initiated alterations to bodily, 161, 186, 194, 196, 242n20; globesity and, 23–24; influence of on metabolic living, 12–13, 21–22; influence of underlying social conditions on, 12, 13, 20–22, 29, 234; interface of body and environment, 9, 24, 63–64, 236n8; interface of body and substance, 17, 24–25, 140, 160–61, 216, 233; as intermingling of bodies, substances, and environments, 4–6, 15, 97, 226–28; malnutrition and obesity as two extremes of malnourishment, 14–15; metabolic illness as product of, 5, 62, 145–46; multifaceted, complex character of, 6, 23–26, 106, 109, 120, 146–47, 213; of food, 37, 89, 113–15; state of being absorptive, 6, 160–61, 249n10; temporal manifestation of by human body, 31–34, 147, 228–29, 232–33

Actor Network Theory (ANT), 243n4, 251–52n7

addiction: case of Poorvi, 166–67; food, 162–68; morals of responsibility and, 25; Sedgwick's "Epidemics of Will" essay, 25–26. *See also* willpower

adiposity, 17, 31, 38–39, 56, 59, 61, 241–42n17

adulteration: act of, 114, 119, 245n7; as incentive for brand loyalties and purchase of expensive packaged foods, 120–22, 123–24; case of Wilfred (fisher), 230; commonplace occurrence of in urban India, 113–16, 120, 124; food export as incentive for India to combat, 123; Food Safety and Standards Authority of India (2009), 126; foods typically adulterated, 118–19; incentives for, 113–14, 118, 245–46n9; interview with Almas (fashion industry director) concerning, 117–21, 122; legislation and regulation to prevent, 123, 125–26; linguistic references commonly used for, 245n7; long-term, generational impact of, 115; media discussions and coverage of food, 120–21, 123–25; by nexus, 24, 114–16, 118, 120–21, 123, 245–46n9; nutrition labeling as means of combating, 123, 126; of beverages, 120–21, 230; of dal, 100; of drugs, 245nn7–8; of fish, 108; of foods, 108, 118–19; of fruit, 114, 118, 120; of ghee, 113–14, 124; of loose (bulk) foods, 113–14; of milk, 113–14, 116, 118, 120, 245–46n9; of packaged foods, 122–24; of spices, 120; packaged food touted as free of, 24, 109, 119, 123–26, 140; potential of to cripple or kill, 120–21; practices against common

adulteration (*continued*)
foods and spices, 118–19, 124; Prevention of Food Adulteration Act (1954), 125;
Professor Munir on, 113–15, 121; proposed
punishments for those convicted of,
115, 125; rackets and criminality, 124–25;
scandals, 114–15, 120, 122–24, 246n12;
trans fats in processed foods, 112–13, 114;
vs. food preservatives, 116, 136; vigilance
against as household imperative, 109–12,
115, 118–24, 139. *See also* foods; food safety;
processed foods
agency, responsibility, and authority: agents
of absorption, 6; agents of blame, 110,
114; in diet enforcement, 187–89, 202;
following metabolic surgery, 200–201, 204,
220; of a device in ANT, 243n4, 251–52n7;
of patients, 13, 21, 25, 149, 157–60, 168,
184–86; of metabolism, 10, 146, 161, 166,
194, 199–201, 203, 218; surgical intervention as exercise of, 196, 198, 203
Alter, Joseph, 245–46n9
amputation: among diabetes patients, 145–
46, 173, 178–79, 183; circulatory problems
as precursor to, 179, 182; demarcation, 177,
179, 181, 182; Dr. Samant (diabetologist)
on, 177–83; failure of bodily absorption as
precursor to, 147, 177, 182; foot problems
and care among diabetics, 177–82; gangrene, 177–78, 182; limb, 147; neuropathy,
145–46, 177–78, 181; ulcers, 180, 181, 182
Anjaria, Jonathan Shapiro, 111
anthropometric measurement, 39, 42–43, 56
Appadurai, Arjun, 71, 73–75, 243n1, 243n4,
244n11, 251–52n7
*atyachaar* (tyranny by medicine), 218, 221–23,
232
Ayurveda: as complement to biomedicine,
156; as influence on conceptions of body-
environment relationship, 155; approaches
to diabetes through, 171, 176; approaches
to obesity through, 155–56; approaches to
metabolism through, 183, 237n12, 242n18;
diet control through, 163, 200, 219; overlap
of food and drugs in, 109, 245n6, 248n8;
remedies, 58; treatment centers, 21. *See
also* biomedicine; medical systems

bad copy, 36, 44–48
Balasaheb. *See* Bal Thackeray
Bandra: anthropological research done in, 7,
18–19, 93, 141, *224*; Carter Road, 1, 3, 15,
145, 158, 176; cold storage stores in, 141;

cosmopolitan character of, 18, 141–42,
169; hutments in, 19, 20, 85, 87, 117, 225;
location of neighborhood of in Mumbai,
1; as neighborhood containing village of
Manuli, 7; plague crosses of, 1–2, 1–4, 7,
15, 29, 225, 235n1, 251n3; rations stores for,
102; socioeconomic profile of, 18–19. *See
also* Manuli
Bangalore, 70, 96
Barad, Karen, 237n13, 238n16
bariatric surgery: as possible treatment for
diabetes, 213; "Bariatric Edge" patient
information materials, 208, 209; case
of Chandra Sahu, 212; case of Purnima,
210; case of Rajinder Sethi, 211; information and counseling for patients, 190–91,
209–11; media coverage of patient cases,
210–13, 214; patient qualifications for, 41.
*See also* metabolic surgery
Barker, David, 33, 56, 59, 242n20
Bateson, Gregory, 237n13, 239n33
Berlant, Lauren, 63–64, 242–43n24, 250n3
Bernard, Claude, 11–12
*bhat. See* rice
biomedicine: allopathic medicine, 154, 156; as
rationale used to market processed foods,
95, 109, 114, 151, 160, 245n8; heart-healthy
rationale used to market processed foods,
130, 132–33, 139; limitations of, 14, 21,
26, 146, 167, 248n4; metabolic disorders
defined through, 13; overlap of with food,
politics, and culture, 24, 72, 95, 154, 175,
184–85, 250n5; quantification in, 36, 43;
risk management in context of, 36, 48–49,
54, 168, 249n12; role of agency in prescribing diets and drugs, 22, 23, 154–56, 157–58,
185, 248n8; surgery as act of personal
agency, 204–5; tissue-based definitions of
fat by, 38–39; will as proxy for metabolism
in, 25, 194. *See also* Ayurveda
biomoral substances, 185–86
blood: assays, 22, 57, 170; cardiovascular impact of amputation, 179; circulation, 148,
177–78, 181, 182, 198; detoxification treatments, 52; dyslipidemia, 17; manifestation
of hormonal changes as diabetes in, 54;
samples for medical investigation, 20–21,
44; vessels, 148
blood sugar (blood glucose): as marketing
object for food companies, 109, 131; change
to as outcome of metabolic surgery,
195–99; control of hunger as means of
also stabilizing, 94; function of pancreas in

regulating, 17, 147, 173, 182, 232; influence of mango consumption on an individual's, 65–66; levels as markers for appearance of diabetes, 17, 62, 168–70; measurement of HbA1c, 17, 153; monitoring of in obesity and diabetes cases, 94, 151–52, 156, 175–76, 200, 202–3; national surveillance of individual levels among India's populace, 6; use of fenugreek (*methi*) to control, 51, 131, 176; use of metformin to control, 152, 158, 174, 176, 249n11; use of to define metabolic disease, 42, 170–71, 175, 241n13

body: absorptive powers of, 6, 9, 15, 25–26, 161, 226, 233; as processor of substances, 10, 13, 167, 173–74; Ayurvedic understanding of, 154–56, 157; bad copy, 44–48; body mass index (BMI) calculation, 6; brain adaptability, 10, 13, 35, 194, 196, 218, 237n13, 240n5; Canguilhem on body as product, 242n23; consumption and, 5, 14, 184, 186, 194, 226; demarcation by, 177, 179, 181, 182; ideas of temperature effects on, 14, 155, 157; Indian, 38–42, 48, 56–62; influence of *tenshun* on, 36, 39–40, 45, 48–55, 59–60, 62–63; inside-outside boundaries between environment and, 9, 35, 113, 140, 154–57, 176, 229; interaction of with environment, 6, 22, 35, 49, 59–60, 72–73, 222; measurements of, 6, 36, 39, 43, 56, 156, 202; metabolic similarities between visually different bodies, 32–34; metabolism, 9–11, 22, 147, 154, 157–58, 195, 203, 226–28; morphology, 33, 56, 61, 168, 242n23; neuropathy, 177–78, 181; obese, 17, 44, 59, 204, 208–9, 220; pain, 173, 179, 181, 182; plasticity of, 34–37, 48, 57–58, 61–64; porosity of, 6, 11–12, 49, 183, 201, 222; skin, 11–12, 32, 56, 147, 178–82, 186, 220, 239n31; somatic self-analysis, 10–13, 34, 55, 63, 147, 181, 220–21; surgical resetting of, 194, 196–97, 199–200, 204–5, 220–23; therapeutic and self-preserving powers of human, 177–79, 185, 194, 196–97, 199–200, 201; thin-fat Indian paradox, 24, 31–34, 46, 56–57, 60–63, 241n12; Y-Y paradox, 31–34

Body Mass Index (BMI): as means of exposing disease risk, 41–43, 48, 60–62; as medical diagnostic tool, 21–22, 156, 206, 211–12, 216; calculation of, 35, 151; changes to India's guidelines concerning, 23, 35–36, 38–43, 62, 227; development and popularization of, 39, 43, 241–42n17; global standards for diagnosis of weight

status, 35, 40–41; measurement devices for as public conveniences, 37–38; medical insurance regulations concerning, 207–8, 216; National Family Health Survey, 6, 43; shortcomings of, 31–32, 39; vs. body weight as basis for measuring obesity, 17; vs. dual X-ray absorptiometry imagery, 31–32

Bombay: 1859 case of Shakarm, Fat Boy of, 58–59; 1896 bubonic plague epidemic in, 1, 3, 235n1; 1992 riots in, 19, 52, 88; 1995 name change of, 235n1; Bombay burger (*Shiv vada pav*), 78, 80; Bombay duck (*bombil* fish), 7; debate over "Bombay time" and "Indian mean time", 251n3; East Indians ("Portuguese Christians") of, 19, 239n27; function of as global city, 240n36, 244n11; Gateway of India monument in, 89; Sindhunagar (Ulhasnagar) suburb, 81; *vada pav* as symbolic of, 89. *See also* Mumbai

brain: as marketing object for food companies, 139; dementia and brain death through diabetes, 181; food consumption and well-being of, 107, 167; neuronal plasticity of, 35, 240n5; recalibration of with gut following laparoscopic surgery, 194, 196, 218; relationship of gut to, 35, 194, 196

branded foods: addictions and cravings for specific, 45, 122, 167; adulteration of, 112–13, 122; as percentage of food production in India, 131; consumer loyalties to specific, 116, 122, 133, 138; corporate, 88–89; prescriptions for specific, 116, 160; as products of food politics, 24, 70, 77, 82, 83, 88–89, 96. *See also* packaged foods

brand loyalty, 119, 122, 133, 138, 140

bread: as element of *vada pav*, 69, 80, 243n6; avoidance of as medical instruction, 47; brown, 161–62; chapati, 93, 121, 154, 175, 178, 185, 199; enhancement of processed by food companies, 109, 131; inclusion of in diets, 162, 174; *zhunka bhakar,* 76

bulk food. *See* loose (bulk) food

Calcutta (Kolkata), 70, 121, 212, 248–49n8

calories, 6–8, 25, 70–71, 95, 131, 167, 187

Canguilhem, Georges, 222–23, 233, 242n23, 251n6

carbohydrates, 17, 79, 219

cardiovascular disease, 5–6, 17, 41, 49, 52, 53, 126

caste, 6, 14, 24, 42–43, 45, 57, 74

Catholics: Catholic origins of Trinity Hospital, 169; East Indian converts, 19–20, 239n27; Goan, 16; large population of in Manuli, 1, 141–42; Manuli's celebration of birthday of Virgin Mary, 27–28

cells: beta, 17, 147, 182; brain, 35; insulin signal, 17; metabolism as means of maintaining cellular function, 9, 11; plasticity of, 35, 58, 240n5

Centre for Science and Environment (CSE), 112–13

Chennai, 18, 70, 93, 96, 210

children: babies, 55–57; case of Poorvi, 166–67; case of Saurab, 201–3; case of Fat Boy in 1859 Mumbai, 59, 242n19; childhood obesity, 29, 70, 162, 172; confusion of fatness with health in, 47, 167; diets of in India, 40, 51, 70–71, 93–94, 121–22, 126, 162; failure of to play, 29, 51, 172; possible benefits to of epigenetic engineering, 35; Pune Maternal Nutrition Study, 56; school lunches, 94; sedentariness as harmful to, 29, 47, 51; unhealthy snacking habits of Indian, 70–71, 93–94, 122; vulnerability of healthy to metabolic disease, 139, 166–67; vulnerability of to adulterated food, 124–25; vulnerability of to food addiction, 167, 172

cholesterol: as marketing object for food companies, 109, 132; appearance of high in tandem with or ailments, 188; HDL or "good", 7, 113; medical monitoring of individual, 149, 200, 202–3

chronic disease: absorption and, 5, 13, 62, 63; as expression of individual stress, 62; conflation of one's being with having, 13; epidemic of in India, 63, 139, 190, 226, 233; fortification of packaged foods to prevent, 24–25, 239n31; in nutrition transition model of human evolution, 235–36n3; obesity as, 3, 47, 226; problem of motivation to fight, 47, 139; temporal progression of, 23, 147, 173, 178, 181–83, 232

class: association of packaged and functional foods with rich consumers, 51, 121, 127; as basis for vocational distinctions between nutritionists and dietitians, 164–65; body type or morphology as basis for class stereotyping in India, 4, 14–16, 33, 45, 57–58, 61, 245–46n9; caste, 6, 14, 24, 42–43, 45, 57, 74; consumerism as class-associated concern in India, 4–5, 13, 76, 236n4, 243n5, 246n11; cross-class accessibility of metabolic surgery in India, 197, 198–99;

cross-class incidence of metabolic disease in India, 15, 23–24, 33, 46, 55–57, 62, 167; cross-class incidence of stress in India, 40, 49, 52, 54; cross-class vulnerability to food addiction in India, 167; cross-class vulnerability to food adulteration in India, 124; employment as means of upward mobility, 165, 228; employment in food adulteration as means of upward mobility, 118, 245–46n9; Fernandes on state and in India, 236n4; food consumption patterns as indicators of social in India, 6, 74, 112, 153, 166, 236n7, 243n6; India's urban middle as target and reference point for corporate marketing, 4, 76, 90, 110, 133–37, 229; lower-middle population in Mumbai, 16, 52, 112, 157, 167, 169; lower-middle population of India, 15, 24, 55, 135, 137, 165; overconsumption as stereotypical trait of India's urban middle class, 15, 24, 213, 226; poor in Mumbai, 99, 118, 121, 165, 167, 169; poor of India, 15, 46, 113, 236n4, 238n16; sedentary work as stereotypical trait of India's urban middle class, 40, 54; social hierarchy in modernizing India, 14, 110–11, 116–17, 221; stereotyping of social classes in India, 23–24, 45, 244–45n5

Coca-Cola, 77, 78–79, 82, 121, 122

Codex Alimentarius, 125–26

Cohen, Lawrence, 115, 203, 241nn15–16, 243n7

cold storage shops, 141–42, 143

collateral structures and resources, 146–48, 173, 183, 185, 186

commensality, 14, 73–74, 88, 111

conferences attended: concerning metabolic illness, 18, 29, 94–95, 149; concerning metabolic surgery, 206; concerning obesity, 130–31, 155, 193, 218

consumption: commercial appeals to, 15, 115, 131–33; food as precursor to metabolic disease, 15, 161, 226, 228; food patterns, 6, 15, 57, 185, 245–46n9, 246–47n14; gastropolitics of vada pav, 24, 70–74, 77, 87, 89, 92–97, 244n11; influences of Westernization and materialism on, 4–5, 23, 43, 46, 76, 204, 236n4; inside-outside dichotomy of food choices, 111, 114, 120, 126, 139; metabolic surgery as means of resetting bodily patterns of, 25, 204–5, 222; middle class, 13, 226, 236n4; overconsumption, 5, 13, 63, 70, 114, 226, 228; urban consumers, 13, 75, 79, 85, 92, 246n11

cooking. See food preparation

dal: adulteration of, 100, 124; in ration shops, 102; in school lunches, 94; traditional consumption of, 3–4, 102, 121, 136, 175, 200, 245n6

Das, Veena, 20, 244n4

Delhi, 41, 44–45, 70, 82, 117, 211, 229

demarcation, 177–81

Deonar abattoir, 142–44

Dhruv (journalist), 80–81, 92

diabetes: 2008 consensus statement regarding metabolic disease, 41–42; abstinence as inadequate approach in controlling, 47, 50, 165–66; as disease of stress, 49–54, 149, 165–66; as disease of tropics, 55; as genetic or hereditary disease, 33, 50, 56, 59, 170, 175, 206, 242n20; among Mumbai's *koli*, 107; amputation as life-prolonging therapy for patients, 25, 180–81, 183; Annemarie Mol on, 239n31; beta cells, 17; blood glucose measurements, 170; BMI as indicator of risk, 41; case of Anjali, 158–59, 174; case of Aunty (Manuli neighbor; caterer; diabetic), 49–50; case of Eileen (Manuli church worker; retired teacher; diabetic), 52–53; case of Father Matthew (priest; retired school principal; diabetic), 50–51, 122; case of Joseph (diabetic neuropathic progression), 177–78; case of Kapil (newspaper journalist and diabetic), 46–47, 48; case of Muffazal (diabetic progression), 176–77; case of Paul (retired computer technician and diabetic), 175–76; case of Surekha (*koli*), 107; case of Winnie (Manuli neighbor; cook; diabetic), 51–52; circulation slowdown, 181; common, nonmedical conversations and references to, 49, 50, 158, 168–69, 174; comorbid occurrence of, 44, 49, 50, 51–52, 93, 154, 173; control of through diet, 25; curse of "thrifty gene", 33–34, 46, 58; demarcation, 177, 179, 181; dementia, 181; "diabetes pressure", 50; diabetic neuropathy, 145, 177–78, 181; diabetology, 25, 39, 54, 55, 178, 183, 233; diet and foods, 50–53, 65–66, 93, 115, 126, 160, 166–67; Dr. Anoop Misra (metabolic disease specialist) on, 40–42, 53; Dr. Modi (diabetologist) on, 39–40, 48; Dr. Srinivasan (nutritionist; professor; diabetic) on, 163–66; drug therapies used for type 2 diabetes, 25, 152, 158, 171, 197, 249n11; elderly patients, 99–100; epidemic in India of type 2 diabetes, 4, 5–6, 13, 15, 22, 107, 175; food company product targeting of, 131–32,

136, 138; foot problems and foot care among diabetics, 145, 177–82; gangrene, 177–78, 182; identification of individuals at risk for, 42; India as Diabetes Capital of World, 40, 47, 137, 207; infections from minor injuries among diabetics, 177–78, 180; insulin resistance, 17; kidney profiles and dialysis among patients, 170, 173, 175; limb loss among diabetics, 178; low birth weight in babies as indicator of risk of, 56; media commentaries regarding, 46–47, 54; metabolic syndrome as bodily precursor of, 17, 41, 56; multiple, simultaneous therapies as means of controlling, 51; neuropathy, 145, 177–78, 181; obesity and, 40, 154–56, 170, 173, 218, 228, 234; onset of type 2 diabetes among adolescents and young adults, 39–40, 52–53, 172, 232, 238n25; pancreas, 147, 173; patient self-management of, 50–51, 53, 65–66, 93, 122, 171, 175–76; patients in clinic of Dr. Chitre, 168–77; patients in clinic of Dr. Samant, 177–83; pharmaceutical company investments in drugs for, 169–70; physical injuries sustained by diabetics, 177–78; plasticity of human body as means of preventing, 35, 57–58; Poorvi (nutritionist, diabetes clinic) on, 65–66; prediabetic glucose levels, 17; public awareness of threat of, 40, 46–47, 48, 49, 164–65; Pune Maternal Nutrition Study, 56–58; rescaling of BMI measurements for earlier identification of, 41; research by C. S. Yajnik on, 55–58; research by David Barker, 33, 56, 59, 242n20; risk of as influence on nutritional labeling policies, 126; shortcomings of BMI in predicting onset of, 39, 40; "small, fat, and thin" babies as at-risk candidates for, 56; surgical treatments for, 194, 195, 197–200, 203, 206–8, 213–14, 217–18; symptoms of type 2 diabetes, 17, 50, 51, 173, 175; T2DM (type 2 diabetes mellitus), 41–42; temporal progression of, 147, 148, 173, 176–77; type 1 diabetes, 248n1; ulcers, 180, 181, 182–93; in utero damage as cause of, 6; in utero diet engineering to prevent onset of, 35, 57; Westernization as cause of in India, 4, 115, 126, 131, 172; WHO study of in South Asia, 40–41

diagnosis: as justification for pharmaceutical-based medical treatment, 43, 155; as means of medicalizing a bodily condition, 43, 147, 149–50, 222; Ayurvedic, 156; BMI as means

diagnosis (*continued*)
of locating individuals at risk for disease, 35–36, 39, 40, 41; diagnostic diet recall, 152–53, 161; disease thresholds established through, 43, 172, 182–83, 202; lab reports, 66, 151, 152–53, 172, 185; of comorbidities, 39–40, 51, 216, 241n13, 242n22; of diabetes, 51, 173, 178–79; of metabolic illness, 10, 16, 25, 156, 168; ScanTech medical diagnostics lab, 44, 151; self- by patients, 51, 155, 168; *tenshun* as mode of, 51–52, 62; visual manifestations of bodily malfunction, 61, 63, 156; weight scale as tool for medical, 37. *See also* medicalization

diet: adulteration as threat to, 116; agency, authority, and power over an individual's, 22, 25, 26, 156–61, 175, 183–87, 189–90; as medical therapy, 161, 184, 202, 223, 249–50n14; as therapeutic complement to pharmaceuticals, 168–69, 173, 204; as tool for self-redefinition, 185, 201–3; bad eating habits, 47, 71, 151, 160; based on small, frequent portions of food, 157, 189–90; case of Saurab (obesity), 201–3; cholesterol in, 7, 41, 109, 113, 149; daily eating rhythms, 136, 153; dietary recall for patient diagnosis, 150–53, 155, 161, 200–201; dietary treatments for metabolic problems, 42, 146, 149, 160–61, 163, 183, 185–86; dietary trends in human history, 235–36n3; disease-specific diets, 151, 156–57, 160, 166, 170, 178; during childhood and adolescence, 35, 172–73; during pregnancy, 35, 57; engineering of to prevent metabolic disease, 35, 57, 172–73; fiber in, 7, 109, 127, 131, 133, 159, 164; folic acid deficiency in India, 57; food addiction, 167–68; food portions as concern, 153–54; grains in, 37, 127, 133; hunger, 52, 124, 159, 190; integration of into daily regimens, 94, 147, 189–90, 200–201; juices in, 15, 65, 87; Ketkar, 189–90; models, 7, 124, 166; postsurgery, 194, 220–21; prescription of processed foods, 116, 151, 160; preventing overconsumption of fats, 148; preventing overconsumption of rice, 132, 178; preventing overconsumption of sugar, 66, 148, 161–62; shortcomings of in treating metabolic problems, 25, 161, 166, 193–94, 204–5, 212, 219–20; toleration of a prescribed by patients, 52, 66, 94, 122, 186, 187; typical of *koli*, 107; typical of oil rig workers, 231; *vada pav* as basic snack

in Mumbai, 94; Westernization of eating patterns, 45, 127. *See also* nutrition

dietetics: concerns of with metabolic illness, 183; Foucault on as regimen, 194, 249–50n14; vs. nutrition, 163–65

dieting: as means of repairing a metabolism, 148, 186, 188, 223; case of Saurab (obesity), 201–3; food addiction and, 168; limited effectiveness of, 57, 188, 194, 200, 210, 216, 219; as personal empowerment, 184, 189, 201–3; widespread practice of, 6, 16, 99

dietitians: bodily constitution as concern of, 155; food portions and eating schedules as concerns of, 153–54; intellectual and professional interests of, 161, 164–65, 167; prescription of processed foods by, 151, 160; prescriptions by, 7, 150–51, 156–61; proscriptions by, 66, 94; use of medical diagnoses by in creating diets, 150, 152–53. *See also* nutritionists

Dirks, Nicholas, 42–43

Doctor, Vikram, 80–81

Don, W. G., 58–59, 242n19

drugs: as complement to dietary therapy, 148, 150–51, 158–59, 183, 185, 186; agency underlying absorption, 6, 13, 22, 169, 175–77, 186, 189, 230; blur between food and, 24, 109–10, 112, 129, 140, 160, 167–68, 183; diagnosis as justification for medical treatment using, 43, 152–53; Ecks on concept of "eating drugs", 248n8; fake, 245n7; food as addictive, 167–68; functional foods as, 109, 131, 244n3, 245n8; heuristics underlying absorption of, 12, 167–68; injections, 147, 171, 228; limitations of pancreas in tolerating, 147, 173, 182; metabolization of, 10, 182; metformin use for diabetes, 152, 156, 158, 174, 176, 249n11; multifaceted nature of bodily absorption of, 5, 10, 186, 200; Mumbai Food and Drug Administration (FDA), 124, 125, 127–28, 129, 160; self-treatment through pills, 50–53, 93, 147, 158, 170, 173–76, 180–81; shortcomings of as tools to control obesity, 25, 158, 167, 199, 204; use of in treating diabetes, 50, 146–48, 158, 169, 176–77, 178, 249n11; use of in treating hypertension, 50, 174–75; use of in treating obesity, 42, 147–48, 151, 197; use of to sustain benefits of metabolic surgery, 197, 205, 220, 222; Xenical use for weight loss, 151

dyslipidemia, 17

East Indians: ethnographic study of
Bombay's by Elsie Baptista, 239n27; food
traditions of Mumbai's, 19, 50, 239n27; of
Mumbai's Bandra neighborhood, 19
eating. *See* diet; rhythms
eating schedules. *See* work schedules
employment: bakers, 49; in call centers, 8;
case of Chandra Sahu (overweight oil rig
worker), 212; case of Surekha (*koli*), 106–8;
case of Thomas (oil rig worker), 230–31;
case of Wilfred (fisher), 230; in catering,
8, 96, 112, 135; cooks, 52, 112, 123, 198;
domestic servants, 20, 52, 112, 116, 180,
246n10; drivers, 50, 87, 176, 199; efforts by
Shiv Sena to create, 69, 81–82, 85; family
cooks, 52, 110–11, 112; family ownership
of *vada pav* carts, 83–88, 96; fishers, 37,
50, 108, 230, 239n26; *koli* (fisherwomen),
106–8; milkmen, 116, 245–46n9; nature of
as potential impediment to health, 8, 173;
on oil rigs, 7, 212, 231; in pav bakeries, 87;
Qureshi Muslims at Deonar, 143
endocrinology, 11, 17, 31, 145, 169, 172, 233
environment: Ayurvedic understanding of
interactions between body and, 154–55,
157; bodily plasticity in response to, 55,
56–58; epigenetic engineering, 35; fetal,
6, 33; intermingling of body and environment through absorption, 5, 9–12, 222,
226–27, 236n8; Mumbai as urban, 15, 49,
63–64, 72–73; Navaro-Yashin on influence
of, 251–52n7; of illness, 161, 175, 183, 185,
186, 228; role of consumption in shaping,
15, 26, 226–27; sociotemporal influence of
an on a body, 34–35, 49, 231–34; *tenshun*
between body and, 22, 34, 49, 62–63; toxins
and pollutants in, 6, 10, 15, 35, 49
epidemic: bubonic plague in Bombay
(1896), 1, 3–4, 235n1, 238n15; concept
of, 238nn15–16; "Epidemics of the Will"
essay, 25–26; epidemiological transition
model, 235–36n3; of diabetes in India, 4,
6, 47; of diseases of prosperity in India, 4,
47, 54–55, 63, 95, 190, 207; of diseases of
prosperity in U.S., 166; of obesity in India,
4, 21, 42
epigenetics, 24, 32–35, 46, 56, 233, 240n1
exercise: as means of countering obesity, 42,
156, 191, 204, 212; as means of maintaining or regaining health, 7, 155, 157, 172,
183, 188, 223; lack of as cause of childhood
obesity, 29, 47, 51, 172; time and scheduling
constraints as discouragements to, 53, 173;

walking, 16, 153, 171, 188, 189; yoga, 19, 21,
116, 156, 157
export of food, 108, 123, 124, 125, 142

families: attempts by to intervene and to protect relatives, 45, 157, 162, 178, 230; clinic
patients accompanied by, 146–47, 151, 170,
180, 217; family businesses, 18, 29, 71, 75;
family businesses in *vada pav*, 81–85, 88,
91, 245–46n9; family compounds, 7, 28;
Family Health Survey, 6, 43; genetic inheri-
tances within, 23, 33, 50–51, 170–72, 175,
188, 206; meal gatherings, 50, 136, 200;
money and food distributions to poor, 99,
99–100; obesity as cause of estrangement
within, 219, 221; packaged foods designed
for use by, 25, 231; religious observances
in, 27, 154; role of housewife as protec-
tors of, 112, 115, 119–23, 124, 130, 139,
244–45nn4–5; sedentary lifestyles within,
29, 47, 51, 219; sociocultural influences of
on individual metabolisms, 166–67, 188,
200. *See also* households; kinship
fasting: fasting blood glucose, 17, 22, 42, 152,
170, 200, 202; religious, 154, 221
fat: 1859 Bombay Fat Boy, 58–60; abdominal,
39, 56, 61; as cause of individual emotional
withdrawal, 201–2, 216, 220; accumulation
of as process, 45–46; accumulation of as
something to be controlled, 49–50, 71, 95,
147–48, 151, 158, 225; adipose, 17, 38–39,
241–42n17; as feature of stereotypical *koli*,
107; as socioeconomic symbol of prosperity, 16, 28–29, 45; "bad copy" as product of
Westernization, 44–48; bodily conversion
of, 6; and bodily plasticity, 23, 34–35, 56,
61, 166, 170; bodily storage of, 33; children,
29, 51, 70, 162, 172; common local terms for
describing people, 49, 162, 202; comorbid
presence of, 5, 50, 172; dual X-ray absorptiometry imagery, 31–32; measurements
of, 17, 31–32, 35, 43, 56, 156, 241–42n17;
medicalization of, 21, 43–44, 49, 147–48,
174, 204; metabolic obesity contained in
thin body, 33–35, 38–39, 43–44; as product
of individual's socioeconomic environment
and lifestyle, 20–21, 226, 228, 233; stigmatization of, 43–44, 49, 105, 188, 193, 201–4,
238n21; surgery as means of reducing
bodily, 193–98, 207, 212; temporal character
of absorption, 33–35, 36–37, 45–46, 62–63,
231; thin-fat Indian paradox, 31–35, 38–39,
41, 45–46, 56–61, 164, 241n12; "thrifty

fat (continued)
    gene" hypothesis, 33–34; visceral body, 17, 113. See also obesity

fatafat, 45, 162, 193

fats: in endocrinology, 17; legal regulation of in processed foods, 125, 126, 127; trans fats, 21, 112–13, 114, 126, 127; vanaspati ghee, 245n6

Fernandes, Leela, 236n4

film: Bollywood, 87, 174, 189, 247–48n18; Hindi, 18, 124–25, 189, 221–22; Marathi-language, 87

fish: damaging effects to from pollution of Arabian Sea, 15, 49–50; deterioration of Mumbai's supply of, 15–16; economic reliance of Manuli on, 18, 37, 49–50, 108; fishers, 37, 50, 108, 230, 239n26; frozen from Colaba market, 108; local or fresh from Manuli fishers, 108; by McDonald's, 218–19; sales of in Manuli by koli (fisherwomen), 106–8; shellfish, 108; Surekha (koli or fisherwoman), 106–8; traditional consumption of, 3–4, 7, 51, 106, 231

food adulteration. See adulteration

Food and Drug Authority: Commissioner Mahesh Zagade on role of Mumbai's, 127–28, 129; of Mumbai, 125, 160

food carts and stalls: family-owned, 71, 74–75, 83–88, 95–96, 229; locations of in Mumbai, 83, 243n6; municipal regulation of, 79, 128; Shiv Sena, 77–79, 81, 82, 83–88, 95–96

food companies: Enjoy Foods, 127; Maza, 89–92, 96; OilCo, 130–33, 138–39

food-drug overlap, 109, 112, 131, 160, 167–68, 183, 244n3

food marketing and advertising: adulteration as perverted form of, 118–20; adulteration used as tool for, 109, 116, 120–24; branding, 70, 77–78, 82–83, 88, 96, 131; brand loyalty in response to, 119, 122, 132–33, 138, 150, 160; disease-targeted, 133, 136–38; educating consumer as tool of, 132–33, 134–35; ethnographic studies by companies to enhance, 132, 134–35; focus group work to assist, 135–37; food carts and stalls, 84–88, 95–96; functional foods, 109, 130–33; gender-targeted, 133–37, 139; hawking and selling by koli, 106–8; health-targeted, 111, 114, 130, 132, 138–39, 160, 218–19; influence of on children, 8–9, 45, 122, 129, 167; "insighting", 132, 134, 136; labeling of nutritional content as hindrance to, 112–13, 115, 122, 127; logic underlying by

Maza, 89–92; logic underlying by OilCo, 129–38; logic underlying by Shiv Sena, 77–80, 81–82; public service-based, 132; Saffola products by OilCo, 129–30, 133–34, 138–39, 160; sanitation used as tool for, 77, 79, 82, 83, 90–91, 122, 227; standardization and, 82–83, 85, 92; taste as concern in, 77–78, 82–83, 85, 88–89, 91–92, 96. See also readiness

food preparation: as topic of discussion, 7, 20, 27, 116; bakery vs. home-cooked foods, 94; cart vs. home-cooked foods, 70; Codex Alimentarius guidelines concerning, 125; collection and sharing of recipes, 7, 19, 22–23, 27–28, 65–66; cooking as factor of personal dignity, 136; fish, 49, 107; home-cooked vs. "outside" food, 110–12, 122, 140, 161; proportions as concern of dietitians, 153; vada pav recipes, 72, 77–79, 83, 85, 89–90, 96

food processing. See processed foods

foods: authenticity of, 16, 72, 74, 96–97, 245n7; beef, 50–51, 141–42, 169, 231; bhat, 3–4; bulk or "loose", 109, 113–14, 121, 123; chapati, 93, 121, 154, 175, 178, 185, 199; chicken, 27, 50, 67, 91, 141–42, 169; chilies, 78, 81, 82, 86, 90, 119; Chinese, 76, 154, 159–60, 229; dal, 94, 102, 121, 136, 175, 200, 245n6; export of from India, 108, 123–24, 125–42; fish, 49, 50, 67, 108; frozen, 88, 92, 108; fruit, 51, 93–94, 107, 221; garlic, 78, 81; ghee, 3–4, 113–14, 124, 245n6; goat, 142, 144; grains, 37, 127, 133; halal, 141, 143, 246n13; honey, 38, 124, 176; lobster, 108; mango, 51, 65–67, 118; meats, 141–44; Mumbai's cold storage shops, 141–43; Mumbai's rationing system for its poor, 99–103; mutton, 141; noodles, 8–9, 13, 23, 122, 167, 233; pesticides in, 115; pork, 51, 141; quality of vs. quantity consumed, 56–57; religious functions and mandates concerning, 135, 136; temperature effects of various, 157. See also adulteration; oils; packaged foods; snacks

food safety: Food Safety and Standards Act (FSSA), 126, 127–28, 129; Food Safety and Standards Authority of India (FSSAI), 126–27, 128; food safety courts, 126; Meridian surveillance and testing, 128–29; misuse of safety gloves, 128–29; outbreaks of sickness, 129; public scandals, 114–15, 120, 122–24. See also adulteration

Foucault, Michel, 184, 194, 249–50n14

functional foods: development of by food companies, 109, 111, 114, 130–33, 136, 239n31, 244n3; drug-foods, 244n3, 245n8; readiness of Indian housewife to accept, 123, 133, 139

Ganesha, 27–29, 102

gastropolitics, 24, 71–77, 88–89, 96, 243n1, 245–46n9

gender: as consideration in critiques of epigenetics, 242n20; as factor in differentiation between work of nutritionists and dietitians, 164–65; association of masculinity with meat, 231; association of with domesticity, 110–11, 112, 123, 130, 132–34, 136–37, 244–45n4; association of with "inside" and "outside" sociocultural worlds, 110, 179, 244–45n4; association of with patterns of stress, 54, 185, 241n15; associations of absorbency with, 249n10; associations of with *tenshun* and with BP, 241n15; food marketing campaigns based on, 132–34, 137; gendering of foods, 66; housewives as targets of surreptitious preventative health marketing, 133–34; influence of on food consumption patterns, 6, 24, 28, 111–12; medical treatment as factor influencing marriageability, 171, 212, 214

genetics, 23–24, 33, 46, 55–56, 155, 171

ghee: adulteration of, 113–14, 124; dangers of vanaspati, 113; traditional consumption of, 3–4, 113, 245n6. *See also* oils

globesity, 23, 34, 44–45, 48–49, 57, 228, 241n12. *See also* Westernization

glucose: drug therapies for high blood, 158, 174; high blood levels among patients, 65, 66, 152; insulin signals instructing cellular storage of, 17; levels and metabolic diseases, 17, 42, 156, 176, 200, 202; levels in prediabetes, 17; measurement of HbA1c in, 17, 153, 170

glycemic index, 132, 160

Goans, 16, 19, 49–50, 80, 241n14

Gujaratis, 16, 19, 117, 153, 166, 243n3

gut: gut-brain axis, 194, 196, 218; power of, 13, 35, 148, 222; surgical intervention into human, 196, 205–6, 218, 228

halal, 141, 143, 246n13

Hansen, Thomas Blom, 70, 74, 76, 235n1, 243n7

herbal remedies, 51, 131, 176

heredity. *See* genetics

high blood pressure: appearance of in tandem with or ailments, 49–52, 170, 188, 241n13; bariatric surgery as possible treatment for, 208, 211; case of Uncle Salman, 174–75; failure to treat, 53; hypertension as product of unstable work and mealtime schedules, 149; hypertension in India, 4, 40, 49, 115, 241n13, 241n15; impromptu testing of as publicity for food companies, 132; manifestation of in metabolic syndrome, 17, 42, 149; monitoring of, 174, 175; obesity and, 49, 149, 211

Himanshu (food workshop leader), 135–37

Hindi: *chini* (sugar), 176; films, 87; *miliwat* (mixed, adulterated), 245n7; *motapa* (obesity, fat), 49, 202; news coverage of metabolic surgeries written in, 210, 211, 212; prescriptions written in, 93; pulp fiction novels in, 114; *rishta* (arrangement, relationship), 250n2; verbal communications in, 45, 93, 108; vernacular expressions in, 5, 202, 241n14, 244n15

Hindus: 1992 Bombay riots, 19, 52, 88; daily consumption of *vada pav* by some, 93; dietary concerns of as deterrent for using Trinity Hospital, 169; East Indian converts to Catholicism, 19; fasting days, 154, 221; Gujarati, 19, 166; Hindu nationalism, 75–76, 244n11; life paradigms of Hinduism, 14; Manuli's celebration of birth of Lord Ganesha, 27–29; Marriott's model of Hindu life paradigms, 14; Marwari in Mumbai, 16; protein and folic deficiencies among vegetarian, 57; refugees from Pakistan Partition, 80; response of rural to modernization of India, 237n11; Sangh Parivar nationalist coalition, 76; Shiv Sena political movement, 69, 75–76; Shiv Sena *vada pav sammelan* (festival), 77–79; thin-fat babies, 56–57; vegetarianism, 57, 154, 169

HIV, 25, 216–17, 232

homeliness (homely domesticity), 130

hormones: function of pancreas in regulating, 17; glp-1 (glucagon-like peptide 1), 195–96; hormonal activity of belly fat, 39; hunger-regulating, 195–96; as indicators in diagnosis and treatment of diabetes, 152; insulin regulation, 17, 194, 195–96; intestinal, 195, 196; regulation of by metabolism, 9–10; regulation of following laparoscopic surgery, 194, 200, 223; stress as trigger for hormonal change, 54; testosterone levels and balance of, 172 households: collections of things in Bandra, 7; employment of domestic servants by, 52, 246n10; interviews in, 16, 52, 100, 115–16, 139, 174. *See also* families

housewife: as participant in surreptitious preventative health, 133; "processed", 109–10, 132, 134–37, 231; protective role of, 112, 115, 119–23, 124, 130, 139, 244–45n4; as target of marketing readiness, 119, 132, 137, 139

human body. *See* body

hunger: as marketing point for food companies, 138; eating to satisfy hunger pangs, 52, 94, 160; food quality and, 6, 56–57; hidden, 56; malnutrition, 14; manifest, 56; metabolism and, 11; micronutrient deficiency, 56, 58, 194; protein deficiency as cause of, 56; protein intake to prevent, 116, 157, 189; regulation of by intestinal hormones, 195–96; vegetable consumption to alleviate, 149

hygiene, 72, 77, 79, 89, 90, 242n23. *See also* sanitation

hypertension. *See* high blood pressure

identity: and food, 74–75; self-redefinition through diet, 184, 185, 201, 249–50n14; self-redefinition through metabolic surgery, 204–5, 212, 216–23

India: 1896 bubonic plague in, 3–4; Codex Alimentarius, 125–26; colonial, 43, 45; food export policies of, 123–26, 139; low birth-weight babies in, 55–57; postcolonial damage in, 45–46, 166, 245–46n9; precolonial prosperity of, 58

inside-outside: absorption between body and environment, 5, 6, 9, 11–12, 34–35, 72, 147; agency of putting outside in via drugs and diets, 22, 161, 202; *andar se* and *bahar se*, 248n3; body as therapist, 147, 194, 199–200; in context of actor-network theory (ANT), 251–52n7; footwear as symbolic of, 179; Hannah Landecker on, 11–13, 35, 233–34; Lakeoff on divide as critical infrastructure for a population, 248n19; role of household as interface for food, 109–12, 115, 122, 132–33, 136–37, 139–40, 244–45n4; role of metabolism as interface, 11–12, 34, 154, 157–58, 184, 203, 226, 239n31; Westernization as letting outside in, 45–46

insulin: adipose tissue as element in regulation of, 39; as indicator of metabolic

disease, 33; dialysis following diabetes-induced kidney failure, 170, 173, 175; function of in body, 17; insulin resistance, 17; insulin sensitivity, 33, 151; laparoscopic surgery as means of normalizing, 188, 194, 195–96, 198, 201, 216; mangoes and, 66–67; obesity and levels, 170, 216; pancreatic production of, 173; patient's role in management, 53, 66–67, 147, 168–69, 173, 239n31, 249n11; rice and, 53, 107, 132, 228; shots and tablets to regulate, 23, 53, 66–67, 147, 151–52, 168–69, 171; type 2 diabetes, 17

insurance: diagnosis as means of legitimizing medical treatment, 43, 207–8, 213; medical tourism as means of bypassing of coverage restrictions, 215, 217, 218; targeting of stress by health insurance marketers, 54

Internet, 171, 216

interviews: Adil (marketing and public relations, Meridian food surveillance), 128–29; Almas (fashion industry director), 117–21, 122, 176; Alok (*Shiv vada pav* cart owner), 83–88, 96; Diya (obesity patient), 153; Dr. Anoop Misra (diabetologist), 40–42, 53; Dr. Bhatt (metabolic disease specialist), 149; Dr. C. S. Yajnik (endocrinologist), 55–58; Dr. Karke (metabolic surgeon), 199–200; Dr. Kartick (epidemiologist), 59–61, 242nn20–21; Dr. Ketkar (weight loss specialist), 189–90; Dr. Laxman (Head of Research and Development, OilCo), 130–31, 132, 133; Dr. Mehta (biochemist), 58, 242n18; Dr. Modi (diabetologist), 39–40, 48; Dr. Nita (head pathologist, ScanTech), 44–46; Dr. Pillai (veterinarian, Deonar abattoir), 142–44; Dr. Prakash (metabolic surgeon), 209–10; Dr. Sanjay Nagral (medical ethicist), 214; Dr. Srinivasan (nutritionist, professor, diabetic), 163–66; Dr. Vishali (Ayurvedic specialist in diabetes and obesity), 155–56; Kapil (newspaper journalist and diabetic), 46–47; Mahesh (*Shiv vada pav* cart owner), 83–88, 92, 96; Mahesh Zagade (FDA commissioner, Mumbai), 127–28; in Manuli households, 16, 52, 100, 115–16, 139, 174–75; Mr. Anand (Head of Operations, Maza), 89–92; Muffazal (diabetic), 176–77; Nitin (*Shiv vada pav* cart owner), 88, 92, 95; Parth (Marketing Director, Maza), 89, 92, 96; Poorvi (dietitian), 65, 166–68; Satish (quality control, Enjoy Foods), 127; Seema (housewife and mother), 121–23, 139; Sudhir (marketing manager, OilCo), 132–33, 138; Surekha (*koli*, fisherwoman), 106–7; Tejas (quality control, Enjoy Foods), 127

intestines: pancreas, 17, 147, 173, 182, 232; surgical reconfiguration of, 25, 193, 195–96, 198, 205

invitations, 111, 119–20, 130, 139

*jaan* ("life"), 230, 234

Jonas, Hans, 195

journals and newspapers: *British Medical Journal*, 213, 214; *Cochrane Review*, 213, 250n4; *Mint*, 213; *Navbharat Times*, 112–13, 210–11; *Lancet The*, 31–32, 58–60; *New York Times, The*, 120–21; *Times of India, The*, 54, 210, 213, 214

juices, 15, 65, 87

junk foods: burgers, 45, 71, 95, 159, 188; McDonald's, 188, 218; Marathi or Bombay burger, 78, 82; packaged, 121; pizza, 45, 136, 158, 159

Keys, Ancel, 39

kidneys and kidney dialysis, 67, 153, 170, 173, 175

kinship: adulteration of foods as betrayal of, 119; as basis for delineating "inside" from "outside", 110; collateral vs. lineal kin, 148; commensality and, 111; financial assistance based on, 198–99; obligations of housewives to their in-laws, 132, 136, 137, 171; occupations tied to, 86; personal obligations based on, 20. *See also* families

Kolkata (Calcutta), 70, 121, 212, 248–49n8

labeling: as means of ensuring accountability of food processors, 123; exploitation of loopholes in by food companies, 113, 115, 122, 129, 139, 218, 244n3; halal designation, 246n13; legal regulation of food and nutrition, 17–18, 113, 125–27

*Lancet, The*, 31–32, 58–60

Landecker, Hannah, 11–12, 35, 195, 229, 233–34, 236n8, 237n10

languages. *See* Hindi; Marathi

*lassi*, 118

Latour, Bruno, 236n9, 237n13, 240n35, 250n2

Leo (church social services worker) on food and rations in Manuli, 99–100

lifestyle: emulation, Westernization, and bad copy, 36, 45–48, 70–71, 115, 233; influence of on body, 31, 129, 131, 153; lifestyle

diseases, 46, 54, 207; modern urban as cause of poor health, 4, 33, 70–71, 126, 153, 204; sedentary as threat to health, 47, 51, 172, 219

lipids: in blood, 21–22, 33, 39, 200, 202; dyslipidemia, 17

liver, 41, 205–6, 208, 209

Livingston, Julie, 147, 235–36n3, 239n34, 249n12

loose (bulk) food: comparative cheapness of, 100, 109, 121, 131, 138; liability of to adulteration, 113–14, 116, 118, 123

McDonald's: as model for Indian fast food vendors, 24, 70, 90; collaborations of with food marketers in Mumbai, 77–79, 82–83, 91

Maharashtra, the State of: city of Pune, 31, 55–57, 80, 219; food as element of politics of Maharashtrian empowerment, 77, 80–85, 91; Hindu nationalism in, 69, 76, 244n11; *Marathi manoos* (native born Marathi-speakers) of, 69; metabolic disease in, 6; Mumbai's *vada pav* festival, 77–79; rural, 91, 241n12; Sangh Parivar (Hindu nationalist coalition), 75–76; *zhunka bhakar* (traditional porridge and bread dish), 75

malnutrition: as factor in development of metabolic disease, 32–33, 58, 62–63, 164; maternal as influence on fetal development, 33, 56; persistence of in India, 4, 14–15, 62, 120; and plasticity of human body, 48. *See also* nutrition; obesity

mango: *aamras*, 65–66; adulteration of, 118; medical restrictions against consumption of, 51, 66–67; popularity of in India, 65; sugar content of as influence on human blood glucose levels, 65, 66

manufacturing: guidelines for practices, 115, 125–26; textile mills, 76, 81

Manuli: awareness and fears of adulterated food among residents of, 109, 115, 117–23; awareness and gossip within, 121; Catholic families in, 18–19, 141, 177; consumption of processed foods by residents of, 109; convent school lunch program in, 94; cosmopolitan character of, 16, 20, 27–28, 52, 141–42, 241n14; East Indian food traditions of, 19; economic reliance of on fish, 18, 37, 108, 230, 239n26; fieldwork done in, 18; function of as fishing village, 7, 37, 108; Hindu families in, 19; homes in, 49, 50;

Manuli (*continued*)
interview with Almas (fashion industry coordinator) concerning adulteration and readiness, 117–21, 122, 176; *koli* (fisher women) of, 106–8; lobster export from, 108; *mahila mandal* (women's group) of, 20, 100–102; Muslim families in, 19, 20, 52, 117, 169; neighborhood of in Bandra, 7; "nexus" (criminal underworld) presence in, 24, 115; poverty in, 16, 99–100, 117, 169, 225, 230; problem of environmental pollution for, 49–50; ration shop crisis in, 99–103; religious celebrations in, 27–29; simultaneous Catholic and Hindu celebrations in, 27–28; story of Wilfred (fisher), 230–31; *tenshun* as fact of life in, 45, 50, 52; Trinity Hospital as primary medical location for residents of, 145–46, 169. *See also* Bandra

Marathi: *miliwat* (mixed, adulterated), 245n7; *saakar* (sugar), 176; vernacular expressions in, 5

marriageability and sexuality, 21, 171, 202, 212, 214, 221, 249n14

Mary (research assistant): advocacy work by on behalf of her neighbors, 20, 100–103, 117; as source of recipes, 7, 27; assistance of with neighborhood food consumption survey, 19–20; on food adulteration, 117–19, 122–23; function of as coordinator for neighborhood women's group, 20, 100–102; function of as neighborhood social worker, 20, 177; function of as protector of familial food supply, 119–22; home of, 7; kinship and relatives of, 8–9, 174–75, 177–78; metabolic disease crises among family and friends of, 176, 177–78; participation by in neighborhood celebration of birthday of Virgin Mary, 27–28; post-pregnancy diet regimen of, 7–8; ration shop controversy, 100–103

Maza (food company): avoidance of Shiv Sena by, 91; food production at, 92; goals of, 89–91; interviews with Parth (Marketing Director), 89, 92, 96; interview with Mr. Anand (Head of Operations), 89–92; marketing strategies of, 91, 96; standardization of foods at, 89–91, 92; street seller responses to, 92–93; taste of its foods as concern at, 91, 92; transnational ties of, 91–92; *vada pav* by, 89–92

measurement: assays, 57, 170; BMI calculation, 6, 35, 151; body, 22, 56, 156; body age,

202; dyslipidemia, 17; of food portions, 153–54; of HbA1c, 17, 153, 170; scales, 22, 36–37; skin-fold, 56; weight, 17

meat: cold storage stores, 141; consumption of as indulgence, 154; export of from India, 142–43; halal, 143; inclusion of in diets, 169, 231; medical threat presented by, 67, 144, 155; processing, 141–44; in snacks, 49; vendors, 17, 26, 37

media: 1990s coverage of metabolic diseases by, 40; campaigns to educate Indian public regarding metabolic disease risk, 44; coverage of obesity in India, 38, 49, 54; failure of to educate public regarding foot care, 178; glorification of thinness by, 184; health advice columns, 21; Kapil (newspaper journalist and diabetic) on as means of educating public about metabolic diseases, 46–47; linkage between food adulteration and metabolic disease made by, 115, 123–24; promotion by of surgery as solution to metabolic disorders, 204, 209, 213–14; public response to globesity coverage in, 49, 139; reactions by to change in India's BMI scale, 42

medicalization: diagnosis as of a bodily condition, 43; of consumerism and of overconsumption, 43; of foods and their contents, 21, 97, 111–12, 138; of weight and obesity, 43, 48, 56, 204; surgery as of an individual body, 203, 204–5, 223. *See also* diagnosis

medical systems: homeopathy, 21, 146, 155, 163, 176; naturopathy, 156, 166; premised on concept of bodily "humors", 14, 154, 157; Unani, 17, 154. *See also* Ayurveda

Meridian (testing and sampling company), 128–29

metabolic disease: 2008 Indian consensus statement regarding, 41–42; absorption as basis for understanding, 5, 9, 63–64, 73, 227–29, 233; appearance of among young people, 39–40, 53, 172, 178–79; appearance of throughout all socioeconomic strata, 15; bodily plasticity that obscures detection of, 34–36, 38–39, 43–44, 63; cardiovascular disease as comorbidity of, 5–6, 13, 41, 49, 52, 126; cases of specific patients displaying comorbidities, 149, 158–59; comorbidities, 39, 44, 49–52, 93, 159, 170–72, 208; diagnostic categories, 149–50, 152; Dr. Anoop Misra (diabetologist) on, 40–42; Dr. C. S. Yajnik (endocrinologist) on, 55–58; dyslipidemia, 17; epidemic of in India, 4, 14, 42, 47, 207; factors that can produce, 12–13, 15, 23, 32–33, 36, 105; fat, adiposity and, 33–34, 38–40; food company targeting of, 109–10, 119, 123–24, 126–27, 133; foods as culprits in producing, 65–67, 105, 109, 111–19, 125–27, 153–54; genetic predisposition to, 32–35, 170, 171, 188; lifestyle as influence on, 45–48, 59–61, 149, 153, 171–73; malnourishment and, 14–15, 32–33; malnutrition and obesity as two extremes of malnourishment, 14–15, 228; metabolic syndrome, 17, 41–42, 149, 208; progression of in an individual body, 173, 176–78, 181–82, 186; self-monitoring of patients having, 66, 146, 156–59, 175–76, 201–3; *tenshun* as cause of and contributor to, 48–55, 59–60, 62; treatment of, 34–35, 150–62, 170–71, 183, 194, 214, 223; willpower and, 25, 199, 204–5, 221

metabolic living: absorption as influence on, 9, 11–13, 21–22, 26, 222–23, 227–29, 233–34; blur of food and drugs characteristic of, 24, 109–10, 112, 129, 140, 160, 168, 183–85; definition of, 12, 21–22, 238n21; endurance, 9, 114, 147–48, 204–5; gastropolitics as major influence on, 73, 96–97, 109–12, 114; invitation in relationship between food and home, 111, 119–20, 130, 139; temporal aspects of, 57–58, 62–64; therapeutic features of, 10, 145, 147–48; willpower as basis for, 194, 204–5, 221–23

metabolic surgery: as form of agency, 193, 198; *atyachaar* following, 218–23, 232; case of Neha, 193–94, 218–22; case of Purnima (post-surgical failure), 210; costs of, 198, 198–99; Dr. Karke (surgeon) on, 199–201; Dr. Prakash (surgeon) on, 197–99, 209–10, 216, 220; gastric bypass surgery, 193, 195–96, 198, 209, 212, 217, 219; intestinal change through, 25, 193, 195–96, 198; laparoscopic surgery, 193, 198, 205, 209, 212–13, 218, 223; negative experiences with, 210; reattachment following, 168, 194, 201, 222–23; reconfiguring of organs through, 25, 193, 195–96, 198, 250n1; rejection of dieting in favor of by many patients, 223; sleeve gastrectomy, 198, 206, 213, 216. *See also* bariatric surgery

metabolism: as absorptive interface between body and environment, 9–12, 22, 24–25, 57–58, 62–63, 161, 226–29, 233–34; addiction as threat to health of, 166–68, 230; agentive powers and responsibilities of

those who possess a, 149, 151, 153, 157–62, 175, 183–86, 200–201, 220–22; agentive powers of, 10, 161, 185–86, 194–95, 199, 203; as biological system, 9–11, 195–96; as therapeutic site for body, 10, 146, 157–58, 166, 194, 199–201, 203, 218; at-risk, 63, 66, 173, 183, 194–95; Ayurvedic understanding of, 154–56, 157; balance of as somatic concern, 10, 17, 58, 147–48, 154, 157, 159, 161–62; balance of hormones as concern, 172, 176–77, 194, 200; bioscientific definitions of, 9–10, 26; bodily plasticity and, 35, 57–58, 62–63; cellular function and, 9, 11; city as possessor of a, 70, 71–73, 89, 234; disorders of, 40, 53, 63, 159; energy and as somatic concern, 11, 59–60, 138–39, 173, 176–77; function of, 9–10; gut-brain axis connected through, 194, 196, 218; in social theory, 10–11, 237n13, 237nn10–11; interest of dietitian in, 164; interest of nutritionist in, 162–63; Landecker on, 11–12, 35, 195, 229, 233–34, 236n8; metabolic similarities between visually different bodies, 31–34; "to metabolize", 10; Mol on balance of, 203, 239n31; personhood and concepts of being a metabolism vs. having a, 13, 23, 149, 195, 226, 228, 231–32; protein and, 9–10, 17, 41, 57, 116; speed of as somatic concern, 10, 149, 154, 158–59, 182; stress as source of damage to, 48–55, 63–64, 228; surgical resetting of, 195, 199–201, 208–10, 219–23; temporal nature of, 11–12, 23, 24, 153, 173, 182, 228–29, 231–34; thin-fat Indian paradox, 24, 32–34; treatment and renewal of, 25, 146, 148, 158–62, 173, 183–86; willpower and, 194–95, 199, 203–5, 219, 221–23, 228

metformin, 152, 156, 158, 174, 176, 249n11

micronutrient deficiency, 56, 58, 194

middle class: as participants in India's food industry, 90, 135; as targets of food company marketing, 110, 135–37; class boundaries in India, 110–11, 165; dietary deficiencies within India's, 57, 62; metabolic disease within India's, 15, 57; obesity in India's, 24, 57, 213; overconsumption by urban of India, 4, 5, 13, 76, 226, 236n4, 246n11; sedentary work patterns of India's, 54, 153, 173, 201; *tenshun* within India's, 54; vulnerability of to adulterated foods, 124

milk: adulteration of, 16, 113, 114, 116, 118, 120; Amul brand, 116, 157; Ayurvedic classification of as sweet, 155; consumer purchases of preserved boxed milk as milk (*continued*)

preferable to probably adulterated, 116, 118; consumption of for protein and for satiety, 116; dilution of by adulterers, 111, 116, 120; dilution of by rural milkmen, 245–46n9; low-fat and skim, 66, 157; Nestlé brand, 118; prescription of packaged, 116; *thandai*, 157; use of cardamom and pistachio in, 157; use of sugar powders to flavor, 167

Mintz, Sidney, 74, 245n8

Misra, Anoop, 40–42, 53

Mol, Annemarie, 203, 239n31, 242n22, 250n1

Monteiro, Carlos, 105–6

morals: biomoral substances, 185, 186; food addiction, 167–68; influence of on bodily behaviors and lifestyles, 48, 238n21; measurement as means of establishing guidelines for bodily conditions, 36; metabolic disease as condition that cannot be controlled by, 161, 168, 185–86; of individual responsibility for diet control and weight loss, 25, 161, 184–85, 202; underlying prescriptions and proscriptions, 25, 184–86; use of as marketing tool by food companies, 110, 114, 124, 140

Mumbai: 1992 riots in, 19, 52, 88; 1995 renaming of Bombay, 231n1; 2008 terrorist attacks in, 197; abattoir of Deonar, 142–44; Almas (fashion industry director) on food adulteration in, 117–19; as absorptive environment, 6, 12–13, 15, 145, 231–32, 234; as environment characterized by poor hygiene, 89, 239n31; anthropological fieldwork conducted in, 16, 39, 156; as sociocultural environment, 110–11; as stressful urban environment, 15, 241n15; Catholic population of, 1, 18, 141; children in, 8–9, 70–71, 94, 121, 122, 162, 167; cosmopolitan character of, 16, 88, 141–42, 240n36, 244n11; decline of textile mills in, 76; diabetes in, 65–67, 107, 145–46, 164–67, 172, 175–79, 181–83; East Indian population of, 19, 239n27; food adulteration reported in media of, 114, 117–19, 124–25, 245n7; food company targeting of entire social strata of, 133; *Ganesh Chaturthi* celebration in, 27–28; gastropolitics of, 73–76, 95–97, 243–44n10; Hindu population of, 16, 19, 20, 69, 82, 88, 154; "inside"-"outside" dichotomy toward food in, 110–11; interviews with Thomas (oil rig worker), 230–32; interview with Mahesh Zagade, FDA Commissioner

for, 127–28; *koliwada* (fishing village) of Manuli in Bandra neighborhood of, 18; mangoes as fruit of, 66; medical and healing options available in, 21, 156, 164–66, 178, 187, 190, 197, 205; medical tourism in, 215–18; middle class residents of, 243n5; Muslim population of, 16, 19, 20, 88, 117, 141–43, 154, 169; Navi Mumbai (New Bombay) suburb, 44; obesity and treatments for obesity in, 24, 70, 197, 213–14, 219, 223; packaged fast food sales in, 89, 90, 239n31; pollution in, 15, 28, 49; processional *murtis*, 28; Professor Munir on food adulteration in, 113–15; public roadside health checkups in, 132; public scales in, 37, 227; regional sociopolitical significance of, 69; Shiv Sena political party in, 69, 75–76, 79, 83; Sindhis in, 80–81, 243–44n10; street foods of, 24, 69, 73, 89, 243n3; textile mills of, 76, 81, 82; Trinity Hospital in, 145–46, 169; *vada pav* of, 24, 69–70, 74–76, 79–82, 243n3; Virgin Mary celebration in, 27–28. *See also* Bombay

Muslims: 1992 Bombay riots, 19, 52, 88; among settlers in Bandra displaced by 1992 Bombay riots, 19, 88, 117; availability of halal meats for Bandra's, 141–42, 154, 169; Gujarati, 16, 117; Qureshi at Deonar abattoir, 143–44

Narain, Sunita, 113

Navaro-Yashin, Yael, 75, 243n4, 251–52n7

*Navbharat Times*, 112–13, 210–11

Neel, James, 33, 240n2

neighborhood: awareness and gossip within Manuli, 121; hutments, 19, 20, 85, 87, 112, 225; ration house petition, 102

neuropathy: in diabetic body, 145, 177–78, 181; in diabetic brain, 181

New Delhi, 18, 38, 120–21, 211

nexus, 24, 114–16, 118, 121, 123, 245–46n9

North Indians, 87, 241n15, 245–46n9

nutricentric persons, 183–84, 185

nutrition: 1859 Fat Boy case of perverted, 58–60; assertions of positive nutritional value of *vada pav*, 79; clinical, 163, 165, 183; condemnation of negative nutritional value of *vada pav*, 93; consumption of nourishing, wholesome foods, 57, 70–71; diagnosis and treatment of metabolic illness through, 25; dietary prescriptions for processed foods, 116; fortification of processed foods, 24–25, 123–24; functional foods, 131–32,

137, 244n3; individual initiative as influence on, 94, 156–58, 159–62, 165, 183–85, 200–201; influence of local standards on perceptions of, 6; intrauterine, 31, 33; labeling, 17–18, 113, 115, 122, 123, 126–27; mango madness, 65–67; as means by which an entity converts environment into itself, 11–12, 161; nutritional content of home vs. outside food, 110, 124, 245n5; of children, 93, 94, 162; overnutrition, 14, 58; packaged foods, 116, 119, 122, 131–32, 137, 140, 168; and physiology of weight gain, 33; plasticity of human body in responding to changes in, 57–58, 235–36n3; postsurgery, 205, 220; Pune Maternal Nutrition Study, 56–57; shortcomings of vegetarianism, 57; social services support for food purchase, 99; thin-fat Indian paradox, 32–34, 56–58, 60–62; undernutrition and hunger, 14, 200; vs. dietetics, 163–65. *See also* diet; malnutrition

nutritionists: dietary prescriptions from, 7, 116, 162–63; educational programs for training, 163–64; encouragement by for patients to consume nourishing, wholesome foods, 70–71; intellectual and professional interests of, 163–66; interview with Poorvi, 65–67; nutrition counseling sessions with patients, 151–62, 180; prescriptions regarding diets for children, 93; proscriptions against *vada pav* by, 24, 93; Rashmi (Bandra metabolic disorders clinic), 93–94, 150, 152, 153–54, 159–61, 163–64; role of in treating metabolic disease, 146, 150, 162–65, 168, 183, 248n2; Usha (Bandra metabolic disorders clinic), 149, 150, 152, 154, 156–64. *See also* dietitians

obesity: 2005–6 Family Health Survey, 5–6; 2008 consensus statement regarding, 41–42; abdominal fat, 39; adiposity, 17, 31, 38–39, 56, 59, 61, 241–42n17; as disease of stress, 39–40, 54, 61–64, 149; as metabolic disease, 40–41, 215–16, 219; as product of "bad copying", 45–46; as product of poor eating habits, 54, 70–71, 172; as risk of life, 63, 209, 210, 211, 225; association of PCOD with, 94, 149–50, 157, 159, 170; Ayurvedic approaches to, 155–56; bariatric surgery, 41, 191, 208–14; belly fat, 38–39, 46, 56, 173; biopower and, 184; BMI measurement as means of determining, 17, 23–24, 36–43, 241–42n17; body weight as indicator of,

36, 39; case of Anjali (diabetes patient), 158–59, 174; case of Diya (public relations worker), 153; case of Mrs. Qadeer (obesity yo-yo), 157–58, 159; case of Neha (medical *atyachaar*), 218–21; case of Peter (medical tourist), 215–17; case of Purnima (postsurgical failure), 210; case of Fat Boy in 1859 Bombay, 58–59; cases of Amy and Dina (medical tourists), 217–18; childhood, 29, 47, 70–71, 172; comorbid occurrence of, 5–6, 17, 39, 44, 49, 149, 211, 219; cultural traditions and, 28–29, 45; diabetes and, 17, 149, 170, 172; Dr. Anoop Misra (metabolic disease specialist) on, 40–42; Dr. Karke (surgeon) on, 199–201; Dr. Modi (diabetologist) on, 39–40; Dr. Prakash (surgeon) on, 197–99; Dr. Vishali (Ayurvedic physician) on, 155–56; dyslipidemia as determinant of, 17; epidemic of in India, 4–6, 21–23, 42, 49, 71, 207, 211–12; euphemisms for in Hindi, Gujarati, and Marathi, 49, 244n15; food addiction and, 25, 166–67; food company product targeting of, 129–33, 138, 139; gastropolitics and, 24, 70, 95; genetic or hereditary nature of, 170; globesity, 23, 34, 45, 48–49, 57, 62, 228, 241n12; heart disease, hypertension and, 149; ideas concerning causes of, 23, 25; identification of individuals at risk, 42; Ketkar diet, 188–90; Lauren Berlant on, 63–64; as malnourishment, 14–15, 58, 63; measurements to determine, 17, 41–42, 56; media coverage of, 38, 40, 46, 54, 70–71, 105–6, 210–13, 225; medical tourism in India to cure, 214–18; as metabolism controlling human body, 204, 215–16; mistaking of a fat child as being a healthy child, 47; nutrition and physiology of weight gain, 33; nutrition labeling as means of fighting, 126–27; onset of among adolescents and young adults, 39–40, 162, 172; plasticity of human body as means of preventing, 35, 57–58; plasticity of human body as signaling conflict and risk, 48, 56, 61–62; in poor populations as commonality, 14–15, 16, 211; Poorvi (dietitian) on, 166; processed food consumption as cause of, 105, 166; public health concerns over, 70–71, 73, 95, 126, 212; Pune Maternal Nutrition Study, 56–58; research by C. S. Yajnik on, 55–58; research by Dr. Ancel Keys, 39; research by Karen Throsby, 204–5; sedentary lifestyle as cause of, 40, 47, 54, 172; side-effects of

obesity (*continued*)
treatments for, 166, 197; "small, fat, and thin" baby as at-risk baby, 56; street food consumption as cause of, 70–71, 73; surgical demonstration of laparoscopic sleeve gastrectomy by Dr. Pitt, 205–7; surgical treatments for, 193, 195, 197–98, 199–201, 207–13, 250n4; thin-fat Indian body, 33–34, 56–58; in utero diet engineering to prevent onset of, 35; *vada pav* consumption as cause of among Mumbaikars, 70–71; weight-loss businesses, 21; Westernization as cause of in India, 45–46; WHO research on obesity and metabolic disease in South Asia, 40–42; willpower and, 201–2, 204–5, 215–16. *See also* fat; overweight individuals; malnutrition

Obimet (metformin), 158, 159

observations: encounter of Mrs. Qadeer with Usha (obesity), 157–58, 159; food-addicted adolescent, 167; information session by Dr. Prakash (metabolic surgeon), 197–99; at metabolic disease clinic of Dr. Bhatt, 149–63, 169, 175, 180, 248n1; patient interactions with Dr. Karke (metabolic surgeon), 200–201; sleeve gastrectomy performed by Dr. Pitt, 205–7; at Trinity Hospital foot clinic of Dr. Samant (diabetologist), 145, 148, 173–74, 177–83, 232; at weight loss clinic of Dr. Ketkar, 187–89, 190

Ohmann, Richard, 119

OilCo: business activities of, 130, 132; market research methodology of, 131–33, 138, 139; Mr. Chanda (CEO), 130, 132; Saffola products to address obesity and diabetes, 131; surreptitious preventative health approach of, 133

oils, 125, 129, 130, 132, 160. *See also* foods; ghee

organs: intestines, 25, 193, 195–96, 198, 205; kidneys, 67, 153, 170, 175; liver, 41, 205–6, 208, 209; multiple contributing to metabolic function, 9–11, 25, 172, 207–9; pancreas, 17, 147, 173, 182, 232; as part of metabolic system, 9–11, 172; protection of by adipose tissue, 32, 39; reconfiguring of through laparoscopic surgery, 25, 195, 196, 207–9; skin, 11–12, 32, 56, 147, 178–82, 186, 220, 239n31; thyroid, 49, 149, 152, 157, 159, 171, 219

overweight individuals: BMI definition of in India, 6, 23, 35, 38, 41, 42, 43; children,

71, 162, 172; comprehension of threat of metabolic illness among, 40; concerns of medical patients who are, 154, 168; consumption of rice among, 132, 153; dietary treatments for, 185; election of metabolic surgery by, 25; food addiction among, 167; risk of diabetes among, 173; risk of heart attack among, 188; surgical treatments for, 186, 193, 197, 198, 210, 213, 221. *See also* obesity

packaged foods: adulteration of, 122–23, 124; as means of intensifying relations between homes and corporations, 119–20, 129, 135–37, 139, 157, 232; claims regarding unhealthy nature of, 11, 24, 166; codex regulation of logos for, 126; expensive cost of, 109, 121; inclusion of in medical care, 116, 151, 160; junk foods, 45, 121, 167; Kurkure snacks, 122–23; marketing of by food companies, 25; milk, 116, 118, 124; promotion of as solutions to physical disorders, 123–24, 129, 131, 133, 138–39; Quaker Oats, 119; readiness and, 119, 139; snacks as, 24, 160; symbolically filtering nature of, 119–20, 227; Treptin biscuits, 160. *See also* branded foods; foods; processed foods

pancreas, 17, 147, 173, 182, 232

Patel, Geeta, 130

Patell, B. F., 2–3, 4

patients: absorption of drugs by, 12; abstinence from proscribed foods as challenge for, 65–66, 93–94, 165; agency and responsibilities of, 21, 25, 66, 147–48, 157–58, 161, 171; amputation, 178–79, 181–82, 249n12; awareness of disease risk among, 40, 168, 170, 173, 183; Ayurvedic understandings of body as influence on, 154–55, 157; bodily evolution of metabolic disease, 173, 176–77, 178, 179–82, 199; bodily resetting among metabolic surgery, 195–96, 200–201; case of Aditi (metabolic surgery), 200; case of Amy and Dina (medical tourists from U.S.), 217–18; case of Anjali (diabetes), 158–59, 174; case of Diya (obesity), 153; case of Mr. Bala (metabolic comorbidities), 149; case of Mrs. Qadeer (obesity), 157–58; case of Muffazal (diabetes), 176–77; case of Neha (laparoscopic gastric bypass surgery), 193–94, 218–22, 223, 250n2; case of Paul (retired computer technician), 175–76; case of Peter (medical tourist from U.S.A.), 215–17; case of Saurab (obesity), 201–3;

case of stubborn thyroid patient, 156–57; case of Uncle Salman (diabetic), 173–74; change in archetype of metabolic disease, 39–40, 178–79; clinic environments for metabolic disease treatment, 145–50, 161, 187–91; compliance by, 173–77, 183–86, 199; concurrent use of allopathic and homeopathic treatments by, 154–55; daily scheduling of medications and therapies by, 147; dead tissue and appendages, 179–82; demarcation, 181–82; diabetic, 170–71, 172, 173, 178–82; dietary review and nutrition counseling sessions for metabolic disease, 150–55, 156–61; dispersed coordination to achieve metabolic balance, 203; foot care among diabetic, 178–79, 180–82; habits that must be changed as challenge for, 154, 156–60, 161–62, 168, 183; impatient and uninformed, 156–59, 161–62, 170, 171–72; Internet as influence on, 171, 216; lab reports, 66, 151, 153, 172, 185; medical tourists, 214–15; metabolic disease counseled by Dr. Chitre, 170–73; metabolic disease counseled by Dr. Samant, 178–79, 180–82; metabolic disease diagnoses, 149–50, 152, 170–71, 182; metabolic postsurgical, 200–201, 205, 208, 213; metabolic surgery, 193–96, 198–99, 203, 204–5, 210–11; motivation as challenge for chronic disease, 47, 158, 159–60, 186, 199; neuropathy, 177, 180–82; noncompliant, 151, 185, 200–201; obesity, 201–3, 211–12; pain, 171, 173, 179, 181, 182; PCOD, 170; protests and complaints by, 156–60, 200; sedentary lifestyles and lack of exercise among metabolic disease, 153, 155, 157, 170, 172–73, 183; self-diagnosed understandings by, 155, 168, 173, 185; therapy and risk, 183–84, 199, 210–11, 214; thyroid, 155–56; Trinity Hospital endocrinology unit, 169–73, 180–83

pharmaceuticals. *See* drugs
phenotype, 33, 40, 58, 242n21, 242n23
pills. *See* drugs
plague crosses, 1–3, 7, 15, 29, 225, 251n3
plasticity: as ability of an organism to shape itself in response to its surroundings, 34–35, 58; bad copy, 36, 45–48; bodily, 23, 35, 48–49, 58, 62–63, 240n5; bodily as possible epigenetic solution to heritable disorders, 35; cospatial domain or third space, 48; human at point of conflict between modernization and tradition, 48;

influence of *tenshun* on, 48–49, 55; metabolic, 36, 38, 46–47, 57, 61, 63; misleading nature of, 43–44; neuronal of brain, 35; nutritional change as means of manipulating of body, 57–58; obesity as clash point between metabolism and *tenshun,* 55–56, 61–62; of thin-fat Indian, 34–36, 38, 43–44, 48, 60–63, 241n12; sighting of, 36, 43–44, 61–63

pollution: absorption of by human body, 21–22; damage to Manuli's fish supply by, 18, 37, 49–50; dangers of to home food, 111, 123; in Mumbai, 15
polycystic ovarian disorder (PCOD), 94, 149–50, 157, 159, 170
porosity: of home to food from "outside", 109–11, 136; of human body, 6, 158, 201; *tenshun* as product of negative, 49, 63; that exists between body and environment, 9, 73, 97, 222, 223, 227, 231–32
portion sizes, 127, 153–54, 189, 228
potatoes: as basic element of *vada pav,* 69, 77, 80–84, 91–92; abstinence from by diabetics, 53, 170; adaptation of by food companies, 82–83, 91–92; medical prohibitions against consumption of, 47, 170; Radcliffe Salaman's history of, 96; sociopolitical significance of in India, 244n11; traditional consumption of, 49, 80, 82, 122, 243n6; use of to adulterate ghee, 113–14
poverty: as threat to India's middle class, 246n11; availability of medical care for poor, 169, 199; crime as product of, 118; in India, 165; India's poor as victims of bad processed food, 113, 121, 167, 238n16; obesity in poor populations, 14–15, 16, 211; plagues of, 3
pregnancy, 7, 35, 55–57, 171, 187
prescriptions: absorption of food and drugs, 12, 13, 160, 186, 200; dietary, 94, 151–52, 157–60, 168, 178, 185, 202; drugs commonly used to treat diabetes, 249n11; for exercise and muscle development, 42, 156; as exercises of power and agency, 22, 159–61, 184; food company efforts to induce moral prescriptions for their products, 110; linear, long-term, 147–48; of packaged foods, 116, 151, 160; postsurgery maintenance, 222. *See also* proscriptions
preservatives, 88, 92, 116, 136
processed foods: as absorption point between body and market, 24, 105–6, 111, 135, 139; consumption of as means of

processed foods (*continued*)
avoiding adulterated foods, 109, 139–40; consumption of as act of being fed by an outsider, 110–12, 114, 139–40; contribution of to global obesity, 105–6, 111, 126–27; food processing as physical and moral act, 114, 119; food workshop for marketing, 135–37; meat processing, 142–44; of food companies and multinational corporations, 91–92; potatoes, 91; processing of fresh fish by street vendors, 107–8; as site where foods and drugs overlap, 109–12, 138–39, 183; snacks, 91, 109; sociocultural significance of in home, 109–11, 121, 123–24, 136, 139, 231. *See also* adulteration; packaged foods

proscriptions: against *vada pav*, 93, 94, 151, 184; dietary, 157, 159, 160–61, 168; as exercises of power and agency, 22, 184. *See also* prescriptions

protein: as concern of endocrinology, 17; deficiency in India, 57; high-protein diets, 166; in packaged milk as means of producing satiety among patients, 116; lipoprotein, 41; in manifest hunger, 56; powders and shakes, 132, 157, 158, 197, 220, 247n15; relationship of to metabolism, 9–10; use of to enhance foods, 160, 189, 218–19

public health: ambivalence of authorities toward processed foods, 109, 139; attitudes of Mumbai authorities toward *vada pav*, 70–71, 73, 95; foot health as concern for authorities, 179; gastropolitics as complicating factor for authorities, 72–73, 75; global concerns of, 40–43, 55–56, 105, 156; influence of stressful environments on, 15; media support of metabolic surgery as solution for obesity epidemic, 212–13; risks of "being" vs. "having", 13; stereotypes and realities as determinants of policies, 23–24, 47, 204, 226, 236n6; use of BMI measurements in assessing present and future, 43

Pune, 31, 55, 57, 80, 219

Pune Maternal Nutrition Study, 56–57

Quetelet, Adolphe, 39

Radhakrishnan, R., 48, 241n12

Ramadoss, Anbumani (Union Health Minister), 126

Rashmi (nutritionist), 93–94, 150, 152, 153–54, 159–61, 163–64

rations: as political issue in Mumbai, 24, 100–103; Mumbai's public distribution system, 100; prices, 20; ration cards, 100–101; ration shops, 99–102

readiness: food workshop, 135–37; interview with Almas (fashion industry director) concerning, 117–21, 122; marketing logic underlying, 119. *See also* food marketing and advertising

reattachment, 168, 194, 201, 222–23

rhythms: conflict of local with global, 241n12; consumption and familial as concerns of food companies, 133; daily food of Bandra, 15, 106–8; daily food of individuals, 7, 231; daily food of patients, 94, 153, 186; stress as influence on daily, 53, 171, 242–43n12. *See also* time

rice: abstinence from by diabetics, 53, 132, 178; adaptation of by food companies, 130, 132–34, 138–39; as standard element of Indian cuisine, 3–4, 51, 59, 100, 102, 107, 121; as traditional element of Indian cuisine, 127, 131, 136, 200, 230, 231, 245n6; *bhel puri*, 243n3; consumption of to alleviate hunger, 52, 94; "functional" of food companies, 109, 130; *modak*, 28; non-consumption of as personal sacrifice, 153; *poha*, 45, 79; portion sizes consumed by patients as medical concern, 153–54, 160, 228; rice-based diets, 7; and weight management, 132, 133–34, 153–54, 160

risk: as marketing tool for food companies, 110, 133; awareness of in consumption of food and beverages, 70, 71–72, 91, 92, 110, 113, 168; definition and exposure of populations at risk for disease, 35–39, 41–44; genetic factors, 57, 231; individual awareness of health, 10, 48–49, 63, 116, 120, 133, 171; neuropathic, 145, 178–79; of adulterated food, 114–16, 118–20, 121–22; of diabetes, 17, 173; of metabolic disease, 6, 38–39, 44, 63, 183; of obesity, 63, 151, 173, 208–9, 210; of processed food, 110, 113, 126–27; of surgical complications, 211, 213; public health assessment and management of disease, 6, 13, 43, 126–28, 246–47n14; "risk behaviors", 183; surgical vs. disease-embedded, 198, 199, 208–9, 210

Rose (Manuli neighbor; caterer), 49–50, 53

Rosenberg, Charles, 43

Roy, Parama, 73–74, 236n8, 244n13

Saffola: marketing of products, 129–30, 133–34, 138; product usage in homes, 139, 160; Saffola Arise rice, 138

Salaman, Radcliffe, 96

sanitation: as gastropolitical issue, 77, 89, 90, 92–93; food safety, 128–29, 129, 136. *See also* hygiene

scales: public for measurement of body weight, 22, 37; sociocultural significance of, 36, 227; as tools that expose temporal quality of body plasticity, 62–63; for weighing fish, 37

Schlosser, Eric, 89

Sedgwick, Eve, 25–26

sexuality and marriageability, 21, 171, 202, 212, 214, 221, 249n14

Shiv Sena: attempts by to control public space via food, 76, 79, 83; Bal Thackeray (founder), 76–77, 79, 81, 82, 84, 244n11; corporatist tactics and collaborations of, 78–79, 83; gastropolitical acts of, 76, 82–83; gastropolitical acts of based on *vada pav*, 69, 75–76, 77–80, 81–83, 91, 95–96; job creation and job "reservation" by, 69, 76, 78; perception by of non-Maharashtrians as outsiders, 69; political connections of to Hindu nationalist coalition, Sangh Parivar, 75–86; protection of *Marathi manoos* as priority of, 69, 83; "protection" of vendors by, 81, 84; role of in modernizing Mumbai, 76, 78, 244n11; *Saamna* daily newspaper of, 78; Shivaji Park *vada pav sammelan* (festival), 69, 76, 77; Shiv Sena *vada pav* cart of Alok and Mahesh, 83–88, 95–96; Shiv Sena *vada pav* cart of Nitin, 88, 92, 95; socioeconomic goals of, 69; Uddhav Thackeray, 77–79, 82; violence by, 76, 79

Sindhis, 80–81, 243–44n10

slaughter: abattoirs and slaughterhouses, 141; cold storage shops, 141–42, 143; "emergency", 143; "ground", 142, 143, 144; halal meat, 141, 143, 246n13; inspection and tagging of animals, 142, 144; interview with Dr. Pillai (Deonar abattoir), 142–44; legal guidelines for animal, 142; "line", 142, 143, 144; Qureshi Muslim traditions, 143; veterinary care prior to animal, 142

snacks: *aloo boonda*, 82; bakery, 49; *chaat*, 15, 229; constant daily consumption of, 136, 160; consumption of by children, 70, 93, 122; consumption of unhealthy, 70, 94, 95, 160, 230; cookies, 28, 129, 160; food politics and, 76, 79; ice cream, 15, 155, 199; *idli* and *dosa*, 76; nutritionally enhanced, 160, 189, 208; packaged foods, 24, 109, 122–23, 130, 132, 160; *poha*, 79; as sociocultural symbols,

73, 76, 79, 82; street food, 73, 243n3; *vada pav* consumed as, 70, 73, 80, 93–94. *See also* foods

South Asia: food substance, exchange, and propriety in, 14, 17, 73–74, 110, 111; overlap of food and drugs in, 109, 112, 131, 160, 167–68, 183, 244n3; understandings of body, medicine, and healing in, 12, 238n20, 241n13, 248n4, 249n10; understandings of metabolism in, 9, 13, 38, 39, 40, 236n8, 237n13

spices: adulteration of, 120; chili powder, 109, 119, 120, 227; conflicting associations of with foods, 52, 75, 80; standardization of, 85, 92, 136; in *vada pav*, 75, 80, 81, 83, 85, 96. *See also* adulteration

standardization: as goal of food companies, 24, 92, 93; by Shiv Sena of its *vada pav*, 77, 79, 82–84; McDonald's as symbol of mechanized food, 24, 91; of foods as goal of Maza, 90–91; of taste, 85, 89, 92

standards: Codex Alimentarius, 125; global food, 112–13, 123, 125–26, 127; global for defining obesity, 35, 42; global medical as defined by WHO, 55; Indian public health, 95; India's decision to abandon global BMI model, 35–42, 43; legal food safety of India, 126, 246–47n14

starvation, 14, 56, 58, 74

street food: as gastropolitical issue, 72, 73–74, 75, 79, 87, 88, 96–97; as ethnographic object, 74, 89, 92; as public health concern, 71, 72, 73, 128; consumption of by children and students, 70, 71; food company replications of, 89, 90–91, 92; harmful nature of, 70; of Mumbai, 69, 243n3; unhygienic nature of, 70, 90

stress: absorption of by individual, 21, 36, 48–49, 62; as link between food and fat accumulation, 21, 49, 50, 54, 165; function of as foundation for disease, 23, 51–54, 60, 62; gender- and class-related patterns of, 54, 171, 185; indigestion as bodily means of registering, 237n12; urban environments as sources of, 15, 36, 52–53, 62–64, 228. *See also tenshun*; tension

sugar: consumption of through fruit, 51, 66–67, 187; content of in brown bread, 161–62; dietary regulation and restrictions to control, 51, 52, 65–66, 131, 148, 165–66, 175; medical monitoring of in body, 49, 54, 147, 149, 152, 170, 185–86; medical threat presented by, 21, 65–67, 167–71; *modak*,

sugar (*continued*)
27; restorative properties of, 176–77; sugarcane, 55, 87; use of in festive food items, 27; use of in processed foods and beverages, 89–90, 121, 136, 167; use of to adulterate foods, 118

surgery. *See* amputation; bariatric surgery; metabolic surgery

tablets. *See* drugs

taste: as major concern for food companies, 130, 131–32, 135–36; changes to of food that is not fresh, 88; conflict between food hygiene and, 72, 91, 92; government regulations as threat to of processed foods, 127; inadequacies of in processed foods as challenge for food companies, 160, 162; sociocultural associations of with place, 74, 78, 81–83, 91–93, 96; standardization of, 85, 89, 91–93, 96; trans fats as means of preserving of processed foods, 112–13

temporality: as characteristic of metabolism, 24, 153; in context of thin-fat Indian, 33, 40, 62–63; pancreas as influence on bodily, 17, 147, 173, 182, 232; and plasticity of human body, 34–35, 36–37, 62, 186, 231–32; stress as product of tension, 53. *See also* time

*tenshun*: as illustration of porosity of body, 36, 48–49; expressions of, 49–55, 60, 62, 63, 225, 228, 242n20; ubiquity of in South Asia, 241n13, 241n15. *See also* stress

tension: as semipermanent state of stress, 53, 241n13; as trigger of bodily change, 48–51, 55, 62; event-caused, 51–52. *See also* stress

Thackeray, Bal, 76–77, 79, 81, 82, 84, 244n11

Thackeray, Uddhav, 77–79, 82

therapy: absorption and, 10, 146, 183; agency and authority in, 156–59, 185, 186; approach to of Poorvi, 166–68; body as source of its own, 194, 196–97, 199–200, 201; collateral character of medical, 148, 184–85; diagnosis as initial key for, 150, 152; importance of time in, 147, 151, 173, 182–83, 186; knowledge as key to successful, 168, 183; metabolism as site for receiving, 166, 183, 185–86, 203, 219; nutritional, 150–51, 152, 157, 161, 248n2; for obesity, 193–94, 197, 205; pancreas as major point of concern in clinical, 147, 173, 182, 232; pharmaceutical, 197, 198; role of willpower, 166, 185, 186, 190–91, 218; shortcomings of in treating metabolically-driven obesity,

158; simultaneous application to one body of multiple forms of, 23, 146, 150, 156, 161, 183; surgical, 194, 197, 199, 203, 205; therapeutic pipeline, 147–48; tolerability of, 147, 171–72, 184

thin-fat Indian: as cultural figure, 56–58, 164, 231, 241n12; as process rather than as product, 46, 60–61; coexistence of morphological thinness with metabolic obesity in, 33–34; and controversy over BMI measurements, 60–62; globesity and, 241n12; impaired insulin sensitivity in, 33; in epigenetic science, 24, 46, 56–58; "thrifty gene" and, 33–34; visual manifestation of, 60–61; Y-Y Paradox of, 32–33, 34, 36, 38. *See also* Y-Y paradox

"thrifty gene" hypothesis, 33–34, 46, 58

Throsby, Karen, 204–5

thyroid: appearance of thyroid problems in tandem with or maladies, 49, 159, 171, 219; eyes as indicators of a malfunctioning, 156–57; hypothyroidism, 149–50, 152

time: absorption and, 23, 226, 231–33; amputation as means of manipulating, 249n12; as influence on household readiness, 232; change in conceptions of epidemics through, 238n15; "clock time", 250n2; in development of chronic disease, 23, 147, 173, 182, 199, 202, 218; food consumption and, 154, 226, 233; Foucault on diet as means of manipulating, 249–50n14; historic debate concerning "Bombay time" and "Indian mean time", 251n3; Kartik's "life is shit" hypothesis of, 59–60; labor and, 54, 149, 153, 173, 231; lack of as threat to health, 52–53, 54, 59–60; management of by patients, 153, 175–76, 220, 222; scheduling of medications, 147; somatic, 147, 233; transition of thin-fat body through, 34–35, 40, 57, 62–64, 219, 231–32; *world clock* idea of, 232–33, 251n3. *See also* rhythms; temporality

*Times of India*, 54, 210, 213, 214

Trinity Hospital: endocrinology clinic at, 168–76; infection, demarcation, and amputation, 177–83; metabolic disease treatment at, 100–101, 145, 148, 232

ulcers, 180, 181, 182

Usha (nutritionist), 149, 150, 152, 154, 156–64

*vada pav*: as basis for job creation, 69, 81–82, 85, 86, 90; as cause of metabolic disease,

70–71, 93–95, 202; as healthy snack, 79, 82–83; as "lifeline" for Mumbaikars, 70, 74, 86–87, 88, 94, 243n6; as symbol for *Marathi manoos*, 77, 81–82, 83, 84, 87–88; as symbol of Mumbai, 74, 79, 89; bakery-produced, 94; branding of, 70, 82, 83, 88–89, 95, 96; carts and stalls, 77, 78–79, 82, 83–88; consumption of by children, 70–71, 93, 94; description of, 69; Dhruv (journalist) on, 80–81, 92; as focus of gastropolitics in Mumbai, 24, 69–70, 71–76, 78–79, 82–84, 89–91, 95–97; hygiene of cooking and eating, 77, 86, 89, 91–93; interview with Vinod (Shiv Sena–affiliated municipal representative) on, 81–83; Mahesh and Alok (cart owners) on, 83–88, 92, 95–96; Maza brand, 89–92, 96; media coverage of, 70–71, 78; medical proscriptions against, 93–94; Nitin (cart owner) on, 89, 92, 95; origin stories concerning, 79–81; packaged versions of, 70, 88, 89–92; preparation of, 84, 85–86, 87, 92; public health author-ity animus toward, 70–71, 93, 94–95; Shiv Sena's sociopolitical exploitation of, 75–76, 78–79, 81–83, 85, 95–96; Shiv Sena *vada pav sammelan* (*vada pav* jamboree), 69, 77–79; standardization of, 79, 82–83, 90–91; street food alternatives to, 76, 82, 84, 87, 243n3; taste of, 77, 82, 83, 88, 92; Thackeray family association with, 76–79, 81, 82, 84; transnational corporate involvement with, 78–79, 82, 91; Vikram Doctor on history of, 80–81

vegetables: for children, 93; consumption of in India, 107, 127, 136, 153, 159, 175–76; frozen, 91; high cost of, 84

vegetarianism: as dietary tool for treatment of metabolic disorders, 52; incidence of folic acid and protein deficiencies through, 57; practice of in India, 127, 154, 157, 158, 166–67, 244n13; vulnerabil-ity to deterioration of vegetarian street food, 91

water: abattoir, 142–44; as ingredient for adulteration or dilution of liquids and foods, 114, 116, 118–19, 120, 245–46n9; and food sanitation violations, 129; legal regulation of packaged (bottled), 125; sampling of by lab testing companies, 128; therapeutic use of, 38, 176

weight: BMI and body, 39, 43, 62; body as means of determining obesity, 17, 39; fluc-

tuations in, 157; scale recordings of body, 22, 36; thresholds for body, 39

well-being: of individuals, 133, 181, 183–84; of populations, 9, 13, 61, 72, 137

Westernization: "bad copy" Indian body as product of, 44–48; call center employment, 8, 29, 47, 173, 201, 202; damaging effects of, 4, 45; influence of on Indian consumption patterns, 23, 45, 70–71, 91–92, 166, 167, 190; as spread of prosperity, 4, 244–45n4; work schedules that produce stress, 54, 149, 153, 171. *See also* globesity

willpower: attempts by food companies to manipulate of individual, 168; case of Neha, 203, 218–23; case of Peter, 215–17; case of Saurab, 201–3; concept of reattachment and, 168, 194–95, 197, 221, 222, 228, 232; failure and, 194, 204–5; nutrition- and diet-based assumptions concerning, 161, 165–66, 193, 195, 203–4, 216; obesity construed as failure of, 12, 23, 168, 204, 227; relapse and, 248nn6–7; surgery as means of resetting body-brain relationships, 25, 191, 194–95, 197, 203–5, 221. *See also* addiction

women: absorptive capacity of female body, 249n10; as bariatric surgery patients, 211; career choice restrictions (case of Almas) on, 117; consumption of street food among, 87; cooking as factor of personal dignity among, 136; education for, 163, 165; employment, 8, 37, 52, 92, 106–8, 112, 123; employment for in professions, 117, 163, 165, 172; engineering diets of pregnant to avoid next-generation metabolic illness, 35, 55, 57; familial cooking responsi-bilities of working, 7, 20, 54, 112, 123, 139; homeliness (homely domesticity) and, 130; *koli* (fisher women), 37, 106–8; lifestyle ailments among, 54, 107, 171; magazines for, 7, 29, 54; as marketing targets for food companies, 132, 133; in market research focus group, 135–37; marriageability as concern among, 171, 212, 219, 221; neigh-borhood *mahila mandal* (women's group), 20, 100–102; obesity experienced by, 16, 54, 107, 159, 187–88, 210–11; odd eating hours of working in call centers, 8; poly-cystic ovarian disorder (PCOD) among, 159; pregnancy, 7, 35, 55–57, 171, 187; product loyalty among, 132; Right to Information Act (2005) as protection for, 101; stress among, 54, 171, 241n15; thyroid disorders

women (*continued*)
   among, 159, 171; trans fat as threat to
   health of, 113
work schedules: damage of to individual eating schedules, 149, 153; integration of diets
   into, 147; plight of Diya (obesity patient),
   153; plight of Mr. Bala (comorbidities
   patient), 149
world clocks, 232–33, 251n3

World Health Organization (WHO), 40–42,
   55–56
World Trade Organization (WTO), 125, 126

Yajnik, C. S., 31–32, 36, 38, 55–59, 62, 141n12
yoga, 19, 21, 116, 156, 157
Yudkin, John, 31–32
Y-Y paradox, evidence of, 31–33, 34, 36, 38, 55,
   58–60, 63